Praise For Massage For Dummies

"Touch is a powerful tool in any relationship, and learning to use that power with wisdom, compassion and skill is what *Massage For Dummies* is all about. I recommend this book for everyone who would like to make the art of massage a part of their lives."

—John Gray, author, *Men Are From Mars, Women Are From Venus*

"The only bad thing about this book is that Steve Capellini no longer works at a spa where I can get his revitalizing massage. Learning how to get the benefits at home through *Massage For Dummies* is the next best thing to being in Steve's hand."

—Bernard Burt, author of *Fodor's Healthy Escapes* and Senior Editor *Spa Management Journal*

"I have long recommended massage as an important ingredient of a holistic, self-nurturing lifestyle. Finally, there is a book for the average person that gives you everything you need to know about giving and receiving massages. I highly recommend this book."

—Jack Canfield, co-author of the *Chicken Soup for the Soul* series

"I've received massage from experts around the world and have become somewhat of an expert in the art of receiving. Steve Capellini is definitely the 'best of the best,' and I've been one of the most loyal clients for over twelve years now. If readers of *Massage For Dummies* come away with even a small fraction of the skills and knowledge he's shared with me over the years, they'll be well on their way to some of the most incredibly healthy, relaxing, and spiritually nourishing experiences of their lives. Enjoy!"

—Phyllis Sandler

"Massage therapy hits the big time!!! What a wonderful approach to the art and science of massage. *Massage For Dummies* blends factual information with a good sense of humor. Even though we've been in practice for over twenty years, we couldn't put it down. We highly recommend the book to laypeople as well as those in the field."

—Dan & Tekla Ulrich, Suncoast School of Massage, Tampa, Florida

"*Massage For Dummies* is an easy read: delightfully funny, thought-provoking without any work on the part of the reader. There is a wealth of information that is almost automatically absorbed. Steve is a born teacher. The authors use humor and wit to help you understand the many facets of massage. They help you visualize the material and see the advantages of touching and being touched. With a single pen swipe, they destroy myths, create mirth, and foster curiosity. The book is well-designed for easy access to technically sound material, and can be used as a reference, quick read, or a teaching text for a wide audience. I have over twenty-five years in this business, and I was entertained, laughed a lot, and appreciated the authors' techniques and competent teaching methods."

—Nancy W. Dail, LMT, Director, Downeast School of Massage

P9-DER-395

"Capellini and Van Welden literally take their readers by the hand and gently lead them into the delightful practicalities of massage. Sensitive and fun, this book is like a good rub."

—Gil Headley, Ph.D., Rolf Institute Adjunct Founder, Somanautics, Inc.

"As a massage therapist and school owner for a total of sixteen years, I highly recommend this book for the student, professional, and novice alike. It's easy to comprehend, entertaining, informative, and most of all, it's fun! Readers at any level will find themselves developing skills faster than they ever imagined."

—Jody Stork, owner, Space Coast Massage & Allied Health Institute, Melbourne, FL

"As a new millennium approaches, the essence of our being human will truly be defined as our ability to *feel* and experience the fullness of life in the face of an increasingly depersonalized world. *Massage For Dummies* not only legitimizes, but goes the furthest of any book, in demystifying massage, whether as a receiver or giver. A careful reading will guide you in how to integrate massage and its incredible benefits into the 'here and now' of your everyday life."

—Deborah A. Smith, Spa Director and Founder of Smith Club & Spa Specialists

"*Massage For Dummies* is not just for the novice (or Dummy), but for the professional massage therapist as well. The information is invaluable and presented in a light and humorous style. Steve — whose Spa Certification Workshop, The Royal Treatment, has opened doors for massage therapists everywhere — is truly a massage and spa genius."

—Gerald Levine, LMT

"Massage is a great medicine, and with the help of *Massage For Dummies*, all of us can have healing hands — or at least know how to find them."

—Margaret Pierpont, coauthor, *The Spa Life at Home*

"My congratulations to Steve Capellini and Michel Van Welden for writing *Massage For Dummies*. I enjoyed reading this book from cover to cover. *Massage For Dummies* is a practical guide for anybody who would like to enhance their skills in massage, from the novice to the 'professional body worker.' The authors deliver their message with intelligence, passion, and humor. I will enthusiastically recommend this book to my clients or to anybody who seriously wants to learn about massage, its origins, and applications, yet have fun doing so."

—Michael F. Livingston, LMT, Personal Therapist to Jimmy Buffett and Brian Wilson

"What a treat! You feel massaged just reading this book. Superb professionals in their field, the authors demystify this oft-misunderstood arena. They convey essential information on every aspect of bodywork in a warm, humorous, and inspiring way. This book is truly inspired — and inspiring. Not only is it full of excellent scientifically-based information, it is a joy to read. Read it, you'll love it!"

—Hyla Cass, M.D., author, *St. John's Wort: Nature's Blues Buster* and *Kava: Nature's Answer to Stress, Anxiety, and Insomnia*

"With lots of deep (k)needed information and long smooth strokes of humor, Steve entirely entertains, expertly educates, and masterfully manifests for any reader the essential facts, fictions, functions, and fun of massage, touch, and bodywork."

> —John Paul De Vierville, Ph.D., M.S.S.W., T.R.M.T, Owner/Director Alamo Plaza Spa, San Antonio, Texas; Co-Chair Education Committee, International Spa Association

"It's about time that people understood the medical benefits of massage. [This] book presents practical ways that *everyone* can decrease stress and prolong their lives by something as simple and elegant as therapeutic massage."

> —Pamela M. Peeke, M.D., MPH, Assistant Professor of Medicine, University of Maryland, Division of Complementary Medicine

"Discover the life-enhancing information provided for you in this remarkable book. Steve Capellini and Michel Van Welden have done an outstanding job delivering the message of self-healing, and in doing so, have created a valuable resource for all to use."

> —Suzy Bordeaux-Johlfs, Kohala Spa Director, Hilton Waikoloa Village, Hawaii

"Here is a rare mix: one of massage therapy's most knowledgeable, experienced, and sensitive practitioners happens to be a fine and funny writer! Breath deeply and enjoy learning from a master."

> —Patricia Weinman, Massage Connoisseur

"I found *Massage For Dummies* to be a wonderful and funny guide to massage, whether you're a massage therapist or first-time recipient. . . . Steve brings his passion for the massage profession along with a journalist's perception to print. A must for everyone's library to put touch in your life everyday."

> —Lynda Solien-Wolfe, LMT, NCTMP, Massage Therapy Public Relations Specialist

Praise for Getting the Most out of Massage by Steve Capellini

"A beautiful book at the right time. . . ."

> —Bernard S. Siegel, M.D., author, *Love, Medicine, & Miracles*

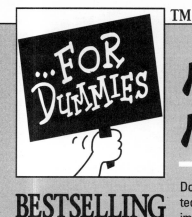

TM

References for the Rest of Us!®

BESTSELLING BOOK SERIES

Do you find that traditional reference books are overloaded with technical details and advice you'll never use? Do you postpone important life decisions because you just don't want to deal with them? Then our *For Dummies®* business and general reference book series is for you.

For Dummies business and general reference books are written for those frustrated and hard-working souls who know they aren't dumb, but find that the myriad of personal and business issues and the accompanying horror stories make them feel helpless. *For Dummies* books use a lighthearted approach, a down-to-earth style, and even cartoons and humorous icons to dispel fears and build confidence. Lighthearted but not lightweight, these books are perfect survival guides to solve your everyday personal and business problems.

> *"More than a publishing phenomenon, 'Dummies' is a sign of the times."*
>
> — The New York Times

> *"...you won't go wrong buying them."*
>
> — Walter Mossberg, Wall Street Journal, on For Dummies books

> *"A world of detailed and authoritative information is packed into them..."*
>
> — U.S. News and World Report

Already, millions of satisfied readers agree. They have made For Dummies the #1 introductory level computer book series and a best-selling business book series. They have written asking for more. So, if you're looking for the best and easiest way to learn about business and other general reference topics, look to For Dummies to give you a helping hand.

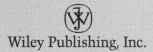

Wiley Publishing, Inc.

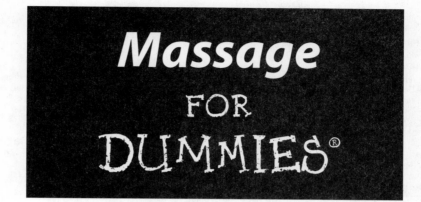

Massage FOR DUMMIES®

by Steve Capellini and Michel Van Welden

Foreword by Robin Leach

WILEY

Wiley Publishing, Inc.

Massage For Dummies®

Published by
Wiley Publishing, Inc.
111 River Street
Hoboken, NJ 07030
www.wiley.com

Copyright © 1999 by Wiley Publishing, Inc., Indianapolis, Indiana

Published by Wiley Publishing, Inc., Indianapolis, Indiana

Published simultaneously in Canada

No part of this publication may be reproduced, stored in a retrieval system, or transmitted in any form or by any means, electronic, mechanical, photocopying, recording, scanning, or otherwise, except as permitted under Sections 107 or 108 of the 1976 United States Copyright Act, without either the prior written permission of the Publisher, or authorization through payment of the appropriate per-copy fee to the Copyright Clearance Center, 222 Rosewood Drive, Danvers, MA 01923, 978-750-8400, fax 978-646-8700. Requests to the Publisher for permission should be addressed to the Legal Department, Wiley Publishing, Inc., 10475 Crosspoint Blvd., Indianapolis, IN 46256, 317-572-3447, fax 317-572-4447, or e-mail permcoordinator@wiley.com

Trademarks: Wiley, the Wiley Publishing logo, For Dummies, the Dummies Man logo, A Reference for the Rest of Us!, The Dummies Way, Dummies Daily, The Fun and Easy Way, Dummies.com, and related trade dress are trademarks or registered trademarks of John Wiley & Sons, Inc. and/or its affiliates in the United States and other countries and may not be used without written permission. All other trademarks are the property of their respective owners. Wiley Publishing, Inc., is not associated with any product or vendor mentioned in this book.

LIMIT OF LIABILITY/DISCLAIMER OF WARRANTY: WHILE THE PUBLISHER AND AUTHOR HAVE USED THEIR BEST EFFORTS IN PREPARING THIS BOOK, THEY MAKE NO REPRESENTATIONS OR WARRANTIES WITH RESPECT TO THE ACCURACY OR COMPLETENESS OF THE CONTENTS OF THIS BOOK AND SPECIFICALLY DISCLAIM ANY IMPLIED WARRANTIES OF MERCHANTABILITY OR FITNESS FOR A PARTICULAR PURPOSE. NO WARRANTY MAY BE CREATED OR EXTENDED BY SALES REPRESENTATIVES OR WRITTEN SALES MATERIALS. THE ADVICE AND STRATEGIES CONTAINED HEREIN MAY NOT BE SUITABLE FOR YOUR SITUATION. YOU SHOULD CONSULT WITH A PROFESSIONAL WHERE APPROPRIATE. NEITHER THE PUBLISHER NOR AUTHOR SHALL BE LIABLE FOR ANY LOSS OF PROFIT OR ANY OTHER COMMERCIAL DAMAGES, INCLUDING BUT NOT LIMITED TO SPECIAL, INCIDENTAL, CONSEQUENTIAL, OR OTHER DAMAGES.

For general information on our other products and services or to obtain technical support, please contact our Customer Care Department within the U.S. at 800-762-2974, outside the U.S. at 317-572-3993, or fax 317-572-4002.

Wiley also publishes its books in a variety of electronic formats. Some content that appears in print may not be available in electronic books.

Library of Congress Cataloging-in-Publication Data:

Library of Congress Control Number: 99-64908

ISBN: 0-7645-5172-8

Manufactured in the United States of America

10 9 8 7 6

3B/RV/QS/QU/IN

About the Authors

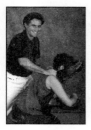

Steve Capellini: You may be thinking to yourself, "What makes HIM so special that he should write this book on massage?" Perhaps what most specifically qualifies me is the inordinate amount of time, amounting to many thousands of hours, I've spent cooped up alone in a room with just one other person, touching them all over their bodies and getting paid for it.

What could be more fun? Or more weird? I hope I've got the communication skills to get across to you the reasons why an otherwise sane human being would spend such a large percentage of his life in such a strange manner.

And in addition, to give you an idea of some more specific qualifications, here's a rough chronology of my life in touch:

1977: Received first massage ever, from high school girlfriend Grace, and knew that something important had just transpired.

1983: Attended 108 hour massage class in Los Angeles and became certified. Had to take V.D. test at local health clinic in order to receive license (a local prostitution ordinance).

1984: Massaged members of the cast and crew of a movie being filmed about Ernest Hemingway in Pamplona, Spain, during the famous running of the bulls. Yes, I ran.

1985: First regular massage job, at a spa in Florida, giving 25-minute full body oil rubdowns to cigar-smoking "good ole boys" for $4 an hour.

1986: Rethought career choice. Started working at a friend's landscaping company.

1987: Was called into work at a new spa in Miami, the Doral. Massaged Dr. Ruth Westheimer, who gave me the "secret" of aphrodisiacs.

1988: Became supervisor of the massage and spa treatments department at the Doral, in charge of 40 therapists.

1989: Became a traveling spa trainer, hiring staff and overseeing openings of spas in Vermont, Jamaica, on cruise ships, and more.

1992: Started teaching workshops to massage therapists and business owners. Massaged Red Cross volunteers and army personnel in aftermath of Hurricane Andrew.

1997: Began publishing books on massage and spas (this is the third one).

1998: First child born. Waiting until he's a year or two old before teaching him how to massage Mommy and Daddy.

1999: Continuing to rub, teach, and write.

Michel Van Welden, PT, NT, received his training at the Physical Therapy Institute of Paris, specializing in orthopedic and neurological rehabilitation, as well as sports medicine and the treatment of burn victims.

For 26 years, he practiced both in hospitals and in his own private clinic. Working hand in hand (no pun intended) with plastic surgeons, he helped develop Plastic Physical Therapy, which increases the positive results of plastic surgery procedures. He also assembled a procedural manual and produced a video about lymphatic drainage and has taught his technique to therapists throughout France and around the world.

Since arriving in the U.S., he has become an "expert on the skin," who, in May 1998, substantiated the first derivative claim ever approved by the FDA for the treatment of cellulite using a patented massage device. All the other stuff you see on infomercials about cellulite is a lot of malarkey.

Mr. Van Welden is currently a consultant and acting Director of Research for two American clinical research projects studying the effects of massage on cute little pigs. These are underway at UCLA and Vanderbilt University, believe it or not.

Michel is also a wild and crazy outdoorsman. He has run to the top of Mount Kilamanjaro seven times. He also became the record holder for long distance running along the Great Wall of China, covering 1,500 miles, half of the wall's length. His greatest achievement in the sports field, though, was in helping dozens of other people discover their own potentials by leading fitness trips to the Great Wall, Kilamanjaro, the Andes peaks, and other destinations.

Mr. Van Welden is married and is the father of three children. He lives in Fort Lauderdale, Florida.

He can be contacted by email at michelvp@worldnet.att.net.

Dedication

I dedicate this book to the coolest little massage partner ever, Brandon Sunthorn Capellini, born August 3, 1998.

Acknowledgments from Steve Capellini

I thank Atchana, my darling partner and wife, who received less massages because I was so busy writing these past months. The rest of my family was equally supportive and enthusiastic too: Mom & Dad, Tina, Bala & Adi, Jim & Lalitha, Rob, Suzanne, Chris, Ari, & Nicole. And of course the Thai side of the family: Umpun, Lek, Pat, Rangsan, Tina, & Rolando. And the father-in-law I never knew, Sunthorn Chuaindhara; he lives on in our hearts.

I appreciate my co-author Michel Van Welden for his help and for being so dedicated to his worldwide massage research.

I'm very grateful to Carol Susan Roth, who believed I was right for this project and made it all possible through her dedication and hard work, and to Lori Huneke for introducing us.

Thank you to stellar literary agents, Michael Larsen and Elizabeth Pomada, who've been steadily supporting my writing and helping me grow.

All the folks at Wiley have been a pleasure to work with because they are smart and they have vision and they like massage! I really appreciate being treated as part of the team, especially at BEA, and I'd especially like to thank Tami Booth for her support, encouragement, and hard work on this project. I also thank Kathleen Welton for remembering me from two years earlier; Tim Gallan, a brave soul who endured major surgery while right in the midst of editing this book; Christina Turner; Karen Young; Kristina Pappas; Mimi Sells; Jonathan Malysiak; Steve Berkowitz; Charles Berkstresser; Roland Elgey; Sarah Woodman & Ana Noetzel for creating killer trade show events; David Scott for staying in touch from Australia; and John Kilcullen for proudly proclaiming "Free massages! Only in America!" at the Book Expo. You've got a great team, and you know how to throw a party!

Also, there are so many friends and clients from the massage and spa world who've helped with this book too: Jai Varadaraj for all her help from India; Lynda Solien-Wolfe for her guerilla massage marketing and the great Massage For Dummies chair; Don Payne; John Fanuzzi; Carole Spellman; Ed Wilson; Iris Burman; Dan & Telka Ulrich; Pat Weinman; Harvey & Phyllis Sandler; Dave Kennedy; Amory Rowe; the Dail family up in Maine for their unparalleled hospitality; and especially Nancy Dail for her technical review of this book; Steve Chagnon; Vincenzo & Susy Marra; Giovanni Grippando; Regina Kipnis; Ellen Wickersham; Connie Johnson; Jim Berenholtz; Mark Siciliani; and Carol Ann Ferrol.

Also, I thank the co-creators of the book: Kathryn Born, for the illustrations; Peter Barrett for the photography; and his assistants Alfredo and Ava, and of course the models, Fardan Karibee, Josephine B. Hortenbrink, Jason Barger, & Linda Vongkhamphra.

Acknowledgments from Michel Van Welden

For my Mom, for all that she did for me, including going through sciatica pain to show me the way of my future. Thanks.

To all the patients who knocked on my door to receive a massage and ended up sweating in Africa or in Bolivia.

To Steve Capellini for not thinking that all French are arrogant, carrying their baguettes and bottles of wine everywhere they go, and for offering me the pleasure of sharing the success of this book.

To Sebastien and Jordane my sons, for all the support they bring to their too often gone away, Dad.

To Jocelyne who taught me how to speak to pigs about massage, and convince them that the guy with the white coat and a strong French accent was not the butcher. And for the love she brings me every day.

To Dr. James Watson, plastic surgeon at UCLA, and Dr. David Adcok plastic surgeon at Vanderbilt University, for all the hours spent together in the lab and in the Plastic Surgery Department trying to understand a non -surgical technique.

To Tami Booth for giving me this extraordinary opportunity — to be published in the USA. And to Carol Susan Roth for making it possible.

Publisher's Acknowledgments

We're proud of this book; please send us your comments through our online registration form located at www.dummies.com/register.

Some of the people who helped bring this book to market include the following:

Acquisitions, Editorial, and Media Development

Senior Project Editor: Tim Gallan

Acquisitions Editor: Tami Booth

Copy Editors: Tamara Castleman, Donna Love, Elizabeth Kuball

Technical Editor: Nancy Dail, Director, Downeast School of Massage

Editorial Coordinator: Karen Young

Editorial Manager: Seta K. Franz

Editorial Assistant: Alison Walthall

Production

Project Coordinator: Tom Missler

Associate Project Coordinator: Maridee Ennis

Layout and Graphics: Amy Adrian, Angela F. Hunckler, Kate Jenkins, David McKelvey, Barry Offringa, Brent Savage, Jacque Schneider, Janet Seib, Michael A. Sullivan, Brian Torwelle, Mary Jo Weis

Illustrator: Kathryn Born

Photographer: Peter Barrett

Proofreaders: Paula Lowell, Nancy Price, Marianne Santy

Indexer: Liz Cunningham

Publishing and Editorial for Consumer Dummies

Diane Graves Steele, Vice President and Publisher, Consumer Dummies
Joyce Pepple, Acquisitions Director, Consumer Dummies
Kristin A. Cocks, Product Development Director, Consumer Dummies
Michael Spring, Vice President and Publisher, Travel
Brice Gosnell, Associate Publisher, Travel
Suzanne Jannetta, Editorial Director, Travel

Publishing for Technology Dummies

Richard Swadley, Vice President and Executive Group Publisher
Andy Cummings, Vice President and Publisher

Composition Services

Gerry Fahey, Vice President of Production Services
Debbie Stailey, Director of Composition Services

Contents at a Glance

Cartoons at a Glance

By Rich Tennant

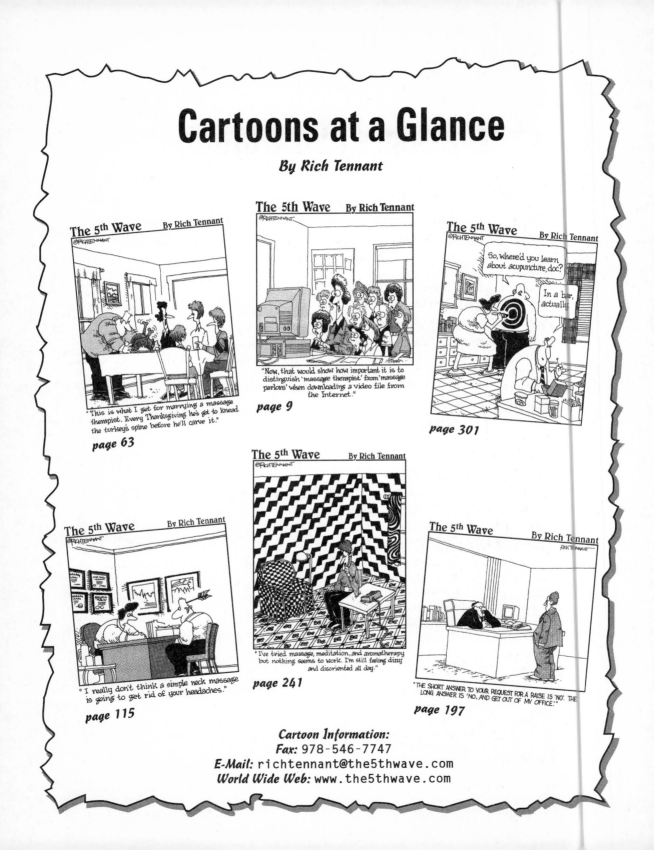

page 63

page 9

page 301

page 115

page 241

page 197

Cartoon Information:
Fax: 978-546-7747
E-Mail: richtennant@the5thwave.com
World Wide Web: www.the5thwave.com

Table of Contents

Foreword

When done right, it can free your body, invigorate your spirit, and refresh your soul. I'm of course talking about massage. Logging 20,000 miles a year may have made me somewhat of an expert on the lifestyles of the rich and famous, but it also taught me to value some of life's simple pleasures, like massage. Whenever I arrive at a new destination, be it the Oriental Hotel in Bangkok, Thailand, or the Canyon Ranch Spa at the Venetian in Las Vegas, the first thing I do after I check in is escape to a good massage. It's the only cure for whatever ails you. Being a devotée of the art of a good massage, my mania isn't confined to just when I'm traveling. I have a massage table in my home in Jumby Bay, Antigua, and SueHua, my Chinese masseuse, is a daily treat. . . .

Perhaps the best thing about massage is that absolutely everyone can enjoy it, recreating one of the greatest pleasures of the jet-set crowd right at home. And now, finally, there's a way for all of us to learn the secrets from one of the great masters of massage, Steve Capellini. This book reveals dozens of healthy tips to help you achieve inner harmony, peace of mind, and an entirely new level of well-being, whether you're receiving your massage at a great luxury hotel on the island of Maui, or on your very own living room floor.

Massage is truly one of the greatest gifts that is a delight to receive and a joy to give. Have fun as you read along and practice because you may even make a few new friends.

Robin Leach

Introduction

For those of us who've already discovered it, massage is just about the niftiest thing on the planet. Better than chocolate. Better than pizza. It's a great way to feel better, look better, treat people better, and treat yourself better, too. It's one hundred percent good for you, with no artificial additives or ingredients, and it's easy to do. In fact, one of the best things about massage is that you don't need a lot of fancy expensive equipment in order to get one or give one. All you really need to get started is a human body. Got one? Great! Then you're ready to go.

First, let me introduce myself and explain what qualifies me to teach you about this subject in the first place. I've been massaging people for a living since I was 23 years old. That's more than 16 years and well over 10,000 massages. I've trained other massage therapists around the world at resorts, in workshops, and in massage schools, and I've written a few books on the subject.

But there's something more to it than that. If all I were offering you was technical experience, analytical knowledge, and rah-rah enthusiasm, I wouldn't blame you for approaching this book with indifference or even boredom.

Yet another book about the beauties and wonders of massage strokes and maneuvers? Wax on, wax off. Yawn.

The Massage Adventure

What I hope to offer you is more than technique, more than know-how, even more than increased pleasure and greater health in your everyday life. What I will be trying to get across in all of the pages to follow is a new way to *be*. I've transformed my own life into an ongoing, unfolding massage adventure and would be most sincerely honored to act as your guide along a similar journey of inner and outer exploration. There's a big, wild world out there, and there's an even bigger, wilder world inside your own body and mind. Massage is an excellent vehicle through which to explore both.

Touching other people with the intention of making them feel better and improving the quality of their lives is one of the most worthy ways to spend one's time as a human being. Massage, in this sense, is more than a job. It's a calling, a cause, a mission. I realize, of course, that this may sound a tad overzealous. Not everybody feels this way, which is good because if they did feel this way, then they'd all be massage therapists like me, and there would be nobody left to do other important jobs like delivering office furniture, piloting commercial airplanes, and making incorrect predictions about the stock market.

But regardless of their "real" jobs, whether they know it or not, everybody in this world is a living, breathing massage sponge. Take you, for example. Right now, before you get to the next paragraph, take a moment to become aware of your body. Where are you? What is touching you? A chair on your bottom? A bed on your whole backside? A carpeted floor pressing against your feet? Somewhere, something is touching you, unless you are reading this introduction to *Massage For Dummies* in free fall during a skydiving expedition (in which case your clothing and the harness over your shoulders are still touching you, not to mention the friction of the air rushing by). In fact, this entire world is reaching out and massaging you 24 hours a day, seven days a week. Gravity is the grip, and everything else is the hand.

Those people with a more spiritual bent may even be tempted to say that "God" or the "Supreme Being" or the "Ultimate Massage Therapist" is touching us all the time, as reflected in mystical songs throughout the ages, such as the ancient Gregorian chant, *Omnis Mundus In Manus Habeo*, which, roughly translated, means "He's got the whole world in His hands. He's got the whole wide world. . . ."

You're not alone

The world is filled with millions of people who have already started their own massage adventures. In fact, in the U.S. alone, approximately 28 million people have received a professional massage, and that number is growing quickly. Millions more have exchanged massages on a non-professional basis with friends and family. Insurance companies are starting to reimburse for it, doctors are including it in their practices, and practically every hair salon in every city is turning into a day spa and offering massage to clients. You've probably seen massage on shows like *Lifestyles of the Rich and Famous*. It's everywhere, and yet, if you're like most people, you still haven't received a massage, and you have quite a few questions about how it works and what it can do for you. If that's the case, then this is the book for you.

You don't have to be a hippie

Let me reassure you right here at the beginning that I'm not going to ask you to do anything you're uncomfortable with. In fact, if you want to receive a massage while wearing a formal, ankle-length ball gown or a football uniform complete with pads, that's fine with me. It may cut down on the effectiveness of certain massage techniques, but I'm not here to tell you what your style should be. I'm here to help you feel comfortable about including massage in your life in whatever ways you see fit.

In this book, you're going to find lots of ways to make massage a part of your day-to-day activities so that it becomes as natural as brushing your teeth, driving your car, or peeling the stickers off sales items you buy as Christmas presents. And in order to help you accomplish this, I've enlisted the help of a pretty impressive character, my co-author, Michel Van Welden. First of all, you should know that Michel is a man. In France, where he's from, many men are called Michel. He's a physical therapist and naturopathic therapist who's traveled the world teaching other therapists and physicians about massage. An expert on physiology and the skin, he has been personally responsible for getting the FDA in this country to sit up and pay serious attention to the effects of certain kinds of massage. The way he accomplished this was through several highly complex laboratory experiments studying (I'm not making this up) the effects of massage on pigs. I defer to Michel's clinical expertise on many crucial issues, and my hope is that his scientific knowledge sets your mind at ease regarding the effectiveness and safety of massage. Throughout your average, everyday paragraphs in this book, though, it will be me, Steve, acting as your guide. Together, Michel and I have created a book that goes beyond any other of its kind to offer you everything you need to know to change your life from a dull, drab, non-massage existence into an exciting massage adventure.

This Book Is for You If . . .

As I stated earlier, this book is for anyone with a body, which should qualify almost every single reader. Disembodied spirits and poltergeists may find it difficult to get the correct amount of friction necessary to perform effective massage maneuvers and should therefore abstain. Certain people in particular will quickly discover the most obvious benefits in reading these pages; you know who you are, and this book is especially for you if . . .

- ✔ You've ever wanted to touch another person with grace, compassion, and caring.
- ✔ You want to share a new level of communication with the people you're close to.
- ✔ You want to increase your well-being and reduce many types of pain.
- ✔ You have a desire to enhance various aspects of your life, including athletic performance, job efficiency, and even your love life.
- ✔ You have a handicap of some kind and would like to discover how in fact massage is the therapy of choice for many people with physical limitations.

  ✔ You want to pursue this adventure more seriously and are perhaps thinking about becoming a massage pro yourself.

  ✔ You think knowing how to give a good massage may be a neat way to get more dates.

So How Do I Get Started Already?

By now you're probably saying, "Alright, Steve. You've convinced me. My muscles are sore and I'm ready to get going. How do I get started with this whole massage thing anyway?"

The best way to use this book is to choose the subject that interests you most and then jump right in at that point. Many of you may be eager to start giving a massage right away, in which case, you can zoom ahead to Part III. I highly encourage you to read all the material in the sections leading up to the how-to stuff, however, instead of simply flipping through the photographs and list of instructions. The attitudes and intentions with which you approach massage are, after all, what make the biggest difference in terms of what you get out of it.

For those of you who like to approach your reading in a systematic fashion, you will find that each part of the book builds upon the one before it in what is, I hope, a logical manner, so that by the end, you can come away knowing just about as much as you'd ever want to know about massage, unless of course you start pursuing it as a passion and profession in your life as I have, in which case, the learning never ends.

How This Book Is Organized

Here are the subjects that you find spread out before your eager eyes and fingers as you use this book:

Part I: Discovering Massage for Greater Health and Happiness

In this part, you find the background information you need to understand how the massage techniques actually work, and where they came from in the first place. You can discover all kinds of interesting things about your skin and what's beneath it, for example, and what it is about massage that helps your whole body feel better. If you're up to the task, you can test your touch-ability in a specially designed quiz. You can also encounter important vocabulary words and, perhaps most importantly, finally find out what all those massage gizmos at The Sharper Image are all about.

Part II: The Art of Receiving Massage

What, there's an art to receiving too, you ask? You mean I can't just lie there like a blob and let someone else do all the work? That's correct. Massage, in this respect, is like the tango, and you know what they say about the tango. In this part, you develop the fine art of "tuning in," which allows you to fully enjoy the benefits and pleasures that await you with massage. I describe how you can invite healthy pleasure into your life, choose the right style of massage for you and your body, choose a good massage therapist, and start receiving massages just like the pros do, with all the trimmings like proper breathing, meditative awareness, and other advanced techniques for basically blissing out.

Part III: The Art of Giving Massage

This part is the "meat" of the book, so to speak, with all the pretty pictures that you may be tempted to flip to immediately and never draw your attention away from again. Resist this temptation, oh hedonistic reader! In fact, go ahead right now (if you haven't already) and flip forward to the photos and then come back after a couple of minutes. Go ahead. I can wait.

There, satisfied? Now promise that you'll look through the other important sections of Part III as well. Make no mistake about it: To give a good massage requires some effort and energy, and you'll do well to prepare mentally beforehand so you don't burn yourself out. You may also discover vital information about when and how not to massage people, including yourself.

Part IV: Massage at Work

If you're suffering from some of the typical aches and pains of office workers and computer users everywhere, rush directly to Part IV. In this part, I give you simple massage moves that you can apply to your own aching body right at your desk, and I offer an entire chapter on how to relieve sore, tired feet with a special kind of massage known as reflexology. (Don't worry, I define that strange sounding word soon enough.) Hint: You may even be able to use this part of the book as evidence to help convince your boss to pay for professional chair-massage right in the work place. You'll see what I mean.

Part V: Living the Good Life: Massage for Every Body

In the fifth part, you can take your pick from a smorgasbord of offerings, reading through the chapters that intrigue you in whichever order you choose. Whether you're an athlete, a pregnant woman, a world traveler, or whatever, you're sure to pick up a ton of useful info here that you can use to integrate massage into your life.

Part VI: The Part of Tens

The last part contains lists of ten quick ways you can improve your life with massage, including suggestions for great places to take massage classes, outstanding locations to receive incredible massages, quick massage tips to ease stress, ways to offer massage as a gift, and, for you pet lovers, massage techniques designed especially for pooches and kitties.

Massaging the Icons

Throughout this book, I place lots of little round things in the margins, calling your attention to various details in the text. These pictures are called *icons,* and I have included some particularly pertinent ones for people learning the ropes of the massage world. To wit, you have your:

The Massage Tale icon lets you know there's a real-life massage story from an actual person in the adjacent paragraph. These stories may leave you happy, misty-eyed, or thoughtful, depending on the subject matter, but they all go to prove how powerful an influence massage can be in your life.

This one signifies that some sagacious and perhaps famous individual is contributing various words of wisdom on the massage subject at hand, words which usually highlight my own brilliant remarks.

The Tip icon clues you in right away to the presence of some especially important information. Perhaps I'll reveal a secret technique for massaging your way into Harvard Business School, for example. Perhaps not. You have to check the tip to be sure. At the very least, you may find some quick and easy pointers to make your reading experience as pleasurable as possible.

The practice of massage is not without its potential dangers. For example, once, after receiving three massages in one day as part of my job interviewing therapists for positions at a new spa, I turned into a human noodle and kept banging my knees into furniture. Seriously, though, there are certain things you have to watch out for when practicing massage, and there are various reasons why you should not offer massage in certain circumstances (what we professionals call *contraindications*). You can catch them right away when you see this icon.

Not wanting to make you feel like you're a wallflower just observing the massage-dance of life from the sidelines, I'm going to do my best to explain in plain English everything you need to know on the subject. When, out of necessity, I use some massage terminology that seems foreign or unnecessarily complex to you, I warn you first with one of these little icons.

Sharing the Adventure

Massage, ultimately, is a way to share with others and to express yourself in a direct, hands-on way, and I hope this book plays a big part in helping you discover this. If you'd like to share some thoughts about what you learn on your own massage adventure, you can contact me in care of IDG Books Worldwide, or you can visit me on the Web at www.royaltreatment.com and send e-mail to steve@royaltreatment.com. I'll be most pleased to hear how your journey is going.

So What Happens Now?

I can feel you getting a little antsy. You wanna get your hands on somebody already, don't you? Well, as I said earlier, you can always skip ahead. In fact, now that you're a little jazzed up about all these great benefits you can get from massage, this may be a good time to flash forward to Part III. Give yourself a little treat by mastering one or two moves, either for yourself or a partner, spend an hour happily practicing your new skill, and then come back and read the first few chapters, in which you find out the answers to such burning questions as, "What famous inventor of psychoanalysis used massage in his practice to calm patients?" Hint: His last name rhymes with void.

Part I
Discovering Massage for Greater Health and Happiness

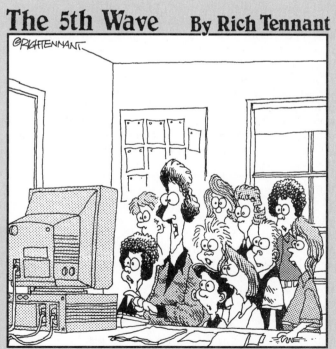

The 5th Wave   By Rich Tennant

"Now, that would show how important it is to distinguish 'massage therapist' from 'massage parlors' when downloading a video file from the Internet."

In this part . . .

As you explore this first part of this book, you may begin to get a sense that's there's something really *big* out there that you've been overlooking, almost as if an elephant were living in your backyard, right over there behind the clothesline, but you'd somehow failed to see it. Yes, it's true: The parallel universe of massage has existed right beneath your nose all along, and millions of people around the world have enjoyed its benefits and pleasures for untold centuries. So, you might ask, if massage is so darn popular and everyone loves it so much, why haven't I been informed?

Don't feel bad. You're in the majority. Most people have no clue about the rich tradition that massage has to offer, and that's because they were never taught by their parents, or their peers, or a respected teacher in grade school. Learning massage is kind of like learning geometry, or your ABCs. If no one teaches you, how are you supposed to find out?

There are certain controversies that still swarm around the whole issue of massage, most of them based on ideas held-over from the Victorian age. In this first part of the book, I'm going to completely quash all such concerns into little tiny bits, leaving you with a jaw-agape appreciation for the tremendous benefits massage can have for you, your family, and friends.

Whether you're already somewhat familiar with massage and are raring to go, or you're a trembling neophyte, slightly intimidated by the very concept of touching another person, or being touched, Part I will quickly usher you into a new world filled with the millions of us who already know and enjoy the many benefits of massage.

Welcome to the club.

Chapter 1

Not Just a Rub: How Massage Can Improve Your Life

In This Chapter

▶ What makes massage work

▶ Types of massage and how they help you

*W*hat does massage really do for you anyway? Sure, it feels incredible to receive one, and it looks nice to watch beautiful people massaging each other on how-to videos, but what's going on beneath the surface? Is it worth it to actually fork over your hard-earned cash to have someone rub your skin for an hour? Should you spend your precious time and energy learning how to give a good massage yourself? Is massage really effective, or is it just an unnecessary, flashy indulgence, like fish eggs on toast?

MASSAGE TALE

Well, being a massage junkie myself, I find it difficult to imagine why anybody would *not* want to get a massage, anytime, anyplace, for any reason at all or no reason at all. For me, massage has just always seemed like such an obviously good thing to do, starting way back in 11th grade when Grace came over to visit at my parent's house one afternoon, and nobody else was home. Being a typical seventeen-year-old, I was hoping that we were soon going to engage in some good old-fashioned hanky-panky, and when Grace told me to loosen my belt and lie down on the carpet, I began singing Handel's *Messiah* silently to myself.

Grace touched me then, on the small of my back, and I'll never forget the sensation. "This is a massage technique that somebody taught me," she said. "How does it feel?"

"Ah, it feels, um, kind of, uh, unbelievable!" I said, and unbelievable was exactly the right word. Grace was doing something clearly non-sexual, and I could not believe that anything non-sexual could feel so good. I could not believe that there was a way to be so intimate with somebody and yet not get in trouble with her father, if he were to find out about it. In short, I could not believe that something that was neither illegal, immoral, nor fattening could be so sumptuously pleasurable.

I asked Grace to keep doing what she was doing, and as she did so, I began devising, right there with my face buried in my parent's green shag carpeting, a future lifestyle that would include the absolutely highest number of massages possible.

This early experience pointed out a fundamental truth about massage therapy, but one that is often missed by those people who judge it before they even give it a try. That truth: There is a difference between sex and massage therapy. There, I said it, right here in Chapter 1, and I'm glad. Some people out there will forever be mixing the two up, which does a disservice to everybody else, especially those people who have shied away from massage over the years because of a perceived less-than-pristine image.

I discovered, in that youthful, eye-opening experience, that massage does indeed feel unbelievable, and that discovery was a great place to begin. Now, more than 20 years later, after studying massage and teaching massage and experiencing the myriad facets of massage both in the U.S. and in other countries, I've been introduced to other, deeper reasons for including it in my life, reasons with profound implications for improved health, well-being, and even longevity. These are the reasons I'd like to share with you in this chapter and throughout the book.

Basic Benefits of Massage

If I were to go into some of the stories about how massage has helped people change their lives, heal themselves, become rich and famous, and so on, you probably wouldn't believe me right away, because, after all, we're still in Chapter 1. So I'm going to start out slowly and offer you some of the simplest, everyday ways that massage can help you, some of which still may come as a surprise to you.

Here, then, not ranked in any particular order, are some basic benefits of massage that perhaps didn't pop straight into your head the first time you thought about it. Massage . . .

 ✔ Helps relieve muscular spasm and tension

 ✔ Raises immune efficiency

✔ Improves circulation

✔ Promotes the healing of tissues

✔ Increases healthy functioning of the skin

✔ Engenders profound relaxation

✔ Offers emotional reassurance

✔ Improves appearance

I'd like to take these points one at a time and let you get comfortable with them.

Helps relieve muscular spasm and tension

As you can see in Figure 1-1, there is a definite physical difference between muscles that are relaxed and happy and muscles that are tensed up due to stress, overuse, injury, and more.

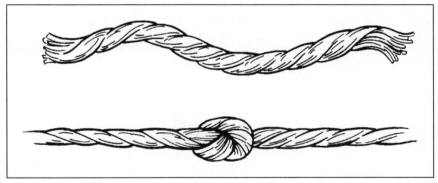

Figure 1-1:
The limp rope is your muscle. The knotted rope is your muscle on stress.

But there's more to it than that, believe it or not. Regardless of how wickedly clever my rope analogy is, the human body is much more complex. In fact, it's so complex that nobody has completely figured it out yet, even though countless researchers have spent a lifetime trying to do so. A whole bunch of really interesting things about the body have been discovered, however, along with how it responds to various types of stimuli, including massage.

For example, one of the most direct effects of massage is to help loosen the tension we experience as knots, kinks, and spasms in our muscles. This is achieved in a number of ways:

✔ The application of pressure creates awareness that there is indeed tension in a particular area, and the person receiving the massage can then begin to consciously release that tension.

✔ Through the application of friction to the area, a *thermodynamic* effect takes place, warming and softening the tight, hard tissue.

✔ By stimulating *trigger points*, the local nerves are soothed, allowing a release of contractions.

Raises immune efficiency

Did you know that there is a vast system of vessels running through your body, roughly parallel to your circulatory system, and that this system is filled with a fluid that is responsible for carrying away and eliminating many of the organisms, bacteria, viruses, and other microscopic bad guys that might otherwise attack you? Yes, it's true. This is the *lymph system*, otherwise known as the Canadian Mounties of your body.

Your lymph system has *nodes* at various strategically located areas throughout your body, and these nodes have the job of capturing the invaders and processing them before eventual expulsion through your *excretory system*. Now, you may be wondering, how the heck does this lymph fluid get pumped through your body anyway? Funny you should ask. I've devised a test to discern your knowledge on that very subject.

Holy anatomy quiz, Batman!

That's right, but it's just a one-question quiz, so don't let your anxiety levels rise too high over it. Here we go:

Question: How does the body pump the critically important lymph fluid through its lymph vessels, keeping your inner ocean clean and healthy?

a. The heart pumps the lymph, just like it pumps the blood.

b. The centrifugal force from riding various carnival rides is the best way to get the lymph fluid moving.

c. Fear caused by sudden, unexpected physical proximity to vampires or werewolves causes the lymph vessels to contract, circulating the fluid.

d. Movement, muscular contraction, and massage therapy are the ways lymph fluid is most effectively moved through the body because the lymph system has no pump of its own, such as the heart.

Right! The answer is d. By helping your body circulate this lymph fluid, massage aids in the elimination of noxious invaders (*toxins*) from your body.

Our neglected muscles

Even though you have over 600 muscles that take up approximately 60 percent of your body weight, they sometimes get neglected, especially when it comes to your average physician.

For example, many times after serious trauma, such as a car accident, physicians perform appropriate procedures to save the life of the injured person and to repair any gross damage. Then physical therapists take over to help restore as much use and feeling to the affected areas as possible. What happens, though, when that person returns to his physician or physical therapist six months later complaining of chronic pain? If no further operations are warranted, and continued physical therapy doesn't seem to help, there are only two choices as far as most physicians are concerned:

- Prescribe drugs
- Counsel stoicism

That's right, the only two choices are to either mask the pain or learn to live with it. In the massage model, though, something restorative can be done with that 60 percent of your body known as *soft tissue* to bring about relief.

There are other factors at play, too, in massage's effectiveness as an immune booster. As reported in *LIFE* magazine (August 97), studies in orphanages have shown that infants and children deprived of touch experience stunted growth, both emotionally and physically. Further study showed that touch promotes the release of human growth hormone (HGH), which is essential to our development. If a child is not touched sufficiently, his or her development will be stunted, and susceptibility to disease will be increased, with potentially catastrophic results. Many of the untouched children in orphanages have died for lack of simple contact.

Improves circulation

This is the reason that the cigar-smoking octogenarians who frequented old-fashioned health spas used to give for receiving massage: "It's good for the circulation!" they'd say. And they were right.

Students in massage school are taught to always massage in the direction of circulation, toward the heart, whenever they're applying enough pressure to move the blood underneath the skin. The reason for this is that your veins have little one-way valves in them that keep blood from going back in the wrong direction. So obviously it's not a good idea to push the blood back against these valves, potentially harming them. In fact, when these valves don't work properly on their own, the blood seeps backward and pools up, causing the appearance of varicose veins, which are a *contraindication* for massage, but I'm skipping ahead to Chapter 10 already. Sorry about that.

You have the idea: Some massage movements physically push the blood around in its vessels and can therefore, when done properly, push it in the right direction, improving circulation.

Massage also draws more blood to the surface of the body and into areas of relatively poorer circulation, thus bringing with it much-needed oxygen and other nutrients for the tissues.

Promotes the healing of tissues

This benefit is primarily a result of the previous two. By helping to bring nutrient-rich blood into areas that are recovering from any type of problem, and by helping to cleanse these same areas of toxins (by stimulating the lymph system), massage promotes quicker healing.

Also, certain types of massage stretch and soften tissues in traumatized areas, helping them regain natural elasticity and strength faster.

But beware: You definitely don't want to rush straight in and massage your cousin John's swollen knee after his recent surgery unless you've been trained in bona-fide massage classes and know what you're doing.

Increases healthy functioning of the skin

The skin is where massage has its most pronounced effects. In fact, I've devoted the whole of Chapter 3 to it. So let me just say here that massage includes several actions that leave the skin silky, vibrant, and fully functioning in both directions. By that I mean it promotes the shedding of dead cells while also encouraging the absorption of moisture, nutrients, vitamins, and other vital elements, especially when the massage is given with the aid of creams, oils, and lotions created for just that purpose.

In this sense, massage helps the skin "breathe." Just as our lungs breathe both in and out, inhaling and exhaling, healthy skin must breathe in both directions, too, and massage can help with that.

Offers emotional reassurance

In a famous experiment conducted by some truly sadistic researchers, some unfortunate little monkeys were brought up in cages with surrogate mothers. Each monkey had two mothers in the cage with him. One was a rag doll and the other was a hard wire shell. The uncomfortable wire mother had a nipple with real milk coming out, but the rag doll mother had no nipples and no milk. The researchers shocked the monkeys, then they sat back with smug-researcher-expressions on their faces to see what would happen. In every case, when they were desperate for comfort and safety, the monkeys scampered straight over to rag-doll-mommy, regardless of the fact that she had never provided any other kind of food or sustenance beyond the fact of being soft and cuddly.

This brings us to an important realization as far as humans are concerned, too: Almost every person alive, when shocked, would rather squeeze a rag doll than a hard wire shell with a nipple attached. This bit of information, I've found, makes a fascinating ice-breaker at cocktail parties.

Extrapolating from this data, the researchers were able to conclude, with a good degree of confidence, that tactile sensations are the most important factors involved with emotional comforting.

Massage, by offering a sustained, intentional, caring form of tactile stimulation, is one of the best ways to impart emotional reassurance, and emotional reassurance just may be the number one need of humans in the twenty-first century. We modern urban dwellers are all a bunch of shocked monkeys searching for Mom, basically. And massage is the ultimate rag doll.

Engenders profound relaxation

Dr. Robert Benson of Harvard wrote in *The Relaxation Response* that by repeating certain breathing and concentration exercises, people could greatly reduce their levels of stress. Massage, by its very nature, induces a similar response. It's a mini-vacation that you can take right there inside your own body. No need to buy expensive plane tickets or submit yourself to the hassles of taxi rides and hotel rooms. Just close your eyes and let someone else send you to your own virtual Tahiti.

If you receive a massage and don't relax, it's the same thing as going to Tahiti and not enjoying the scenery, the warmth, the water, or the colorful little umbrellas in the cocktails. In other words, it's up to you. Nobody can force you to relax while receiving a massage, just as no one can force you to enjoy the South Pacific, but you'd have to be kind of crazy not to.

Improves appearance

The combination of all the preceding benefits leaves just about anybody who receives them looking better than they did before they started, and in that way, massage can improve the appearance of even the most stubbornly unattractive person. You know the type: the man with the big crease down the middle of his forehead, or the woman with her mouth pulled taut like she just chewed an entire lemon. Most of what we deem unattractive is simply poor attitude, and the people with the strangest looking faces and bodies can still be very attractive, especially if they are . . .

- ✔ Tension-free
- ✔ Healthy
- ✔ Flushed with the rosy glow of good circulation
- ✔ Quickly recovering from any painful conditions
- ✔ Covered with silky "breathing" skin
- ✔ Confident and emotionally assured
- ✔ Profoundly relaxed

Who can resist a person like this?

The Massage Menu

There are literally hundreds of types of massage practiced around the world, many of them with wonderfully evocative names like *tui-na* and *lomi lomi*. This is not the section in which I'm going to explain each of those massage *modalities* to you, however (a fairly extensive explanation of several major styles is the focus of one section in Chapter 5). Instead, what I'm doing here is explaining the generic types of massage, broken down into categories based on the observable effects they can have in your own life.

Think of this section like the menu in a restaurant. Each category (breakfast, lunch, dinner) consists of distinctly different dishes, and yet the foods used to prepare the dishes can be the same. So the same eggs used to make your omelet at breakfast can be used in your egg salad at lunch or your dessert after dinner. It's the same with the following categories of massage. Any particular massage technique can be used to create various effects.

When you head into Chez Massage, you can order a-la-carte or request a pre-arranged sampling of offerings, like on a prix-fixe menu. The following do not present a completely exhaustive list, but they cover all the main entrees and several side dishes as well:

Relaxation massage

This category may be the most familiar to those of you who have not delved into the world of massage before. It's the type of massage you see on TV. For example, in one of the older James Bond movies, Sean Connery poses as a massage therapist in a European spa and rubs some information out of one his enemies (a beautiful Russian enemy, of course). The impromptu maneuvers he made up at that point consisted of simple, straightforward rubbing and sliding. A trained massage therapist delivers quite a bit more effectiveness than Sean did, but in essence, the purpose of the relaxation massage is, duh, to relax. This is particularly helpful in these instances:

- ✔ For stress relief, when the daily grind is just too much and the simple act of lying down and having someone pay solicitous attention to you for an hour is enough to make a big difference.
- ✔ For pampering, which is fine, as long as you don't feel guilty about it.

Sports massage

Just ask the world-class athletes who travel with their own personal massage therapists. They'll tell you what a difference a massage can make. Many Olympians and high-level players in all sports are true believers, but they are not the only ones who use massage as part of their training. Even amateur athletes and weekend warriors incorporate it whenever they can, specifically, pre-event, post-event, and for ongoing training.

Rehabilitative massage

This type of massage helps the body repair itself. Many people have found that it was the key factor in helping them heal quickly and get back to normal activity levels as soon as possible after injuries and after surgery.

Doctors are people, too

You may notice that on several occasions in this book, I allude to physicians as people who are not quite up to speed with reality when it comes to the very provable value of massage therapy. In fact, I've already said something to that effect in this chapter.

So I just want to make something clear before you get the wrong idea: I think doctors are great. I respect and admire doctors and consider several to be friends. Sure, there are some jerk doctors just like there are jerk massage therapists, but all-in-all, physicians are some of the most responsible, educated, humane, helpful humans on the planet, doing all kinds of good work.

When you hear me say anything less than complimentary about physicians or *allopathic medicine*, it's not the people themselves I'm referring to so much as the system we've created in which they work. Unfortunately, our present situation does not allow for doctors to spend the time with each individual patient that they'd probably like to. At the same time, many of them are realizing the value of massage and have even begun including it in their practices. In fact, a September 1998 survey of medical schools published in the *Journal of the American Medical Association (JAMA)* revealed that 64 percent of medical schools offer courses in complementary medicine, including massage, which is the most popular alternative *modality* taught.

Miriam Wetzel, Ph.D., director of curriculum development at Harvard Medical School, says that therapeutic massage is part of the school's training. "I would like to see the medical community recognize that there is a difference between therapeutic massage and something that's just relaxing," she says.

In France, where my co-author Michel Van Welden received his training, physicians look at massage in a wholly different light. "What we do is respected as part of the medical model all across Europe," says Michel. "Physicians there have no qualms about referring particular cases to massage therapists. In fact, the word we use in France for massage therapist is *kinesiotherapeut,* which really signifies a combination of massage therapist, physical therapist, and holistic practitioner who utilizes a number of healing tools, such as aromatherapy and herbology. There are 25,000 of them in France, which is an area the size of Texas. Most of them have their own clinics, and they are very highly regarded by physicians and patients alike."

Some of us in the alternative health world have given doctors a bum wrap for too long. I say let's move forward toward an *integrative medicine* that includes their expertise and ours together. This is already happening as witnessed by the quickly growing number of health clinics and hospitals with practitioners from many disciplines: M.D.s, acupuncturists, massage therapists, nutritionists, herbalists, and others.

Esthetic massage

We all want to look as good as we can, and massage can help. Through a combination of several of the benefits mentioned earlier in this chapter, massage softens your skin and gives you a healthy glow. It is also used to improve the appearance of certain skin irregularities such as cellulite, with varying degrees of efficacy. People include massage in their beauty regimen for its ability to promote a youthful appearance and as an auxiliary treatment to enhance the effects of other beautifying procedures, such as plastic surgery and facials.

Energy-balancing massage

If massage were a map of the world, energy-balancing would be China. Yes, that's how big it is. Because energy is invisible, it's easy to dismiss it as unimportant, as far as our bodies go. But for a moment, imagine your body without energy. That's right: limp as a cooked noodle, flat as a pancake, blah as all get-out. Many of the massage styles I go over in Chapter 5 are based on an understanding of the body's energy systems, focusing on how to balance and enhance our inner invisible energy. These techniques can basically be categorized as either ancient systems, such as acupressure, or modern systems, such as cranio-sacral work.

Massage for increased awareness

Most of us inhabit our bodies without giving it much thought. We walk around in them and sit around in them and lie around in them, all on automatic pilot, relying upon the old patterns and habits we picked up in childhood. Sometimes, we're negatively influenced by injuries and other traumas that turn these unconscious habits into potentially debilitating conditions. We feel "stuck" in certain postures and can't get out. A massage can help you become aware of how you're holding onto certain patterns of tension and thus let you break them, and it can help you gain self-confidence through releasing old, negative body images.

Spiritually oriented massage

Depending on your frame of mind, any massage can be a spiritual experience, regardless of whether you receive it in an ancient Asian temple or the treatment room of your local health club. All you need are two people focused on awareness, breathing, releasing, and compassion. This spiritual aspect of massage can be used in the following ways:

✔ For meditation, when the sensitive sharing that takes place between two people in a good massage leads you to quiet your mind and remember some of the more important things in life.

✔ By ministers, nuns, and other clergy members who use this "laying on of hands" as a means to express compassion and in some cases to invoke healing.

✔ By practitioners of Eastern traditions such as Taoism and Buddhism. Buddhist monks in Thailand, for example, often learn the art of massage and practice it in their temples.

Massage for emotional growth

Allowing yourself to be touched with caring, therapeutic intentions takes a high degree of maturity. Several types of massage have been developed to access inner psychological issues and bring them to light. This is especially true in specific cases of past emotional trauma involving abuse and negative body-image caused by being overweight or handicapped.

Massage for sensual pleasure

This type of massage can be performed by any two consenting adults who have a relationship of respect and trust between them. It's especially useful for long-term couples seeking new and exciting activities to spice up their lives and for short-term couples looking for ways to slow themselves down and enjoy the moment rather than rush through to you-know-what.

Massage for non-humans

Believe it or not, there are special courses offered to teach people how to massage animals. As anyone who's ever scratched behind the ear of an appreciative pet can tell you, they love it. Certain animals in particular have been the lucky recipients of massage:

✔ Horses, especially race and show horses that are each worth more than the gross national product of the average third-world country

✔ Dogs and cats and other "people with fur" that we live with on an intimate basis

Chapter 2

A Brief History of Touch

● ●

In This Chapter

▶ The development of massage therapy around the world

▶ Massage in today's world

▶ Where massage is going

● ●

This chapter is supposed to extol the virtues of certain Greek physicians who developed massage a couple thousand years ago, and then it's supposed to move on to the beginning of the twentieth century and talk about a certain Swedish man who was the father of modern western massage. And then the chapter should chronicle the . . . ZZZZZZZZZZ.

Was that the sound of your head smacking the table? Are you already getting so bored that you're about to fling this book against the nearest wall in desperation? "Why can't he tell me something fascinating and different?" you're about to scream.

Okay, I can hear the psychic echoes of your potential screams, so this chapter is going to be a teeny bit different than the history chapters in most massage books, the ones that treat the chronology of massage like the dry academic stuff you find in history texts. What could be more unlike the vibrant flesh-and-bones reality of a subject as physical as massage?

Dramatic Moments in Massage History

For your benefit and edification, I'm going to recreate dramatic scenes from various important massage moments throughout history. Much of what follows has been garnished with a large dose of creative license, but rest assured that the information is based upon historical fact. Only the boring parts have been deleted to protect the innocent reader.

Shaman Bob — hands-on healer

Thousands of years ago, beneath the primeval rainforest canopies of the vast Amazon jungle in what is now part of Brazil, an old *shaman* squatted down by a river, twisting the leaves and stems of a hardy vine between his worn fingers. The shaman's name was unintelligible to modern ears, so we'll call him Bob. His fingers were working the powerful ayuhasca vine, which gave his people visions that helped them to heal. Bob boiled the leaves and stems of the vine in water with other plants, making a thick syrupy tea that he brought with him back into the village.

It was night. The rainforest canopy above was filled with the screeching sounds of life. Arranging the members of the tribe in a circle around a fire he had built, Bob gave them each sips of the tea, and they began to twirl and dance and sing traditional songs. Some of them, the ones who needed healing the most, fell into a trance, and Bob approached them.

As the others watched, Bob appeared to literally reach into each person's body with his fingers. Then his fingers would flutter up toward the dark sky above the fire. He would touch them, brush them off, shake their limbs, staying in almost constant contact, and everyone could see (with the help of the ayuhasca) what Bob always saw — blurry spots where each person's body was weak, demons of darkness clinging to a shoulder.

Although Bob used powerful herbs and jungle plants, his primary tool was touch. The difference between a casual touch from another tribe member and an intentional, focused touch from Bob was sometimes the difference between life and death. His touch healed, and everyone knew it.

The Tao of massage

The enigmatic Chinese word, *Tao*, confuses many people. For one thing, why is the word spelled T-a-o when it's pronounced Dow? And for another thing, what's it supposed to mean anyway? Does it have anything to do with the New York Stock Exchange?

Many of you have heard of the *Tao of Pooh* or the *Tao of Physics* or the *Tao of Flower Arranging,* and if you ever read one of those far-out books on Eastern philosophy published in the 1970s — the kind printed on organic-oatmeal type paper — you probably remember the phrase, "The Tao that can be spoken of is not the true Tao." So then, how are you supposed to talk about it?

Regardless of the fact that you apparently can't talk about the Tao, you can still talk about massage, which is exactly what an early Chinese Taoist did around 5,000 years ago. He wrote a book called the *Con Fou of Tao-Tse* (Cun Fooh of Dow Zee) that described the use of medicinal plants, exercises, and a

MASSAGE TALE

Great Greeks go nude

Imagine the Greek sun burning in a clear, blue sky. Below, in the outdoor *gymnazein*, dozens of naked athletes are exercising, each of them so tanned and muscled and healthy that they look like, well, Greek gods. Why naked, you ask? The word gymnasium itself comes from the Greek *gymnazein*, which means "to exercise naked," from *gymnos*, naked. Those fun-loving Greeks, I tell ya.

At any rate, the sun's beating down, all these naked Greeks are running around outdoing each other in feats of fitness, and old Asclepius is over there in the trainer's corner, ready and

waiting each time another Adonis comes running up with a torn Achilles tendon or sore lower back. The natural thing, of course, is to offer massage, along with other herbs and remedies. Supposedly, Asclepius became so proficient at this healing that he could even raise the dead. As a reward, Zeus struck him down with a thunderbolt and killed him.

This tale brings us to one of the very earliest philosophical lessons tied to the practice of massage: If you like to massage naked Greek athletes, try to keep it a secret.

system of massage for the treatment of disease. Because it was one of the first books ever written on any subject, the *Con Fou* really goes to show you just how ancient and important this whole subject of massage is after all.

A Greek man with a mission

Asclepius (as-klee´-pee-uhs), son of Apollo, the Greek god of healing, may have been an actual Greek man who lived around 1200 B.C., but just as likely he was a mythological figment of the Greek imagination. At any rate, he was credited with being the first to combine exercise with massage. He also founded the world's first gymnasium.

The Middle Ages

Nobody massaged anybody else (or was even allowed to touch much) during the Middle Ages, which almost wiped out western civilization. Luckily, a few hardy souls decided, despite vigorous opposition, to sneak off and touch each other in barns, stables, and other hidden places whenever possible, thus assuring the continuation of the human race and allowing people a chance to practice rudimentary massage techniques at the same time. Needless to say, the Middle Ages were *not* a good time to be a professional massage therapist, and many of them suffered extreme deprivations. In fact, some say that a famous book by Victor Hugo, and the Broadway musical

The Hypocritical oath

You may wonder why doctors have to take a hypocritical oath after they finish medical school and before they begin practicing. After all, you trust your physician with your life; why would you want him or her to be a hypocrite?

The answer is simple. They're not taking a hypocritical oath, but rather a Hippocratic Oath, which means that it was first uttered by none other than that great Greek physician himself, Hippocrates (460 – 380 B.C.). In the very first line of this oath, Hippocrates swears by Apollo and Asclepius to uphold the virtues of his healing art,

to not seduce women (or men) in the households he visits as a physician, and to abstain from mischief of all kinds.

Hippocrates also spoke about massage movements, saying that "hard rubbing binds, much rubbing causes parts to waste, and moderate rubbing makes them grow." He recommended massage for many conditions.

So, the man who penned the words that physicians around the world utter to this day was a believer in massage. Go figure.

based upon it, are actually plagiarized versions of an original story about the lives of these wretched medieval massage practitioners. Sadly, the original manuscript has been lost, and the true origins of *Les Massagerables* will forever remain a mystery.

The Swedish scenario

In most places you go in the western world today, when you ask for a massage, you'll receive one form or another of *Swedish* massage. And so, you may ask, *why* is it called Swedish massage? Here are some of the typical answers people have given to that question:

- ✔ People in Sweden were the only ones liberal enough to allow massage to be named after them.

- ✔ The Swedish director Ingmar Bergman liked to receive massage after a hard day on the movie set, and so they named the technique after him.

- ✔ Nobody knows why it's called Swedish massage, but everyone agrees it sounds better than Lithuanian massage or Uruguayan massage.

Actually, Swedish massage is named after a Swedish physiologist and fencing master by the name of Per Henrik Ling (1776–1839), who developed a system of Medical Gymnastics that included the moves we now use in basic massage. He eventually became known as the father of physical therapy. The fact that his original system embraced massage is interesting because physical therapists in the modern world have to a large degree ostracized massage from their repertoire, and there is sometimes discord between them and massage therapists.

Decline of massage in the twentieth century

Due to the infighting amongst massage practitioners, and the sudden, powerful influence of technology in the medical world, massage faded from favor during the early and mid-1900s. Also, the earlier popularity of massage induced some people to try to make a profit from it illicitly. Around the turn of the century, several schools in Great Britain, for example, were turning out poorly trained practitioners, some of whom ended up acting as prostitutes, which was a big downfall for massage. Since the days of Hippocrates, and even further back into the ancient history of China and India, massage had been accepted as a healthy pastime by a sizeable number of people. Now, things were different.

MASSAGE TALE

Massaging Cain and Abel

Perhaps the discord in the massage world can be traced back to the pair of American brothers who were responsible for bringing massage to the United States from Sweden — Charles and George Taylor. The Taylor brothers shared similar interests, obviously; they both became doctors, both went to Europe to learn these new techniques, and they both wanted to spend their lives helping other people. But, as so often seems to happen when people go on a quest to help others, they just couldn't seem to get along themselves.

Coming back to New York in the 1850s, they opened a clinic together, but within a year they dissolved it and went their own ways.

"It's *MY* technique for helping other people feel better," said Charles, adjusting his bowler hat atop his head.

"No way, it's *mine*," replied George, adjusting his identical bowler cap.

"Mine."

"Mine."

And thus started a problem that has persisted to this day, with various massage innovators and practitioners teaching that their way is the best way. George and Charles Taylor were the Cain and Abel of the modern massage world. And, even though massage as a whole is a glorious way to help people feel better on many levels, it has been broken up into sects, with the proponents of certain techniques loudly proclaiming theirs as the best. This book, I hope, will help you cut through all that so that you can gain an appreciation for massage as a whole.

Freud and massage

Sigmund Freud, the inventor of modern psychoanalysis, used massage with his patients. Early on, when Freud wanted to calm and reassure his clients that he was on their side, he used massage maneuvers primarily on their hands. Unfortunately, Freud left massage behind as he further developed his psychoanalytic techniques, perhaps out of a fear that he wouldn't be able to know what was really working, talking or touching. But he was greatly in favor of it from the start. In the modern world, many psychologists are rediscovering the power of massage and incorporating it into their practice with body-centered psychotherapy and somatic therapies.

Throughout the mid-1900s, many massage therapists in the U.S. worked in a YMCA or a Turkish bath house and weren't expected to do much more than pummel their victims (er, clients) with some extraordinarily vigorous maneuvers, usually meant to purge the recipient of excess alcohol and fatty acids ingested the night before. In fact, some spa towns, such as Hot Springs, Arkansas, had massage facilities that were open on Sunday mornings especially for this purpose. The upstanding men of the community came in early to have the effects of Saturday night's revelry pounded and sweated out of them by hardy massage practitioners.

Hippies save massage from extinction

Overall, things weren't going so well for massage in the United States. And the same was true, for the most part, in Europe. Only people with hangovers wanted massage. Of course, on a worldwide level, massage in many areas still retained the same untainted prestige it had enjoyed for centuries. But even in the most remote areas there was a clamoring for things new — vibrating massagers instead of actual massages, for instance — and as technological revolution swept the planet, it left people high and dry as far as contact goes.

The human species was literally getting out of touch.

As always, when society swings too far in one direction, a mounting momentum tends to bring it back toward equilibrium. Somewhere in the 1960s, people began to tire of the soulless sway of machines and technology in their lives, and they started to react against it. These revolutionaries were called hippies, or flower children, and they spread out from San Francisco to cover much of the world, toting with them tie-dyed T-shirts, prayer beads, big black vinyl discs called albums, and home made massage tables.

MASSAGE TALE

Keep in touch, Lorraine

The hippie movement brought people back into touch with themselves, as exemplified by the story of Lorraine, who, in 1968, couldn't decide exactly what to do with her life and so went off in search of something new in California, like so many of her generation.

"I need to get in touch with myself," intoned Lorraine to anyone who asked her what she was doing. Perhaps she didn't realize how precise her choice of words truly was.

Heading her faded yellow VW Bug west, with "Go Ask Alice" playing over and over again on the eight-track tape deck mounted under the dash, Lorraine kept driving and driving until she came to the remote spot on the winding highway south of Big Sur in California that so many people had told her about.

The place was called the Esalen Institute, and it was a mecca for consciousness-raising workshops, research into alternative health, superb massages and massage instruction, and just plain blissing out. People from all over the world came to Esalen to get back in touch, literally, with themselves and with life. Lorraine moved in, stayed for five years, and by the time she left she had found her calling in life and became a massage therapist.

Massage Today

Through the years, massage has had a serious, multiple-personality disorder, kind of like Sybil. Every time you look at it, you're never sure exactly what you're going to see. A Greek physician massaging athletes? A Swedish physiotherapist creating movements to help ease common suffering? A shaman purging evil spirits? A spiritual seeker sending healing vibrations through her fingers during an Esalen style massage at a spectacular seaside retreat?

So many choices

Massage is enjoying such a large renaissance right now, in fact, that at times the market may appear glutted with too many massage therapists. An alternative newspaper in Asheville, North Carolina, for instance, printed a cartoon summarizing the plight of that city's abundance of highly trained, underemployed massage therapists. The cartoon showed an out-of-work therapist standing at a corner holding up a sign: "Will massage for food."

So where does that leave you as you head out the door today, tomorrow, or next week to go seeking your own massage experiences? Well, you certainly have a lot more choices, which I clarify in Chapter 9. You also have a lot more massage therapists to choose from — somewhere between 30,000 and 50,000 new massage therapists in the U.S. each year, for example. And France, which is not a huge country, has over 35,000 practicing *kines*, short for *kinesiotherapeut*, their term for massage/physical therapist. These practitioners are popular, partly because insurance has covered their services since 1974; people in France are used to receiving massage as part of their healthcare.

Although you do have more choices than ever, I think the assumption that we're getting anywhere near a critical mass of massage practitioners in the world is mistaken. There are just too many people around these days to massage — over six billion of them as of August 1999 — and the population continues to expand rapidly.

What you can expect in terms of massage in the year 2000 and beyond is an ever-increasing number of choices, kind of like you find in those designer coffee shops. Whereas before the choice used to be simple — regular or decaf? — now you're faced with an overwhelming array of mochas and frappes and lattes and on and on. This phenomenon has been termed the Starbuckizing of massage.

Touch research

To keep up with all the rapid changes and to document the effectiveness of massage in the midst of all these changes, somebody had to start some serious research into the matter, and that's just what they do at the Touch Research Institute.

If you happen to live in South Florida, and you were to stroll down to the local medical center, you probably wouldn't be too surprised to find some scientific studies being conducted in one of the buildings there. But you may be surprised to find that, instead of an operating room or a clinic, these studies are being conducted in softly lit chambers with flute music playing in the background. And the subjects, instead of undergoing cutting-edge medical technologies, are receiving the age-old techniques of massage therapy.

The Touch Research Institute was founded in Miami in 1992 to study the effects of touch on human beings. Whereas the senses of smell, hearing, sight, and taste all have had their institutes and studies for decades, poor little orphan touch was neglected until the 1990s.

Perhaps touch was neglected because it is just so obvious. When you think about it, nothing is *not* touch; your body is a large antenna feeling everything as it happens to you. The other senses all involve touch in one way or another, too; molecules of various kinds hit you in the taste buds, the optical nerves, the ear drums, and the nasal passages, which set off the sensations that make the senses work.

A massage pilgrimage to Esalen

The pioneering work done at Esalen helped keep massage alive and well after its decline in the early and mid-1900s. Esalen, located in Big Sur, a couple hours south of San Francisco, was founded by Michael Murphy in 1962, and some of the best massage teachers and researchers in the world have taught and worked there. The result of their efforts has been a shifting of the entire paradigm upon which massage is built. No longer simply a remedial form of "gymnastics" to restore movement and ease pain, massage has become a way to increase awareness and sometimes even access the spirit.

If you're passionate about learning what massage can be on this spirit-enhancing level, you may want to make a trip to this massage-mecca yourself. Wherever you are in the world, if you are a massage lover, making your own massage pilgrimage to Esalen will benefit your spirit!

Esalen's location itself is spectacular, perched upon steep cliffs overhanging the Pacific Ocean, where hot springs flow from the mountainside directly into a series of pools adjacent to the massage area. (Esalen's Web site is at www.esalen.org.)

Nudity alert: Beware, Esalen is clothing optional, and nudity is common. Think of it as a great way to get used to viewing the grand masterpiece of the human body.

In 1998, two new Touch Research Institutes opened, one in the Philippines and one in France, which points toward a globalization of studies on massage. How can they get away with testing massage like that, you ask? How can people just lie around feeling good and then call it research? First of all, they don't call it massage, but rather *Tactile Kinesthetic Stimulation,* which, translated, means "massage that someone can receive a medical research grant for." And the studies include extensive psychological tests, blood analysis, double-blind tests (tests in which neither the participants nor the researchers know which subjects have a particular disease or condition and which don't), and a large amount of paperwork. So it's not just a big vacation.

Some of the studies that have been done at the Touch Research Institute include the following groups:

- **HIV patients:** Serotonin and killer T-cells increased due to the massage.

- **Premature infants:** Massaged infants gained weight more quickly and left the hospital an average of six days earlier than non-massaged infants, at an average savings of $3,000.

- **Depressed teenage mothers:** Massage helped them gain self-confidence and provided a way for them to connect with their infants.

- **Children with post-traumatic shock syndrome after hurricane Andrew:** Massage offered psychological reassurance that the world could be a safe place again.

- **Cancer patients:** Researchers are still gathering data about how massage can help with this disease.

The Future of Massage

Many people are familiar with John Naisbitt's book *Megatrends*, which discusses the problems people face as society heads into an increasingly technological world. Naisbitt says that as people get more high-tech, they have to become equally *high-touch* as well. Massage, of course, is one obvious answer to this dilemma.

Following are examples of some high-touch trends that show every sign of continuing into the future as massage integrates more and more into society's high-tech lifestyle:

- ✔ **Diplomacy:** Massage therapists already travel around the world as ambassadors of compassion. This trend will continue as hands-on techniques evolve and cross-cultural communication develops further.

- ✔ **Performance:** More and more performers, athletes, and high-profile individuals will discover the value and relevance of massage. Every professional sports team, for example, will have massage therapists on staff (many do already), creating a trickle-down effect as fans and the general public become increasingly aware of massage through the team's example.

- ✔ **Affordability:** As the world gradually shifts from a manufacturing-based economy to an information- and services-based economy, the demand for massage will continue to grow. Employers and insurance companies will be increasingly willing to pay for massage services, which will benefit the bottom line by reducing absenteeism, stress-related injury, and so on.

- ✔ **Increased sophistication:** Massage techniques (some of which have been around for centuries) will become more and more sophisticated as practitioners from various schools cross-train and add new skills to their repertoires.

Chapter 3

Your Skin: Frontier to the Rest of the World

"We touch heaven when we lay our hands on a human body."
— Novalis (pen name of Frederich von Hardenberg)

Skin is the essence of what makes humans human. How do I know, you ask? I saw it in a *Star Trek* movie, so it must be true. In the movie, a wily alien treated Data, the android, to a taste of being human by grafting a swatch of flesh to his mechanical arm. He already had a brain and a fully functioning body, but the one thing he lacked was sensation. He was just a machine until he had this little patch of skin attached to him, and with it, he became human.

The essence of being human is the ability to feel. "But," you might respond, "I feel things in my mind and with my nerves, too, not just my skin. And besides, can I really trust *Star Trek* as a source of anatomical knowledge?" Well, guess what? In this case, the writers of *Star Trek* happened to be right on the money. Your skin, your nerves, and your mind are really just different layers of the same thing.

Thinking with Your Skin

In his book, *Job's Body*, Deane Juhan, a researcher into the effectiveness of massage and other touch therapies, says, "Depending upon how you look at it, the skin is the outer surface of the brain, or the brain is the deepest layer of the skin."

This assertion, though it may seem absurd initially, can be proven quite easily if you look closely at the development of the embryo. As you know, you start out as a little clump of cells deep in your mother's womb. In the very first days after conception, these cells begin to divide into three distinct layers that will later become your body. The *endoderm* layer of cells eventually forms your internal organs, the *mesoderm* forms the muscles and connective tissues, and the *ectoderm* forms the nervous system and the skin.

As the *ectoderm* cells develop, they gradually turn into your brain, spinal cord, nerves, and skin, which are really all one unit. "Nowhere along the line can I draw a sharp distinction between a periphery which purely responds as opposed to a central nervous system which purely thinks"(Juhan p. 36). In other words, your skin "thinks" as well as feels, and your brain "feels" as well as thinks. It's all one thing. And it starts at a very early age. In fact, at six weeks and less than an inch long, the little embryo can already "feel" light stroking on its upper lip, which causes a withdrawal reaction.

Feeling = thinking

Imagine the following sequence:

1. Imagine a pinprick at a certain point on the skin (Point A).

2. Imagine the sensation that travels up from the sensory receptor near the skin's surface, to the nerve, and then on toward the spine, which it enters at Point B. From there it continues up to the brain.

3. Imagine your brain processing this impulse somewhere around Point C, sending a further impulse to your mouth, which then says "ouch."

So the question is, at what point does the sensation of the pinprick cause you to pull your skin away from the sharp object?

A. At point A, the exact moment the pin pricks the skin.

B. At point B, a nanosecond later, when the sensation enters the spine.

C. At point C, inside the brain itself.

D. None of the above.

This question is tricky. Most people assume that the answer is C, inside the brain, because that's where they think they have the thought, "That hurts." But in actuality the answer is B, when entering the spine, for the following reason:

You pull yourself away from the pinprick as a result of a *reflex arc* at point B, which is an impulse that enters the spine and then shoots right back out again in the form of a reaction. You actually experience the pulling away before your brain catches up to what's happening and you say the word "ouch." Ever notice that? For the same reason, your knee jerks when tapped with a little rubber hammer, without your having time to think about it. So, in this sense, your skin and nerves do the "thinking" for you.

Note: Do not try this pinprick experiment at home on friends or family. I guarantee that they won't appreciate it.

Investigating Your Multi-dimensional Skin

In his book, *Touching: The Human Significance of the Skin,* Ashley Montagu offers many pearls of wisdom, such as: "To shut off any one of the senses is to reduce the dimensions of our reality, and to the extent that that occurs we lose touch with it; we become imprisoned in a world of impersonal words, sans touch, sans taste, sans flavor. The one-dimensionality of the word becomes a substitute for the richness of the multi-dimensionality of the senses, and our world grows crass, flat, and arid in consequence."

Sadly, he's right. People end up ignoring most of what they feel, and as they get less and less in touch with themselves, they become more and more hectic, filling their days with frantic activity rather than just enjoying the sensation-filled miracle of being alive. Instead of hectic, I think people should become more *haptic*. A *haptic* person is especially in tune with her sense of touch, or, as Ashley Montagu would say, has a "mentally extended sense of touch which comes about through the total experience of living and acting in space."

Haptic comes from the Greek word, *haptesthai*, to touch. To start yourself in a haptic direction, you need to know a few details about the skin:

- ✔ You have more than 3 million cells in a patch of skin about the size of a bottle cap.
- ✔ Your skin contains 2 to 5 million sweat glands and about 2 million pores.

✔ Your skin is your largest organ system:

- 2,500 square centimeters in newborns and approximately 19,000 square centimeters (19 square feet) in an adult male.

- An adult male's skin weighs approximately 8 pounds.

✔ Your skin gets strength and form from collagen, which comprises 70 percent of your skin's dry weight.

✔ You have approximately 640,000 sensory receptors embedded in your skin.

✔ Your skin ranges in thickness from $\frac{1}{10}$ of a millimeter on the eyelids to 3 or 4 millimeters on the soles and palms.

✔ Your skin becomes softer in summer and more dense in winter.

Because you have so many sensory receptors in your skin (pain cells are the most plentiful, followed by a variety of pressure sensors, cold sensors, and warmth sensors), it's no wonder you can be so "touchy" if you're "rubbed the wrong way." And no wonder that a caring, calming massage can be so soothing.

All you really have to do to get back "in touch" with your true, haptic self is to tune in to your senses, your skin, and your environment, like you did when you were six years old and mud puddles were sources of unending pleasure. To help you get back to that sacred sensory space, you can try the sensitivity exercises that follow.

Sensitivity exercise #1: The Zen cantaloupe ceremony

Consider, for a moment, the word "cantaloupe." Nice, round word that evokes the picture of the fruit itself in your mind. Perhaps the word even summons up a sweet cantaloupe memory or two. But too often the word itself is a substitute for the fullness of the thing, a crutch people use to classify this or that specific bit of reality, filing it away for easy reference.

If you want to move yourself beyond your mind's habitual categorizing mechanisms, try the Zen cantaloupe ceremony:

1. **Buy or borrow a fresh, ripe, high-quality cantaloupe.**

2. **Find a quiet, private place (where no one can see you and make fun of you) and sit with your cantaloupe placed on a plate within reach.**

   Have a knife handy. Then close your eyes.

3. **Spend five minutes or so just calmly breathing and slowing your mind.**

4. **Slowly, with your eyes still closed, reach your fingertips out until you make contact with the cantaloupe.**

   Do not attempt to pick it up. Just feel the surface in extremely minute detail, as though you're trying to decipher a message encoded in the fruit's convoluted furrows. Pay attention to your fingertips.

5. **Begin to lift the melon up, using your fingertips alone.**

   Spend a minute feeling the weight, shifting it from hand to hand. Then slowly bring the fruit up to your face, rubbing the rough texture against your cheek.

6. **After this thorough tactile encounter with the melon, place it on the plate again, and then slowly and ritualistically lift the knife and begin your incision, slicing out just one sliver, cleaning off the seeds.**

   Open your eyes while slicing but then close them again.

7. **Lift the slice to your nose and take three long inhalations.**

8. **Open your mouth and place the cool orange flesh inside your lips, but don't bite down at first.**

   Let the juices gather on your tongue and savor the sensation.

9. **Let your teeth literally sink down into the fruit, and then let the piece melt in your mouth for a minute before chewing.**

10. **Repeat the biting and chewing until you eat the whole sliver.**

    Breathe deeply for a few minutes again. Then, finally, open your eyes.

If you pay attention to the feelings that you have at each step of the ceremony, you'll discover that cantaloupes have much more depth than just the word "cantaloupe."

Just as the original Zen tea ceremony was used by Samurai warriors in Japan to calm their minds and bring them into the present moment, the cantaloupe ceremony can help focus you on the tactile reality underlying your ongoing reinterpretation of the world through thoughts and words. You can repeat the experience with other fruits, vegetables, and just about any safe, non-toxic foodstuff.

This exercise is a great way to help yourself get into the right frame of mind for giving a good massage. You don't have to think so much. Don't speak. Just touch. Feel. Be with the world you come into contact with, including other people. Performing the Zen Cantaloupe Ceremony is a great way to sensitize your fingers and your mind immediately prior to giving a massage.

Sensitivity exercise #2: The texture of the world

Your fingertips have the largest concentration of sensory receptors of any part of your body. This feature is quite convenient for giving massages, which requires a real sensitivity to the person you're touching.

With their unique sensitivity, your fingers can actually "see" objects, a fact you confirm every time you fish through a purse or pocket, searching for keys. You can develop and fine-tune this capability through a simple attunement exercise called the "texture of the world." The exercise helps you gain a certain sensibility that is crucial for getting and giving good massages.

You need a partner for this experience — someone you trust.

1. **Have your partner gather four or five objects and arrange them on a table, without showing you what they are.**

   See why you have to trust your partner? You don't want someone who may choose bird droppings, tar, rotten dairy products, and so on.

2. **Have your partner blindfold you and sit you in front of the table, within arms' reach of the objects.**

   If you haven't been blindfolded since playing Pin the Tail on the Donkey as a child, be prepared for a startling and powerful experience.

3. **Reach out and touch one object at a time, picking it up and using your fingertips to try to determine what it is.**

   If your partner has been creative in choosing the objects, you should have an interesting experience. Use just your fingertips for this exercise and resist the temptation to get your nose or other senses involved in the process.

4. **Override your mind's tendency to identify the object and then create a visual picture of it, categorize it, and dismiss it.**

   Your mind goes into its automatic pattern the moment you realize what the object is. Instead of giving in to that tendency, continue to explore the object, discovering properties you overlooked before. If you can't guess what the object "really" is, that's okay. In fact, that's good. Just continue to feel it. When your mind can't categorize something, you're forced to perceive it in a new way.

5. **Based on your present tactile encounter alone, rename the objects.**

   A golf ball, for example, may become a dimple-nut. Have your partner write the new names down on pieces of paper and place them next to the objects.

Little skin, lotta feeling

Do you know why little tots seem so extraordinarily sensitive when it comes to touch? Children up to three years old have a total of 80 specialized sensory receptors called *Meissner's corpuscles* per square millimeter of skin, as opposed to 20 in a young adult, and 4 in old age (Montagu, p. 7). That's why babies are so overwhelmed by tickles and touches. They feel more than we do.

---

6. Remove the blindfold and check out your work.

Just being blindfolded greatly alters your perception of the objects. Unable to take them for granted, labeling one a "golf ball" and another a "yellow stick-on note," you will quite likely discover something about your ability to feel, and in the process increase your touch-ability (see Chapter 5 for more on touch-ability).

Layering It On

Your skin, like every other part of your body, is a living, growing, changing thing. In fact, you have an entirely new outer layer of skin every 27 days, which means you're an awful lot like snakes, lizards, and other animals who leave their skins behind periodically. You just shed your skin one skin cell at a time, so it's not so obvious.

The *epidermis,* the outer portion of your skin that keeps replenishing itself and flaking off, is made up of several layers. The bottommost layer keeps reproducing new skin cells, which are then pushed toward the upper layers, collectively known as the *horny zone.* It is called the horny zone because the cells there are hardened, like horns.

So, what you're really seeing when you look at somebody's skin is a whole bunch of dead, hardened cells that are about to fall off. In fact, *exfoliation,* a particular type of spa treatment that I explain further in Chapter 15, assists the skin in this process.

Keep in mind that certain skin conditions make performing a massage inadvisable (see Chapter 10). For now, I'm talking about basic, healthy skin in an average person.

The hazards of breathing

The "dust" particles that you see floating in a shaft of sunlight are mostly dead skin cells from the epidermis that have recently been shed by you and any other people who have inhabited the room. As you breathe, you can't help but inhale some of these flaky cells, thus sucking cousin Bob, Aunt Julia, the refrigerator repair man, and even your own self into your lungs. This situation presents no biological hazard and is usually not a cause for concern because most people don't know about it and therefore don't get grossed out.

Whoops.

Beneath the epidermis lies the *dermis*, which is filled with fat cells, blood and lymph vessels, oil glands, sweat glands, nerve endings, and hair follicles. The dermis also helps to bind the outer layers of the skin to the subcutaneous (which means "beneath the skin") tissues below. In this area, you find some very important cells called *fibroblasts,* which are responsible for producing connective tissues. You owe a great debt of gratitude to your fibroblasts, especially after you break your skin in some way, because these specialized cells are responsible for rushing to the area and filling it with connective fibers, mending you back together. Massage can also affect these fibroblasts to enhance the appearance of your skin.

Getting the Skinny on Your Personal Border Guard

Throughout your life, your skin defines the intimate boundaries of your existence. Skin is the millimeters-thin line that separates you from the rest of reality and allows you to perceive that reality. Here are the six major functions of your own personal border guard, the skin:

- ✔ Protection
- ✔ Absorption
- ✔ Secretion and excretion
- ✔ Heat regulation
- ✔ Respiration
- ✔ Sensation

The importance of getting licked

Have you ever watched a cat give birth? Directly afterwards, mamma cat begins licking her babies all over, with a special concentration in the genital area. The same is true for dogs. And horses. And cows. And aardvarks and antelopes and giraffes. In fact, every species of mammal with the exception of man lick their young immediately after birth.

At first, you may assume that this licking is to clean off the gooey stuff plastered all over the newborn's body. That's partially true, but far more important than the cleaning is the licking itself, the touch of tongue to flesh or fur.

I was in my first massage therapy class, in California, when the instructor stated that massaging a newborn baby's *perineum* (the area between the genitals and anus) with a warm moist cloth was a good idea to simulate the action of licking engaged in by other animals. In other words, he was advising us to metaphorically lick the baby's butt.

At the moment, and for several years afterwards, I thought this California massage instructor was a little too "out there" for his own good. But now, after discovering the importance of this type of stimulation in every other species of mammal, it makes perfect sense. This critical form of early contact jump-starts the newborn's gastrointestinal tract and is perhaps the most primal type of "massage" that we can offer our young.

You can recreate the natural sensations of licking for your newborn by taking a baby-wipe or moist towel and rubbing it gently over the skin in this important area a couple times a day for the first few months of life, starting on day one.

Protection

Whenever anyone tries to pass over the border from Spain to France, say, he or she is stopped by the border guard (usually men in sadly decorative hats, with sour expressions on their faces). The same basic thing happens with your body. Your skin says "Stop and present your papers" to anything big and obvious trying to get inside of it, such as steak knives, harmful bacteria, #2 pencils, and so on. Having the men in the sad little hats there to protect us is a very good thing, as I'm sure you can appreciate when you think about what kind of chaos would ensue were millions of Spaniards to suddenly turn up in your pancreas.

Absorption

Once in a while, you want to allow some people across the border to spend those tourist dollars and improve the economy, right? Your skin can do the same thing through a process called absorption. Your skin can absorb certain cosmetic products, chemicals, drugs, and water in small amounts. Unfortunately, certain items are not beneficial to your body, such as toxins and pesticides. Your skin is equally capable of allowing these terrorists to cross the border, which means you should stay on guard regarding the products you come into contact with.

Excretion and secretion

Your skin can also get rid of toxic elements, like exiling unwanted characters from the country. This process is called *excretion,* and it's handled by those ruffians, the sweat glands. You have several million of these glands, and they eliminate waste products via perspiration.

In addition to excreting, your skin secretes as well, issuing forth an oily substance called *sebum* that coats the skin and helps preserve moisture. Secretion is a good thing, because the skin is about 50 – 70 percent moisture, and you don't want it to dry out.

Heat regulation

Your skin is constantly monitoring the temperature in the environment and helping to maintain your body's internal temperature at an even 98.6°F (37°C) through adjustments of blood vessels and sweat glands, which dilate or contract in response to heat and cold.

If you don't touch me, I'll die

Touch is literally a matter of life and death. The philosopher Bertrand Russell noted the importance of touch, saying, "Not only our geometry and our physics, but our whole conception of what exists outside us, is based on the sense of touch." For this reason, it's urgently important that infants and small children receive an abundant supply of human contact.

In the early 1900s, Dr. Henry Dwight Chapin reported that when orphaned babies were routinely put in homes and left to wither away with essentially zero human contact, a startling 99 percent of them died within one year of admission (Juhan p.43). Those who survived suffered signs of retardation and maladjustment.

To say that the world would truly be a better place if more people received massage — especially as part of their developmental years — is not an exaggeration. Touch is a vital part of human growth, for individuals and for the entire community.

Respiration

Oxygen comes in through the pores of the skin, and carbon dioxide goes out, just like in the lungs, but on a smaller scale. If you're a James Bond fan and saw the classic movie, *Gold Finger,* you may remember the famous opening scene, which featured a woman painted completely gold and then left on a hotel room bed in Miami Beach. In the movie, she died because her skin couldn't "breathe," and a similar fate could happen to you in real life if all of your pores were suddenly blocked.

Sensation

If skin were basically just nature's way of keeping what's inside of our bodies in and what's outside out, life wouldn't be nearly as much fun as it is, and, as it turns out, those guards at the border have a sensitive side beneath their hats after all.

Providing you with a rich, complex variety of sensations is by far the most personally gratifying of the skin's functions, which is something you'll develop an even greater appreciation for as you practice the techniques in the other chapters of this book.

Touching the Skin through Massage

Recently, even the U.S. Food and Drug Administration (FDA) has become convinced that massage offers undeniable results. My co-author, Michel Van Welden, has worked with the FDA extensively and has substantiated some claims for the effectiveness of massage. Following are some of his findings:

- ✔ Scientific evidence points to the fact that massage can positively impact skin tone.
- ✔ Pigs love massage.

It's true. In a series of experiments at Vanderbilt University and UCLA, Michel worked with a team of ace physicians administering a series of massage experiments on some very special subjects: Flopsy, Zeus, and Peewee, three Yorkshire pigs.

The three pigs were chosen for their high moral character and love of luxurious spa treatments. No, actually they were chosen because pigs (even though you may not like to admit it) have remarkably similar skin to humans. Twice a week for 13 weeks the three brave little oinkers received deeply stimulating massages with a device that strongly affects circulation. The FDA eventually approved this device as an effective way to tone the skin and improve the appearance of cellulite. Here are some of the findings of these experiments, as reported in *Newsweek* magazine, November 1998:

- ✔ This type of massage, called Endermologie®, stimulates fibroblasts, which produce collagen.
- ✔ An increase in collagen fibers can improve the elasticity and youthful appearance of the skin.

Michel should know. He's been a physical therapist in France for almost 30 years, and in that country the physical therapists do an awful lot of massage. In fact, each of the 35,000 practicing physical therapists in that country gives an average of 4,374 massages a year, most of them paid for by national insurance. Perhaps that's why the French have a saying, *bien dans son peau*, for someone who is happy and content; the phrase means "good in his skin."

Chapter 4

I've Got You Under My Skin: The Basics of What's Inside

In This Chapter

▶ Discovering your three-dimensional body

▶ Getting a feel for muscles and bones

▶ Exploring the organ systems

*M*ost people would prefer to leave the interior of the human body a mystery, like the ingredients in a Hostess Twinkie. You're better off just enjoying the thing, they figure, and not asking too many questions. This attitude works fine for most applications in life, such as walking around, going to the movies, eating pizza, and so forth, but once you decide to massage somebody, you'll benefit by knowing a little about human anatomy.

Here's why:

✔ You become aware of certain areas that are delicate or sensitive and should therefore be avoided (see Chapter 10 for more information on this issue).

✔ You develop an idea of what's going on internally when someone complains about specific aches and pains.

✔ You discover how certain strokes on the surface are acting on deeper structures, such as the circulatory system, the lymph system, and more.

✔ You come to understand how your touch is affecting the body as a whole.

The purpose of this chapter is to give you a very basic understanding of how your touch is felt, not just on the surface of the body, but into its depths as well.

Michelangelo's inner vision

Have you ever been to Florence and visited the Galleria della Accademia where Michelangelo's famous statue of David stands? Well, let me tell you, it's worth it. You enter and walk down a long corridor filled with half-finished sculptures before you come to the high glass-domed chamber where David awaits. The power of the piece is not just in its mass and detail, but also in its fullness. David seems to be filled to the brim with life, as if he's about to burst out of his skin at any moment.

How did Michelangelo know exactly how each of the muscles and bones were arranged inside the human body in order to recreate such reality? Did he study anatomy at the medical school of Florence? Did he look it up in books?

The fact is that studying anatomy the time-honored way (using cadavers) was illegal during Michelangelo's lifetime, outlawed by the Catholic Church as sacrilegious. Undaunted, the artist found a sympathetic priest who gave him a key to one of the city's morgues where Michelangelo would break in at night to perform illicit autopsies. Even though he had to risk his own life to do it, exploring the interior of the human body proved invaluable to the creation of his art.

To give a massage that feels like a work of art, you'll want know what's inside the human body, too. And these days, nobody's going to arrest you for wanting to find out.

Wow, That's Deep

Perhaps the most fundamental misconception people have as they first set out to massage somebody is that the human body is a two-dimensional object rather than a three-dimensional object. How is that possible, you say? Everyone knows we're not flat. Right?

Well, that's true, but everyone knows that a lake is three-dimensional, too, having depth as well as width and breadth, right? What do you picture in your mind when you think of a lake, though? If you're like most people, you think of the surface of the lake, the visible area of water surrounded on all sides by the shore.

And in a similar way, even though you know there's depth inside you, too, containing all the unfathomable mysteries of tissue and bone, you may still habitually concern yourself with the surface, because that is what you see.

The problem with this two-dimensional way of thinking is obvious if you consider what would happen were you to attempt to walk out to the middle of the lake. Quite quickly, you'd understand about the lake's three-dimensionality. The same applies when you wade out onto the seemingly two-dimensional surface of a person's body as you give her a massage. The mysterious liquid depths beneath the skin suddenly surge up around your fingers, and if you don't know how to swim, you'll drown. Or at the very least, you'll look silly doing the dog paddle as you head desperately back to shore.

You can give a nice, pleasant rubdown without knowing a thing about what you're doing: The mere tactile stimulation of skin-to-skin has positive therapeutic effects; but to give a good massage, one that makes people say "wow, that was incredible," you have to learn how to swim.

Proof That You're Three Dimensional

Here's a way to prove scientifically that you are indeed a three-dimensional being and that all kinds of secrets exist below the surface of your skin. You only need two things to do this experiment: your hand and a flat surface such as a table or desk.

First, turn your hand palm-downward and hold it over the table a few inches high. Then reach down with just your fingertips to touch the surface. And finally bend your middle finger and fold it under your hand until the first two knuckles are flat on the table. Good.

What I'd like you to do now is lift your other fingers up and away from the table top one at a time while leaving your middle finger firmly planted. Go ahead and do this right along with me as you're reading if you'd like. First try the thumb; it lifts downright easily, doesn't it? Way up high. Next try the index finger; not quite as impressive as the thumb but still definitely off the table. Try the pinkie finger; you see how it lifts up about the same or higher than the index finger? And lastly, try the ring finger. Go ahead. I'll wait. What's wrong? Come on! Lift it up already. Can't do it?

Why can't you lift your ring finger? You may have tried this experiment before, but did you ever figure out what's going on? Somebody showed it to me when I was in high school, but it wasn't until I was studying anatomy as part of massage training that I understood what's happening.

The secret is this: Buried within the depths of your forearm are three tiny little muscles, one that lifts your index finger, one that lifts your pinkie finger, and one that lifts your thumb. But you have just one muscle that lifts both the ring finger and middle finger, and so when one of them is held down, the other one can't lift up. Go ahead, try it with the ring finger on the table instead of the middle finger. Same result, right?

This example is just to show the effects of your three-dimensional depths on your two-dimensional surface. It's important to remember this when you're getting ready to massage someone, and I'll remind you to "think 3-D" when you read the chapters in Part III.

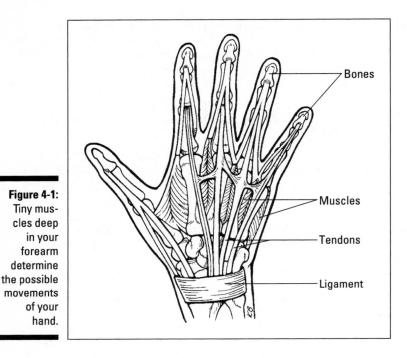

Figure 4-1:
Tiny mus-
cles deep
in your
forearm
determine
the possible
movements
of your
hand.

Bones

Muscles

Tendons

Ligament

Learning to Feel

For a moment, imagine you have a bas-relief map of the world before you in which all the landmarks are raised from the surface. Now imagine an opaque layer of rubber a quarter-inch thick covering the whole thing. Reaching down and touching this smooth surface, can you tell where your fingers are just by feeling? Where's California? Where's the tip of South America? Where's the protruding peninsula of Iberia? Can you determine what it is you're feeling, even without seeing it?

Now, making a leap in your imagination, think of the human body as that covered-up map that you are trying to identify by feeling its contours. This type of feeling-with-a-purpose is called *palpation*. Many professional massage people use palpation to determine what type of massage they are going to give to an individual, based on the way the person's body feels compared to the norm. You can get very sensitive fingers by practicing this, and in the next section, I lead you through an exercise to help you start that sensitization process.

Getting a feeling for palpation

Try this exercise to begin sensitizing your fingers to the various textures, shapes, and landmarks you will find beneath the skin.

1. **Sitting in a chair, with your back straight, turn your head to the right, as if you were trying to look back over your right shoulder.**

2. **Now, reach up with your right hand and, using just the fingertips, feel gently along the front of the neck until you locate the long band of vertical muscle stretching from your collar bone up to the side of your head, called the sternocleidomastoid muscle, which is illustrated in Figure 4-2.**

3. **"Walk" your fingertips up and down this muscle, feeling for where it connects near the center of your collar bone (the origin) and up along the base of your skull (the insertion).**

   Do certain parts feel tighter than others? Is part of the muscle thinner than others?

4. **Grasp the muscle between your fingertips, as if it were a guitar string and you were going to pluck it.**

   Be careful not to dig your fingers into the sensitive front part of your neck.

5. **Still grasping the muscle, slowly bring your head back to center, feeling the softening in the muscle between your fingers as you do so.**

   Repeat the process several times, back and forth.

6. **Walk your fingers down to the base of this muscle and then onto the collar bone, following it along out toward the shoulder.**

   How does the bone feel different than the muscle? In what ways is it the same?

7. **Now walk your fingers away from the collar bone up over toward your back until you reach the top of your shoulder.**

   Use a little firmer pressure to feel along the length of this muscle. Where does it feel harder? Where does it feel softer? Are there any "knots" or "bands" of harder tissue within the more pliable surrounding area?

   Notice whether there are any points that feel more tender when you touch them, and whether these tender points correspond to the "knots".

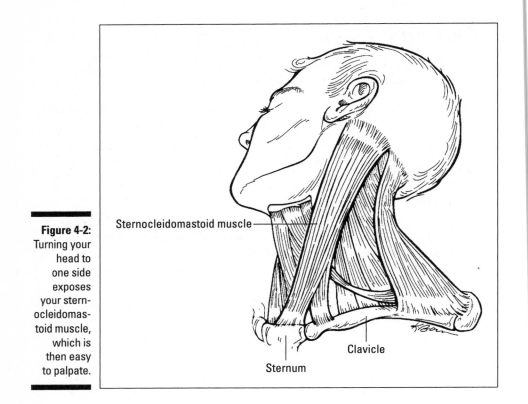

Figure 4-2:
Turning your head to one side exposes your stern-ocleidomas-toid muscle, which is then easy to palpate.

Sternocleidomastoid muscle

Clavicle

Sternum

Take several minutes to do this. Get a feeling for feeling. Let your fingers become familiar with all the permutations of texture, density, and tone that you can find just below the surface of the skin.

Bony landmarks

If you attend massage school yourself one day, you'll learn all kinds of intimidating anatomical terms with which to impress your friends and loved ones, such as "Boy, Cheryl, that's one exquisite medial malleolus you have there."

Cheryl probably won't know that you're talking about her inner ankle bone. And there's a very good chance she won't care either. Therefore, I'm not going to bore you or her by loading you down with all kinds of Latinate words and phrases. Instead, I'm going to do something fun, in plain English, that's going to help give you an idea where things are located anatomically.

Your medial malleolus, or inner ankle bone, is one of at least forty seven "bony landmarks" throughout your body. Now, before you go making any crude comments about bony landmarks, let me assure you that this is indeed what they are called by professionals everywhere. They have compelling names, such as *xiphoid process*, *occipital protuberance*, and *greater tuberosity of the humerus*. I'm going to use laymen's terms, though, and expose you to a few of these landmarks as part of a game. That's right, it's time to play . . . .

The bony landmark game

It can really be a lot of fun getting to know what's where beneath your skin, and, in fact, for many centuries (before the invention of TV) people the world over would sit around the campfire playing the bony landmark game. This was a great way to pass the time between wolverine attacks, and it's an effective method to teach anatomy to the young at the same time.

The game is simple: I describe a particular landmark (see Figure 4-3) for you in terms that you can understand and give you directions on how to locate it through *palpation*. Then, all you have to do is supply me with the common, everyday term we use to describe this landmark. It's important that you actually do the palpation, not just read the words, because that is what will familiarize you with the terrain you massage in future chapters.

Ready?

1. You can find this landmark by holding one hand out in front of you, with your palm facing you. Feeling with the fingertips of your other hand, notice that you have two bones in the forearm, one on the pinkie finger side (the ulna), and one on the thumb side (the radius). Follow the bone on the pinkie finger side all the way from your wrist to its extreme other end. You'll find a bump there, called the *olecranon process*, otherwise known as the _____.

2. Cross one of your feet up and rest it on the other knee so you can examine it. Then feel with both hands along the shin bone (tibia) in the front of your lower leg. Follow it down all the way to your foot and see what happens to it. Feel how it curves back toward you and ends up in a bump at the top of your foot? This is the *medial malleolus*, or _____.

3. Trace your fingers down onto your foot and then back in the opposite direction from your toes onto the *calcaneus*, or _____ bone.

4. Now sit up straight. Reach down along one side of your body until your hand almost slips underneath you. Right at that point you should feel a bone called the *greater trochanter of the femur*, which is otherwise known as the bony knob at the top of the longest bone in the body, the _____ bone.

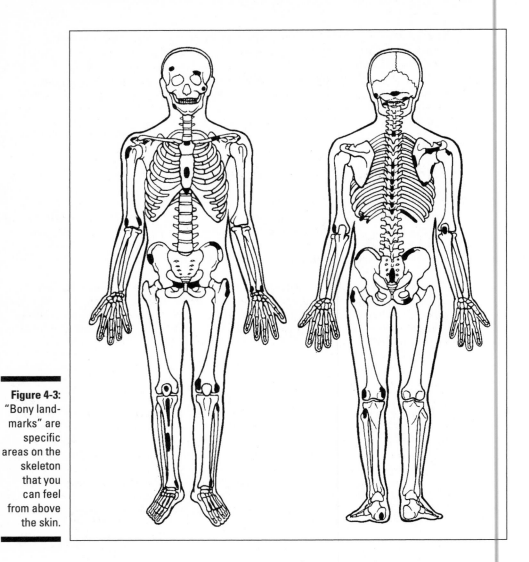

Figure 4-3: "Bony land- marks" are specific areas on the skeleton that you can feel from above the skin.

5. Walk your fingers back up along the side of your body about 6 – 8 inches until you hit the next bony landmark. It should be a sharp ridge that sticks out and that you can follow along toward the front of your body for a few inches. This is the *iliac crest*, also known as the _____ bone.

6. Reaching your hands up to your face, locate your chin and then feel back along the lower ridge toward your ear. It curves up here, forming the *ramus of the mandible*, otherwise known as the point at the angle of the _____ bone.

7. You'll need a partner for this one. Have her lie face-down on a comfortable surface with her back exposed, and then gently lift her arm, bend it at the elbow, and place her hand on her lower back. Let her upper arm rest down along her side. You'll notice that by doing this you cause a big bump to appear on her upper back. Feel along the edges of this triangular-shaped bone, otherwise known as the _____.

Answers: 1. elbow, 2. inner ankle bone, 3. heel, 4. thigh, 5. hip, 6. jaw, 7. shoulder blade.

These are just a few of the many landmarks you can palpate, and this game is meant to get you comfortable with the fact that you can actually feel and affect the structures of anatomy without being a scientist or doctor. When you practice hands-on massage, remember this and use your knowledge to guide you through your partner's body.

Soft tissues

Now that you know how to familiarize yourself with bony landmarks, you're probably wondering about all the other parts of your body that are *not* bony landmarks. After all, you're not going to be massaging bones. It's the *soft tissue* that you'll have in your hands most of the time, and by soft tissue I don't mean Kleenex brand facial tissues. I mean muscles, mostly, and a little bit of connective tissue as well.

Muscles comprise 40 to 60 percent of your total body weight, depending upon your gender and physical condition, and you have over 600 of them, large and small. Each one is compartmentalized in a sheath of *fascia*, which sets it apart and helps it function as a distinct unit, although the truth is that you never use just one muscle to perform any given action. As Mark Beck says in *Theory and Practice of Therapeutic Massage*, "Muscles have anatomic individuality, but they do not have functional individuality." They are always working in groups to create movement. That's their whole purpose for being.

The larger obvious muscles you can see simply through observing a body in motion are called *skeletal muscles*. There are also two other types of muscle tissue: *cardiac* and *smooth*. Cardiac, as the name implies, is the special muscle tissue that makes up the heart. Smooth muscle lines the stomach, intestines, and blood vessels.

The slightest movement of the most mundane part of your anatomy (your left knee, for example) requires the precisely timed and perfectly executed synchronization of many muscles, and there's absolutely no way that you could consciously coordinate all that without going nuts. Imagine Michael Jordan driving in for a lay-up and having to fire off messages to every single one of his separate muscles to do so. It would look something like this:

"Okay, contract the quadriceps, especially the rectus femoris, and simultaneously pull in the psoas, push off the soleus, shorten the gastrocnemius, and extend the web of flexors and the tibialis anterior. Now compensate for the lifted foot by tightening the opposite gluteus maximus and bracing all the muscles in the lower back, too numerable to mention here. Whoops, that threw me off, and . . . whoa!"

And down he'd go, before even moving one step. In fact, it's much more complex than that for even the simplest of maneuvers, and we'd all be helpless to try and stand up, sit down, or walk to the refrigerator if we had to think about it.

So how do we do it? Basically, we learn to move one little piece at a time as we develop during infancy and childhood, laying each chunk of the pattern down in a movement-memory groove, and then building upon it with the next movement. That's why you see babies experimenting with things like kicking their legs out, bobbing their heads around, and bringing small electrical appliances toward their mouths for examination. Every time they do something successfully and then master it through repetition, they file it away, and that's one less thing they have to consciously think about next time. Of course, this is the same procedure that athletes use later in life through their practice as they gradually layer all the perfect little movements they need one upon the next until they no longer have to think about it but rather, "Just do it."

By all of this explanation, I mean to say that muscles don't just flex and contract — they *learn*. What you're holding in your hands when you massage someone is conscious matter. In fact, it's your muscles that tell you where you are in space and time, through special nerve endings embedded in your muscles known as *proprioceptors*. I don't want to freak you out with bizarre-sounding anatomical terms, but there are two of these proprioceptors that are particularly interesting and important, and I want to share them with you.

✔ **Golgi tendon organs** are nerve endings found, strangely enough, in your tendons. They measure how far any particular tendon has stretched, how much pressure it's putting on the nearby bone, and if the tendon's in danger of snapping. It's through these little organs that you are saved from ripping yourself to shreds and pulling all your muscles and tendons right off the bone.

✔ **Muscle spindle cells** are found in the center of muscles, what's known as the "belly," where they perform the important task of constantly communicating the state of the muscle's contraction and movement back to the central nervous system. They are basically scouts on the outpost of your active physical self. Without them, you wouldn't be able to tell where you were going, how fast, or if you were going at all.

Cartilage, ligaments, and tendons

Many people find themselves confusedly referring to various connective tissue structures between the muscles and bones as "tendons" or "ligaments" or "cartilage" without really knowing what the heck they're talking about. Now, I know you're not one of those people, but just in case you have a friend who's guilty of such anatomical faux pas, here's the skinny to set you straight:

✔ Cartilage gives shape to external features like the nose and ears, and it is also found between bones as a cushion at the joints. (Vertebral discs are made from cartilage, for example.)

✔ Ligaments connect bone to bones.

✔ Tendons connect muscle to bone.

Muscle tissue itself is largely insensate, meaning if someone were to cut, jab, or even burn you directly on an exposed muscle, you quite likely wouldn't feel much at all. Your muscles don't so much *feel* massage as they *experience* massage as it retrains them how to *be* more relaxed in stillness, and fluid in movement.

Muscles learn, and massage teaches.

Name that muscle

What often intimidates people when they're first learning massage is the anonymity and invisibility of muscles. Skin is plainly visible: You can clearly watch your own hands make contact with somebody else's body, skin to skin. But muscles? How can you really tell what muscle you're touching when that muscle is covered by the skin? And besides, the muscles are all jumbled together and not that clearly defined, except in professional body builders, whose muscles are so hard and tight that they're almost impossible to massage anyway. So how are you expected to really know what the heck you're touching when you're touching a body?

Glad you asked. This brings us directly to our next little exercise: Name That Muscle. This game is a bit tougher because you need to know the names of the muscles, which you might have forgotten if you weren't paying close attention in high school anatomy class. So, to be fair, I'm going to give you the answers first. Can't complain about that, right? All you have to do is match the right muscle in Figure 4-4 to its description and action. If you're not sure about one, see whether you can use common sense and deductive reasoning to figure out which the best choice might be. It will help if you actually perform the action described in the questions so that you FEEL the muscles you're looking for. After all, feeling is what this book is all about.

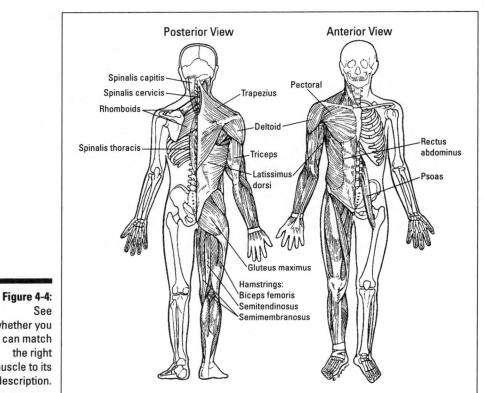

Figure 4-4:
See
whether you
can match
the right
muscle to its
description.

First, here are the answers:

- Pectorals
- Deltoid
- Spinalis
- Rectus abdominis
- Gastrocnemius
- Hamstrings
- Triceps
- Gluteus maximus
- Trapezius
- Biceps

1. Standing with your back against a wall, push against the wall with one heel and reach around to the back of your thigh to feel a tightening in your _____.

2. Place the back of your hand flat on the edge of a desk or table in front of you and then push that hand firmly down onto the desk. With the other hand, feel the underside of your upper arm and discover a tightening in your _____.

3. Standing up tall, lift your right leg out behind you as far as it will go comfortably, keeping it straight. Place your hand on your right buttock to feel a tightening in the _____.

4. Reach across with your left hand and place it on top of your right shoulder, right next to your neck. Now shrug your right shoulder as far up toward your ear as possible to feel a contraction of your _____.

5. Standing up, push onto your tip toes to feel a contraction of the _____ in the rear of your lower legs.

6. Sitting in front of a desk or table, place one hand palm-up beneath the table and lift up, creating a contraction in the _____ muscle of your upper arm.

7. When you lie down to perform a sit-up, the muscles in the front of your body that you're trying to tone through contraction are the _____.

8. Stand in front of a wall and push forward against it with your right hand while touching the right upper portion of your chest with the left hand. The muscles you feel bulging beneath your fingers are the _____.

9. Sitting up straight, reach across with your right hand and place it on the left shoulder, out by the arm. Now lift the left arm straight out to the side until it's at a ninety degree angle from your body, engaging the _____ muscle beneath your hand.

10. You'll need a partner for this one. Have him lie on his stomach, with no shirt on, and then ask him to lift his head and shoulders off the floor with no help from his arms. The two long cords of muscle down along either side of his spine are part of the _____ group.

Answers: 1. hamstrings, 2. triceps, 3. gluteus maximus, 4. trapezius, 5. gastrocnemius, 6. biceps, 7. rectus abdominis, 8. pectorals, 9. deltoid, 10. spinalis.

These three extra credit muscles are more obscure and I don't blame you if you don't know them offhand, but it may be fun to see whether you can decipher which is which.

- Rhomboid
- Latissimus dorsi
- Psoas

1. If you stand up and lift one leg in front of you with the knee bent, you engage a deep muscle that connects your leg bone to your backbone called the _____ .

2. You'll need to observe a partner for this one. Have her sit facing away from you with her back exposed and then gently reach one of her hands up as far as possible along her spine. Her shoulder blade will lift and you'll be able to feel between it and the spine for the _____ muscle.

3. Lift your right hand over your head and reach across with the left hand to grasp your right side below the armpit. The large muscle you feel there is the _____ .

Extra credit answers: 1. psoas, 2. rhomboid, 3. latissimus dorsi.

This is not a test. Repeat, this is not a test. It's just a way for you to become familiar with locating muscles. I refer you to several of these landmarks, bony and otherwise, when you move through the how-to massage chapters in Part III.

Other Body Systems

Don't get the idea that it's just the skin, muscles, and bones that count when it comes time to massage somebody. You also deal with a few other anatomical systems that are strongly affected by your touch as well. These include the . . .

- ✔ Circulatory system
- ✔ Nervous system
- ✔ Endocrine system
- ✔ Digestive system
- ✔ Respiratory system

The next few sections take a brief look at these systems and discuss how they're important when you give or receive a massage.

Circulatory system

The heart is constantly pumping your blood (about 11 pints of it in a 160-pound adult) out through your arteries and into each and every tiny little cell of your body, carrying the nutrients and oxygen that make it possible for you to stay alive. Then the blood travels back to your heart through the veins. On this return trip, the blood has to pass through a series of one-way valves that keep it from accidentally heading back in the wrong direction.

Massage strokes have a direct effect on the flow of blood in the veins, so keep in mind that when you massage someone, your strokes should always be in the direction of venous flow. You wouldn't want to accidentally push the blood back through these valves and therefore weaken them. When a number of the valves weaken and stop working efficiently, blood can pool up visibly and form varicose veins.

As much as half of all your blood is in your skin at any given moment, which accounts for that rosy glow certain people have, and also for the less healthy appearance of varicose veins and other problems. Massage works powerfully on your circulatory system, and for this reason you should always be aware of how your hands are affecting it.

Massage also affects that other circulating fluid referred to in Chapter 1, the lymph. In fact, there is an entire system of massage called manual lymphatic drainage meant to assist the movement of the lymph because, as you may know from Chapter 1, lymph has no heart of its own to pump it along.

Nervous system

As a busy person in the twenty-first century, you don't have any time to fiddle around reminding your heart to beat, your lungs to breathe, and so on. Luckily, your *autonomic nervous system* takes care of all that for you. This system is further broken down into the *sympathetic* and *parasympathetic nervous systems*. The sympathetic nerves prepare your body for action, and the parasympathetic nerves calm you down. Massage is a great way to stimulate the parasympathetic nervous system, thereby lowering the pulse, slowing breathing, and in general, chilling you out.

The largest and longest nerve in the body is the *sciatic,* which many people are painfully familiar with. It runs from the base of your spine down the back of your leg, and when any of its length becomes pinched or trapped between muscles, bones, and connective tissues, it can cause the condition known as *sciatica*. That's the way all nerves work; you don't want to get in their way or piss them off. Massage can help soften the muscles and other soft tissue that surround nerves and sometimes entrap them.

As I mention earlier in this chapter, you also have specialized nerves called proprioceptors that tell you where your body is in space, giving you your sense of depth, position, and movement. Without them, you'd be internally blind, and by making you more aware of them, massage can help you "see" yourself in a new way from the inside out. Chapter 7 has some exercises to get you in touch with your proprioceptors. Look for "The limp arm experiment."

The mind-body connection

Did you ever wonder what the heck people were talking about when they used the term mind-body connection? Is it part of the nervous system you weren't told about in school? Did you think maybe there was a tube or special cable of some kind near the base of your neck that linked your mind and your body, and that you were the only one who hadn't been shown where it was? Well, don't worry; you're not alone. In a far-reaching survey conducted by my wife one day at her restaurant, it was ascertained that only 2.4 percent of normal people understand what the term mind-body connection really means, and those people are new-age geeks.

Typical incorrect responses about what the mind-body connection is included the following:

- That sinking feeling you get when your mind realizes your body did something it shouldn't have

- Nerves

- The neck

Actually, the mind-body connection is simply *awareness.* It's an awareness that permeates way down into every cell of your body, as compared to the awareness of your brain alone. It's the entire *you* consciously affecting every other part of you.

This whole mind/body split problem developed gradually over many centuries and was not really caused by any one individual, but many scholars have pointed to the French philosopher and mathematician Rene Descartes as having had the greatest influence. He's the one who coined that famous Latin phrase, "*Cogito, ergo sum,*" which means "I think, therefore I am." That was in 1637. Well, pretty much ever since then people have been assuming that it was only specific types of electrical activity inside their skulls that proved they indeed existed. What's glossed over in the history books is that Descartes never received a great massage from an expert holistically oriented practitioner. If he had, he certainly would have modified his statement a bit, to something like, "*Cogito et sentio, ergo sum.*" I think *and I feel,* therefore I am."

Endocrine system

Heard of hormones? The glands that make up the endocrine system are what secrete hormones into your body. It's been shown that massage stimulates the release of human growth hormone (HGH), among others, thereby affecting the healthy maturation of your entire body.

Digestive system

Your digestive system is a tube approximately five times as long as you are tall (see Figure 4-5). This tube, along with several digestive organs, has the magical ability to transform whatever enters it into a very special substance known as "you." Massage can beneficially stimulate this process if you're familiar with the various twists and turns this tube follows through your body, especially over the large intestine.

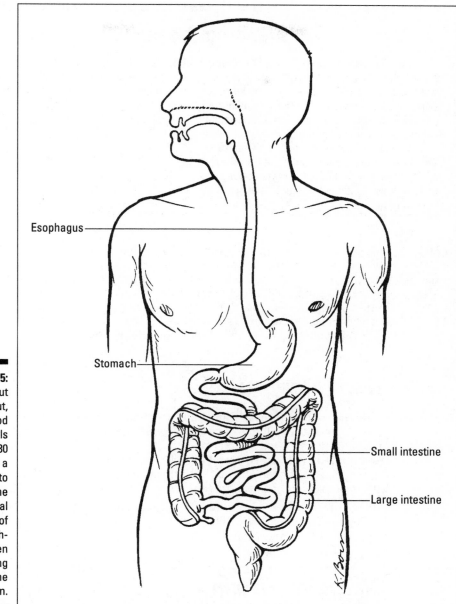

Esophagus

Stomach

Small intestine

Large intestine

Figure 4-5: From input to output, your food travels about 30 feet. It's a good idea to follow the general direction of this path- way when massaging the abdomen.

Cleaning the pipes

If you visit a health food store and search through the herbal potions that line the shelves, you'll find some strange-looking mixtures that promise "internal cleansing." The ingredients in these products have two major actions: absorption and expulsion, and they act primarily in your large intestine, also called the colon. First, certain ingredients (often psyllium husks) absorb much of the matter that tends to get lodged in the many folds of the colon, and then a mixture of herbs comes along to "sweep" it all out. It's similar to the technique favored by many garage mechanics of throwing sawdust on dirty grease before pushing it away with a broom.

This type of cleansing is highly advisable, and some extra massage at the same time may aid the elimination process by stimulating lymph flow.

One landmark along the digestive pathway that many people are able to palpate is the *cecum,* which is a little pouch at the beginning of the large intestine, or *colon.* You can locate it by first touching bony landmark number 5, your right hip bone, and then walking your fingers in toward your belly button a couple of inches. Sometimes this spot makes a liquid-squishing noise, especially after meals. In Part III, I discuss how to use this landmark as a starting point for some abdominal massage techniques.

Respiratory system

Breathing is an extremely important activity for human beings, as can be attested to by the millions of people around the world who have stopped breathing and suffered serious side-effects, even death. Massage is an excellent opportunity to engage in some full deep breathing, as described in Chapter 7. This reconnects you with the source of life. It also fills your blood with fresh oxygen because the first place your blood goes when it leaves your heart is the lungs.

Surprising facts about your stomach

Most of us think of the stomach as a large roundish ball in the center of our abdomens, but actually it's a smallish oval sack up and to the left, tucked mostly under the ribs on the side of your body by your heart. Like the entire intestinal wall, it's lined with smooth muscle. What people are really referring to when they point at the center of their abdomen and say "Look how flat my stomach is" is actually the intestines.

Part II

The Art of
Receiving
Massage

The 5th Wave   By Rich Tennant

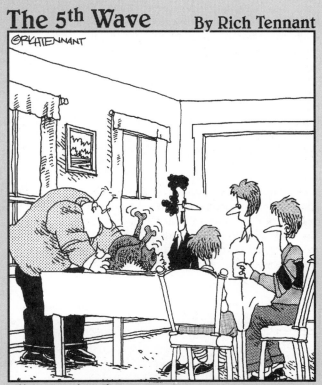

"This is what I get for marrying a massage
therapist. Every Thanksgiving he's got to knead
the turkey's spine before he'll carve it."

In this part . . .

Okay, I can hear you scoffing now: the art of receiving massage? That's like the art of getting rained on. You really don't have to try very hard; just step outside and get wet. Anyone can do it.

Receiving massage? Nothin' to it. No problem. Child's play. Right?

Wrong.

Receiving massage is more like dancing your part in a very intricate pas-de-deux, such as the tango, which, interestingly, means "I touch" in Latin. Both activities, at their best, are extremely interactive. During the tango, if you just stand there and don't do anything, you're going to make your partner look pretty bad. Similarly, when you receive a massage, you've got to communicate with your partner, through both verbal and nonverbal means, in order to get the most out of the experience. Your partner touches you, you react to that touch, your muscles respond accordingly, and then your partner adjusts his touch to suit the reaction, and you go back and forth like this throughout the entire exchange, constantly conscious of each other's presence and movement — two dancers creating one dance.

A good massage is a two-way street, equal parts proper giving *and* informed receiving. That's the focus of this part of the book, in which you'll begin as a freshman in Massage 101 and then graduate just three chapters later with the ability to receive a massage like a real pro. I know, it's tough, but somebody's gotta do it.

Along the way, you'll master the tricky intricacies of massage vocabulary, discover the ten rules for receiving a massage, and get the scoop on all the massage gizmos you see for sale everywhere. I also cover the difference between various massage styles, discuss how to enjoy the pleasures of massage without guilt, and offer techniques for increasing your touch-ability, and lots more.

Chapter 5

A Massage Road Map

*W*hen you first begin to discover massage, you'll undoubtedly encounter some strange new words and some strange new concepts that might confuse you at first. Have no fear! This chapter is your own personal travel guide to help you navigate the sometimes puzzling new terrain in the world of massage. Here you'll find out how to accept the pleasures of massage into your life and how to choose the type of massage that's right for you. You'll even find an English-Massage dictionary at the end of the chapter that will help you speak the language of massage with other people.

Healthy Pleasure

To paraphrase Forrest Gump, sometimes massage is like a box of chocolates — you never know exactly what you're gonna get, but you know it's gonna be good. However, if you eat the whole thing, you're gonna end up feeling guilty and a little bloated.

Many people just can't seem to understand that massage is anything more than . . .

✔ Indulgence

✔ Luxury

✔ Pampering

And therefore they pass when it comes to massage. Some people raise their noses up at its pleasures as if they were too good for it. Others shy away from the experience, calling it expensive and extravagant, as if massage were too good for them.

The Mary Poppins problem

In my opinion, you can trace the debilitating attitude so many people have concerning pleasure back to one particular person, somebody you'd never suspect. Yes, I'm talking about Mary Poppins. In the film, she waltzes around looking all prim and respectable and happy in her tight-fitting outfit, singing, "It takes a spoonful of sugar to help the medicine go down" until eventually people end up believing her. Now, everybody thinks that anything good for him or her should feel bad. No pain, no gain, right? This philosophy pretty much messed up an entire generation. What if sugar *was* the medicine? What if pleasure — not the medicine — made the pain go away?

As one scholar put it, "Recent research supports the view that the deprivation of physical pleasure is a major ingredient in the expression of physical violence" (Juhan p.53). People need pleasure to be healthy, and receiving massage is one of the most natural, healthy ways to experience pleasure without any negative side effects.

The following definition is inscribed on a coffee mug from a massage school in New Jersey: *Mas-sage: (n.) the pleasure that relieves the pain*. That's a good way to look at it. If you think of massage as pleasurable medicine, you will be able to accept it into your life more easily.

The underlying reason for both of these attitudes is guilt. Many people simply have trouble justifying paying for something that feels as good as massage. They also have difficulty justifying having another human pay such lavish attention to them for an entire hour.

Well, this guilt is truly unfortunate, and completely unnecessary, because massage is actually much better for you than chocolate. In fact, it has all of the pleasures without any of the negative side effects. That's right, there's not a single thing wrong with massage.

Massage . . .

- Is calorie free
- Is fat free
- Won't rot your teeth
- Is impossible to overdose on

Well okay, massage does have one catch. Make no mistake about it, once you taste good massage, you're going to want more — lots more. Like chocolate, massage can be addictive. But that's not necessarily a bad thing. You can receive a massage every day for the rest of your life with absolutely no negative side effects.

In fact, beloved entertainer, Bob Hope, has received a massage almost every day of his life for over fifty years. He's dragged a number of massage therapists all over the globe with him while he was off entertaining the troops and making his movies. I had the opportunity to massage him once myself. At the time, he was 87 years old, but because of all the massage he'd received over the years, his skin was smooth and supple, and his muscles were amazingly well toned.

Of course, you may not have the time or money for a massage every day like Bob Hope. But time or money isn't what's most likely to stop you in the first place. It's your attitude.

Testing Your Touch-Ability

The one thing about massage that you really can't avoid is the fact that you have to touch another human body in order to do it. This basic reality is what keeps many people from taking the first step of either getting or receiving a massage. Touch another human? Yuck!

Most societies have quite a few touch-related taboos and complexes, things that may be holding you back from experiencing massage. The following touch-ability survey can help reveal your own, perhaps unconscious, touch taboos, and suggest ways to overcome them. After you know what problems you're dealing with, you can proceed more easily. Be totally honest with yourself. There are no right or wrong answers, only helpful ones.

For each question, fill in the number that most closely matches your feelings.

- ✔ Strongly disagree: 1
- ✔ Disagree: 2
- ✔ Neutral: 3
- ✔ Agree: 4
- ✔ Strongly agree: 5

1. My childhood family encouraged touching and hugging between members. _____
2. I can offer a compassionate touch on the arm, shoulder, or back of someone I don't know, and doing so feels natural. _____
3. When someone bumps me on the street, instead of feeling anger, my first reaction is to brush it off as an accident. _____
4. My natural inclination is to massage animals (at least ones that don't bite), scratching them behind the ears to make them feel good. _____

5. I can touch or be touched by someone I find attractive without having sexual intentions or fantasies about them. _____

6. I prefer to go barefoot outdoors when safe and appropriate. _____

7. I have, on occasion, hugged a tree or draped myself luxuriously over a warm rock in the sun. _____

8. I believe in heart-to-heart hugs that express my affection and openness to people. _____

9. People tell me I have "good hands" and ask me to rub their shoulders when they're feeling stiff or sore. _____

10. In work situations, I offer encouragement and recognition to others with a heart-felt touch in combination with words of praise. _____

Total: _____

The higher the number you come up with, the greater likelihood that touch and massage are something easy for you to accept in your life. If you scored a 50, great! Forge straight ahead into the following chapters, and enjoy. If you scored in the 40s, you're among the most tactile people in the world, and massage is probably a part of your life already. If you scored in the 20s or 30s, you're somewhere in the average regarding touch-ability, and you may want to stop here for a few minutes and consider trying some of the experiences listed below. If you scored below twenty, you're still in the developmental stage of touch-ability, and you will definitely benefit by trying some or all of the following suggestions.

- Pick a parent, sibling, or even a cousin and give that person a hug for no reason.

- The next time an appropriate situation arises, gently place your palm on the shoulder of someone you've just met, offering compassion and solidarity for a moment.

- When someone bumps or jostles you, stop and take a deep breath and look for the hidden cause of your anger. Usually, the anger results because you feel that you're in the "right." Let go of being right and be forgiving instead.

- Spend a full five minutes concentrating on nothing else but massaging the head and ears of a dog or cat (assuming you're not allergic, of course).

- Get a serious, therapeutic massage and concentrate on the inner relaxing of your muscles, just to show yourself that massage involves more than sensual pleasure.

- Take a walk through a park barefoot, feeling the textures of various surfaces — sand, sidewalk, grass, gravel. Notice how your feet feel during and afterwards.

✔ Head out to the woods, a quiet park, or deserted beach and hug a tree, or drape yourself luxuriously over a warm rock in the sun.

✔ Give a heart-to-heart hug that expresses your affection to someone who would truly appreciate it.

✔ The next time someone you know complains of tight shoulders, offer to give him or her a five minute mini-massage. Don't worry about doing it "right." Just focus on caring and compassion.

✔ The next time someone you work with does something right, offer a heart-felt touch on the arm or back in combination with a few words of praise. Examine your intentions before making this sort of contact, to make sure you don't have any subconscious motivations that could later lead to a sexual harassment case. And offer this tactile support in plain view of other coworkers.

So Little Time, So Many Massages

Okay, so you're filled with enthusiasm to go out and experience your first massage; you pick up the phone, call a massage school or clinic in your area, and ask to book an appointment. (See Chapter 8 for details on booking an appointment).

"What kind of bodywork do you prefer?" asks the receptionist.

"Bodywork?"

"Yes. Massage."

"Oh. Just something that feels good," you say.

"Of course. But we offer several modalities. Would you prefer the Swedish, the sports massage, the deep tissue, the Hellerwork, the Aston repatterning, the Thai massage, or the neuromuscular session?"

 "Ah, let me get back to you on that," you say, and you hang up, ready to slip quietly back into your non-massage lifestyle before you even begin.

Don't let this scenario happen to you! Now that you've decided to get a massage, the last thing you want is to get confused by the vast array of choices available and end up not receiving any kind of massage at all.

Be forewarned, this section is just an overview of the types of massage available. For now, I just want to familiarize you with a few of the choices, based upon the three main reasons that people decide to get a massage:

> ✔ To relax
>
> ✔ To feel better
>
> ✔ To improve your body's functioning

Often, your reasons are probably a combination of all three. You may have a little pain in your shoulder you'd like to ease, but at the same time, you want to lower your overall stress level. The three components of massage dovetail with each other; what helps you relax may lessen your pain, what realigns your body may help you relax, and so on.

The spiritual aspect of massage is a fourth component, a wild card that can pop up unannounced during any type of massage. This spiritual aspect is the way that you can use massage to attune to your own inner experience and get in touch — literally — with a deeper sense of self. (See Chapter 7 for more information on this topic.)

So which is the right style for you? Take a glance at the following categories and become familiar with some of the massage styles associated with each.

Massage for relaxation

Stress and tension are real. The human body has developed through eons of evolution to respond to stress and tension by preparing to either fight the obstacle or run away from it. This, the famous *fight-or-flight response,* came in very handy when primitive man was confronted with the occasional, large, dangerous animal. But in modern times, people are faced with a constant, unceasing barrage of tension-inducing stimuli, and they're getting overloaded by it. If you live in a large metropolitan area, for instance, you're being exposed to the equivalent of several dozen grizzly bears and a pack of ravenous wolves every time you venture out into rush-hour traffic.

Reducing the stress and tension in your life is a very good reason for wanting to get a massage. You don't need any more justification than that.

If you're interested in relaxing massage, ask for the following:

> ✔ **Swedish massage:** What most people envision when they think "massage." This method includes stroking, kneading, squeezing, rubbing, and so on.
>
> ✔ **Light work:** As in "not heavy," light work is a generic term for non-intrusive, gentle massage. See the section "Remodeling your body for fun and profit" later in this chapter for information about deeper massage during which the therapist's fingers "intrude" into your musculature.

MASSAGE TALE

When in Hawaii . . .

Once, in Hawaii, I was in the mood for a relaxing massage to help relieve jet lag after a long trip. I was working at a spa there, and one of the massage therapists on staff, a native Hawaiian named Wesley Sen, offered to give me a *lomi lomi massage.*

"Is that relaxing?" I asked as we walked together back to my hotel room.

"Sure it's relaxing," he said.

"Then why are you carrying that pole with you?"

Sure enough, Wesley was carrying a thick, ten-foot long wooden pole in one hand. "It's just for balance," he said. "Don't worry."

Back in my room, Wesley had me lie down on the floor and then proceeded to pray over me in Hawaiian, which sets the mood at the beginning of every true lomi lomi experience. In his prayer, he invited healing forces to be present with us in the room. For the next hour he stood on me, kneeled on me, pressed on me, and tossed my limbs around, all along skillfully keeping his weight partially supported by the pole, one end of which he pushed against the floor to balance himself.

Wesley is not a small guy. I was amazed that he could perform this entire balancing act, using my body as a tightrope, and never once cause me the slightest discomfort. Afterwards, I was more relaxed than I'd felt in many months; the relaxation penetrated way down into my joints and up my nerves into my brain. Also, a pain I'd been experiencing in my shoulder disappeared, never to return again, and my digestion improved noticeably, too.

Skillful, relaxation massage can take you way beyond relaxation, healing what ails you and improving your body's functioning as well. Several massage styles offer relaxation as well as deeply therapeutic results, such as lomi lomi, Trager, Rubenfeld Synergy, and many others.

✔ **Relaxation massage:** Another generic term for nice-and-easy massage, relaxation massage usually refers to a light form of Swedish massage.

✔ **Esalen massage:** Developed at the famous Esalen Institute in Big Sur, California, this massage features many long, flowing, gentle strokes.

Plenty of massage styles leave you relaxed, but the Swedish style is the one you're most likely to run into. Swedish massage is kind of like the Visa or MasterCard of massage, accepted at millions of establishments around the world. It has many therapeutic benefits also, and some of its more advanced moves can be quite vigorous. If your intention is simply to chill out and be soothed by soft fingers, make sure to request light, easy pressure during your Swedish massage.

TIP

Communicate! Even if you're just trading massage with a friend, you have to let the other person know what you want out of the experience.

Rx massage

Many people visit their massage therapist for the same reason they visit their doctor — to fix something that's painful. This type of massage is called *remedial massage,* because it's used as a remedy. Several types of massage, including good-old, relaxing Swedish massage, can have definite remedial effects; but here's a short list of some styles particularly well-known for belonging to the "massage apothecary."

Of course, only well-trained professionals should attempt to give these types of massage.

If you're interested in remedial massage, ask for the following:

- **Manual lymphatic drainage:** This type of massage helps your body flush toxins, such as pesticides and residual chemicals, by stimulating the flow of lymph in your body. It's a very gentle massage that features light superficial movements on the skin.

- **Touch for health:** This treatment, which helps balance your inner healing energies, isn't really a massage at all because the therapist's hands don't necessarily come into contact with the recipient's body. The technique was developed by a nurse on the faculty at New York University and has been taught to thousands of healthcare practitioners.

- **Neuromuscular therapy:** This type of massage works on tight muscles that create the deep patterns of tension that can keep you in pain.

- **Cranio-sacral:** This type of massage adjusts the healthy functioning of your spine and cranium.

- **Deep tissue massage:** This generic term refers to any number of therapies that apply deep pressure and affect the body's connective tissues.

- **Shiatsu:** This massage involves pressure point therapy — to balance the entire body and restore health — on specific points along invisible energy lines in the body called *meridians.*

Shiatsu is the most well-known of several types of massage that work on the *meridians*. It can be quite relaxing, but its primary focus is on restoring health and balance, as are other types of massage that work on these energy lines.

After having a serious car accident, a young man in Ohio began experiencing severe, debilitating pain every day. His doctors told him they had no drugs or surgery that could help him and that he'd have to learn to live with the pain, but his mother decided there must be a better way. She took him to see a massage therapist who treated the young man for several months using neuromuscular and cranio-sacral therapies. The end result was a pain-free young man who has now decided to become a massage therapist himself in order to help other people.

Remodeling your body for fun and profit

Several types of massage have developed over the years that focus on realigning your body, straightening you out, helping you form a healthier relationship with gravity and a more graceful, efficient way of moving. People often refer to this type of massage as *structural bodywork.* You only want to sign up for one of these if you have specific goals in mind (such as improved posture, better athletic performance, and so on.) and, of course, you want a highly trained pro to do the work. The movements involved are quite deep, and the experience is not "relaxing" in the normal sense of the word, but your massage therapist will always keep your comfort foremost in mind.

If you're interested in structural massage, ask for the following:

- **Rolfing:** The most well-known form or structural bodywork, this type of massage was invented by Ida Rolf.

- **Hellerwork:** A unique development of Rolfing, this type of massage was created by Joseph Heller.

- **Aston patterning:** This type of massage is a combination of touch techniques and movement repatterning that helps people move with ease and improve their posture.

- **Myofascial release:** This type of massage is a combination of techniques that combine to "unwind" and release chronic tension patterns in deep tissues, which can cause many painful conditions.

Touch Terminology

Massage has its own lingo, much of which can be somewhat confusing at first. Massage lingo can also be intimidating, for two main reasons:

- Some massage terminology has origins in the medical field and can sound academically dense.

- Some of the words used are just plain weird (and the only people you've heard speak them before are sophisticated, semi-naked celebrities on *Lifestyles of the Rich & Famous*).

Truthfully, though, no insider's massage clique is sitting around in cashmere robes at some exclusive, country-club spa, ready to snicker at you for not knowing what the word "acupressure" means. Most of the massage words you encounter are the result of cultural influences from around the world, with a medical/scientific reference thrown in now and then.

Massage is all about making you feel comfortable in your own skin, and the last thing you want is to have a language barrier make you feel uncomfortable before you even begin. Words you don't know can make you feel like an outsider, which may have the tragic consequence of keeping you from doing what you really want to do when you get a massage — relax and feel better.

Your goal may be to become one of those knowledgeable clients who enters a massage clinic and requests "a bit of cranio-sacral for this headache I've had for two days now, and then some Trager in the hip area to loosen my tight psoas, and throw in some trigger point work on my traps, will you?" Or, on the other hand, perhaps this massage mumbo-jumbo seems completely pointless to you, and all you really want to do is lie down and get rubbed. Even if you belong to the latter group, knowing at least a few of the terms that massage therapists (and those who receive massage) commonly employ is helpful.

This section is a primer on massage lingo to help familiarize you with the terms you may run into when you

- ✔ Contact a massage professional to inquire about rates, services, and so on
- ✔ Visit a massage clinic
- ✔ Read journals, magazines, or books in the field
- ✔ Attempt to explain massage to a friend
- ✔ Ask people to recommend a massage therapist or style for you

Table 5-1 lists several specialized massage words and phrases that at first glance seem deceptively like everyday words and phrases. But don't be deceived. These words, when used in regards to massage, are highly specific and, when used correctly, can lead you to hours and hours of enjoyment, health benefits, and pleasure.

Table 5-1	Massage-English, English-Massage Dictionary	
Word	*Non-massage definition*	*Massage definition*
Rolfed	Past-tense of "to throw up on," a variant spelling of "Ralphed"	Deep massage work on connective tissues that realign the body with gravity
Bodyworker	Mechanic specializing in repairing cars after accidents	A practitioner of massage or similar hands-on healing techniques

Word	Non-massage definition	Massage definition
Structural work	Carpentry, mostly done on house frames	Massage that works on the body's muscles and connective tissues to better align them with gravity
Spa	Hot tub or Jacuzzi	Health facility where people go to learn holistic practices, eat healthy foods, exercise, and receive massages and spa treatments
Ayurveda	Misspelling of a famous brand of natural beauty products found in salons	An ancient healing system from India that uses diet, meditation, herbs, and massage to balance the body
Swedish	Anything from the country of Sweden	The most well-known and widely practiced form of massage in the Western world, consisting of stroking, kneading, applying pressure, stretching, and so on
Trigger point	The fine, pointed end of a pistol's trigger	A tight, tender spot in a muscle that responds well to massage
Connective tissues	Kleenex brand facial tissues all linked together in a box	The web of tissue (primarily collagen fibers) that surrounds your every muscle, organ, and bone, holding your body together
Deep tissue	Kleenex stuck deep between the cushions on your couch	A type of massage that targets the deeper layers of muscle and connective tissue
Energy work	Repairs on the electrical lines of your house	Type of massage that focuses on vital, invisible energies in your body

(continued)

Table 5-1 *(continued)*

Word	Non-massage definition	Massage definition
Adhesion	The sticky mark left on your skin after removing an adhesive bandage	Muscle and connective tissue fibers that are stuck together because of injuries, scars, aging, and lack of movement. Massage can help separate most adhesions, which are sometimes painful, though not usually dangerous.
Drape	Decorative material that hangs in front of a window	Towels, sheets, and so on, used to cover a person receiving a massage
Knots	Things tied in ropes	Tight bands of muscle fibers and connective tissues that massage often softens
On-site massage	Massage given at construction sites	Seated and clothed massage given in special chairs — usually in offices, in stores, or at special events

Bon jour, monsieur masseuse

You walk into a health club and sign up for a massage. A big, burly, bodybuilder of a man walks out, shakes your hand in his massive paw, and tells you his name is John.

"Nice to meet you," you say, slightly awed. "How long have you been a masseuse?"

"I'm not a masseuse!" he thunders, causing you to shake in your sneakers. And once again you have that terrible realization that you've flubbed up the whole masseur/masseuse thing.

"Sorry," you stammer, confused and embarrassed, but inside you're also a little mad. How are you supposed to remember the difference between those silly French words, and who made them up in the first place anyway?

Strangely enough, it was a Dutch man, Dr. Johann Mezger (1839–1909), who decided to use French words to describe the movements of massage, and even the word "massage" itself. The words for someone who performs massage therefore come from the French also:

- A **masseur** is a male practitioner of massage.

- A **masseuse** is a female practitioner.

An easy way for you to remember the correct term is to think of *monsieur* — the French word for Mr. — which sounds like masseur. And an even easier method is to avoid the masseur/masseuse dilemma altogether by using the more modern, non-gender-based term "massage therapist" for males and females alike, which is what most professionals prefer, anyway.

Look Who's Coming to Touch You

ou're no doubt absolutely convinced that massage would make a truly superb addition to your life, and you're just about ready to pick up that phone (yes, that one, right over there), dial one of the contact numbers I'm about to give you in this chapter, and order up your very first session of "touch take-out." Soon, a chipper and thoroughly professional person will show up at your door carrying a monstrous padded folding table. He or she will open the table in the privacy of your own comfortable dwelling. You'll smile self-confidently, take all your clothes off, and then . . . *wait* a minute!

Did I say, "Take all your clothes off?" Well, by golly, I guess I did. Suddenly, this whole, wonderfully abstract concept of massage has become disconcertingly real. And, in spite of your appreciation for the undeniably therapeutic benefits of massage, if that professional stranger were to ring your doorbell right this minute, you may be tempted to say, "Excuse me for a moment, will you? I just have to go get my law degree at Columbia University and then I'll be right with you."

If that sounds like you, don't worry. This chapter's purpose is to make you more comfortable with the people who will be massaging you, including people you already know, with whom sharing massage will be a new adventure.

Stalking the Elusive Referral

One time-honored concept used to battle your fear of a stranger in your home is to assure that the person who shows up on your doorstep to give you a massage is *not* a stranger. You can accomplish this goal in two ways:

✔ Give your cousin Billy several thousand dollars and send him through massage school so you can call him later and make an appointment.

✔ Get a referral.

The second option is by far the more common choice, but that doesn't mean you should entirely dismiss the concept of financing massage school for friends or family members. The world needs more massage therapists! If you happen to be extremely wealthy, do the world a favor and set up a massage-school trust fund. (The investment may even be tax deductible.)

A six-point mental checklist (to go over in your mind before deciding which massage therapist to try)

No matter how qualified and highly recommended a massage therapist may come to you, and no matter what other people say about her, *you* still must decide whether she's the right massage therapist for you. Remember, you're very likely to share a great deal of yourself with this person (massage therapists are like hair dressers on steroids when it comes to the confiding-in factor). And, because your massage therapist will get to know your body better than anyone else except an intimate partner, you have to be willing to trust her. Sometimes, you have no precise way to gauge which massage therapist will make precisely the best "fit" with your personality, and no amount of analytical deliberation will help you decide who to choose.

That said, try using this quick checklist to judge your own gut reaction to the person you're about to spend a considerable amount of quality time with:

1. Does she immediately make you feel like you're important?

2. Does she look you right in the eye and fill you with a sense of utter confidence so that you're already feeling better before she even touches you?

3. Is she someone you'd like to emulate as far as calmness and tranquility go? Like it or not, you will probably look upon your massage therapist as a role model in the relaxation category. A tense, uptight massage therapist isn't setting a good example.

4. Is she "soft" where she needs to be soft (unobtrusive and non-opinionated) and "hard" where she needs to be hard (unrelenting in her serious desire to see you feel better)?

5. Is she someone you feel an immediate sense of empathy with? To use a precise scientific term here, do the two of you *click*?

6. Is she the right sex? The decision on whether to receive massage from a male or female massage therapist is entirely up to you. Many people have no preference, as long as the massage therapist is competent and strong, but others feel more comfortable with one sex than the other in a massage setting. Most massage establishments will give you a choice when requesting a massage therapist. After you get started with the actual massage, you'll probably find that the massage therapist's gender doesn't really matter as much as you may have thought.

Of course, you may be more comfortable going to the "neutral ground" of a professional massage establishment rather than inviting someone unknown into your home. See the section "Visiting a clinic" later in this chapter for more information.

In case you're wondering who to ask for a referral without embarrassing yourself, the following list may come in handy. Actually, you may be surprised at how many people can potentially help you find a massage therapist.

First, you probably should NOT ask certain people to refer a massage therapist, including . . .

- ✔ Certain physicians who are not aware of the benefits of massage and who may think that all massage therapists are "quacks."

- ✔ Your Aunt Gertrude who had a massage once on a cruise and now considers herself an expert.

- ✔ People who are currently under indictment for health-care fraud.

After you cross those sources off your list, you can still find plenty of helpful folks ready to steer you towards the nearest pair of helping hands. Some of those places where you're most likely to get a good referral from include . . .

- ✔ The contact numbers at major massage associations and accrediting organizations (see the section "Organizations That Can Help You Find a Massage Therapist" later in this chapter).

- ✔ Enlightened physicians who are aware of the benefits of massage and who are more than happy to refer you to the ones they work with. In fact, many doctors these days have a massage therapist or two on staff.

- ✔ Athlete friends who receive massage as part of their training.

- ✔ A co-worker or family member who's had a particularly good experience with the massage therapist she's been using for an extended period of time.

- ✔ The "best-of" articles that health and beauty magazines such as *Shape, Self, Mademoiselle, Glamour,* and so on often feature.

- ✔ Your friend Tina, the one who wears the Birkenstock sandals all the time and has that look of blissed-out satisfaction on her face even when she's standing in line at the grocery store checkout counter.

Getting a Helping Hand

You can collectively refer to the four numbers I'm about to give you as "massage central." Among them you'll find the contact information for over 80,000 qualified massage therapists in the U.S. right at your fingertips.

Drum roll please . . . and the contact numbers are:

- ✔ To find a massage therapist who is a member of the oldest nationwide organization, the American Massage Therapy Association (AMTA), call toll free, 888-843-2682, for their Find-A-Massage-Therapist(SM) Location Service.

- ✔ To find the nearest member of Associated Bodywork and Massage Professionals (ABMP), call 800-458-2267.

- ✔ To find a member massage therapist of the International Massage Association (IMA), call 202-387-6555.

- ✔ For a list of massage therapists who have taken the test given by the National Certification Board for Therapeutic Massage and Bodywork (NCBTMB) and are therefore Nationally Certified in all 50 U.S. states, call 703-610-9015.

Of course, among those 80,000+ massage therapists, you're going to find quite a range of skills and offerings, and there isn't one, single tried-and-true means of prequalifying someone. However, you are living in an extremely lucky time, oh fortunate massage recipient, because in the past several years the number of highly skilled and fully trained massage pros has grown at an amazing rate all around the world.

Following is a list of contact numbers for professional massage practitioners in several countries:

- ✔ Australia: Massage Australia, Sydney, tel. (02) 4757 3050

- ✔ France: French Federation of Masseurs Kinesitherapeutes (FFMKR), Paris, tel. 01 44 83 46 00

- ✔ Italy: Federazione Nazionale dei Collegi dei Massofisioterapisti (F.N.C.M.), Rome, tel. 03 94 61 915 499

- ✔ U.K.: The Institute for Complementary Medicine, London, tel. 00 44 171 237-5165

Locating a Massage Therapist

If for some reason you can't locate a massage therapist by simply calling one of the numbers listed previously, you can pursue several other avenues in quest of massage.

Checking the ads

Each locale has its own regulations regarding the advertising of massage, and sometimes the regulations vary from city to city. What may be perfectly legal in Los Angeles, for example, can be verboten in Sioux City, Iowa.

Beware those ads featuring massage therapists with huge muscles, wearing black leather vests with no shirt underneath, staring straight into the camera with a come-hither look in their eyes, especially in San Francisco. These pictures may be a clue tipping you off to the extra curricular intentions of this particular massage therapist, licensed or not. Then again, it could be a fashion statement.

Letting your fingers do the walking

In some areas, massage therapists must include an official massage license number as part of any Yellow Pages listing for massage. According to Dan Ulrich, past president of the Florida State Massage Therapy Association, the inclusion of the license number in Yellow Pages and other ads significantly reduced the amount of unethical massage advertising. Although the license number is not mandatory everywhere, it's a clue that you're dealing with a therapeutic professional. If you don't see a license number or some other professional credentials listed, call and ask for one.

Opening the bureau door

You may occasionally run into ads for massage service bureaus that guarantee you a massage within a specified period of time (usually within a couple hours). The bureaus have a central number that you call, and they send one of the many independent massage therapists on their list out to you at your choice of location. Quite often, these are very up-and-up enterprises run by entrepreneurial massage therapists who have discovered a new way to multiply their effectiveness and their income. At times, though, the quality of the services offered can be a little iffy, because all the massage therapists aren't carefully screened all the time in all the bureaus. So, if you're not personally familiar with the service, and you haven't received a specific recommendation, you're never sure exactly what you're going to get when you call one of these places. Bureaus are most useful when you're traveling and have no other means of contacting a massage therapist.

Getting the most massage for your money

When dealing with your massage therapist, certain tactics can increase happiness for both of you, and in the process, maximize the value you receive from your experience.

✔ **Offer to pay up front for a discounted series of massages:** For example, if the massage therapist charges $50 for a massage, offer $400 dollars for 10 massages. Often, massage therapists appreciate the immediate cash flow and the guarantee of ongoing business. This arrangement is good for their business, and good for your pocketbook.

✔ **Ask for a massage in exchange for referring a new client to your massage therapist:** She will appreciate the new customer, and you deserve the recognition.

✔ **Inquire about rates for longer massage sessions:** Often the price drops proportionally with the length of the massage, and you can receive a 90- minute massage for not too much more than a 60- minute massage. A massage therapist who charges $50 for an hour massage may offer an hour and a half massage for $65 or $70, for example.

Going back to school

Wherever you are, one excellent way to get in touch with a massage practitioner is to call a massage school in your area. There are more schools around than you think — the U.S. alone has over 800. Look in the phone book, under "vocational schools" or "schools, massage therapy." The schools often have a list of graduates in the area that they can recommend, and quite often they offer massage services in a clinic in the school.

One excellent deal that many people take advantage of is known as the *student massage clinic.* In this setup, the students receive part of their training by working on real massage customers, under supervision, of course. Student massages go for only fraction of the normal cost, usually only ¼ to ⅓ the going rate of a professional massage in the area. More often than not, the students are already quite good at what they do, and dollar for dollar this option is one of the best bargains in massage.

Keep in mind that you may be asked to fill out a detailed feedback form after the massage, for training purposes. Also, the student clinics usually take place in a big room with curtains separating the massage tables. Quite often, an instructor stops in to observe the student in action. So if you're a super-private individual who doesn't like to have other people around when you're getting a massage, the student clinic is probably not for you. Also, if you have a specific health problem that you'd like to address with massage, it's best to visit a licensed professional. For relaxation and stress relief, though, student massages are usually as effective as more expensive professional massages because the students are trying extra hard to please you (and pass their coursework at the same time!).

Pampering Your Massage Therapist

After you choose a massage therapist and begin to develop a working relationship with him, a few endearing personality quirks may begin to surface. Some massage therapists work barefoot, even in the winter, for example. Others hold a giant quartz crystal over your body before the massage. And some tape a bunch of magnets under their massage table to "align your energy" while they work on you. Try not to take your massage therapist's idiosyncrasies too seriously. They're just trying to do the best job they can. It's just that some of their methods may seem a little, um, colorful at first. Refer to rule # 9, "You're the boss," in Chapter 7 for advice on letting your massage therapist know what you're comfortable and what you're not comfortable with.

As a general rule, massage therapists are a finicky and extremely sensitive lot. They're somewhat like pure-bred cats, and although their job description calls for a great deal of touching, they also need to receive strokes themselves (often to that most delicate muscle, the ego). If you become an expert at scratching behind the ears of your massage therapist's self-image, you can coax a better performance from him, and your relationship will be a happier one all around.

The following are some simple points to remember whenever you're dealing directly with your massage therapist:

- **Always offer encouragement first before you criticize:** For example, if your massage therapist is applying a little too much pressure in a particular area, definitely let her know about it, but first say something like, "What you were doing a minute ago felt really great. You can lighten up the pressure a little right now, though."

- **Always, always, always praise the massage your therapist just gave you immediately after you receive it, even if this is the seven hundred and eighty-ninth massage you've received from her:** The immediate gratification of this simple act is powerful. It's the same reason all an actress's friends rush backstage after the play to heartily laud her skills. The ego muscle is most delicate directly after the big performance, and for a great massage therapist, every massage is a type of performance.

- **Always communicate clearly about exactly what fee you expect to pay for exactly which services:** Pricing of massage services may be a sensitive issue. Be clear on the answers to the following questions before you begin:

  - Is the charge for an hour and fifteen minute massage higher than that for an hour massage?

  - Does the massage therapist have a cancellation policy?

  - Does your massage therapist reimburse insurance claims?

Licensing Touch

Being a wise consumer, when you head out looking for a massage pro to rub you the right way, you'll want to ask yourself that all-important question: Is she licensed? The problem here is that not all good, professional massage therapists in all areas are licensed. In the U.S., only half the states even require licensing for massage. Some states require no license at all, and in others the licensing is county-by-county or city-by-city. So even someone who is very highly trained and takes her job very seriously may be license-less, through no fault of her own.

Internationally, licensing rules for massage therapists vary widely from country to country. Some countries, like Singapore, for example, have little or no regulation, while in other countries, like France, massage therapists are part of the medical community and operate out of their own medical clinics. The best course of action in foreign countries is to ask someone you trust to recommend massage. Also, you can read through Chapter 17 for some more suggestions.

The rules concerning massage licensing are too complex and changeable to list here. They differ from area to area and time to time. In fact, in Santa Monica, California, where I first started working as a massage therapist, the actual laws on the books stated that nobody could open a massage clinic within 500 feet of a church, and in order to receive your city license to practice, you had to take a test certifying that you were free of all venereal diseases. Go figure.

If you want information about how massage practitioners are licensed in your area, you can call the board or department in your state that regulates massage therapists. If there is no such regulating board, check with a local massage school to see what kind of education and certification is normal for practitioners in your area.

The best thing to do when you're trying to determine the professional status of any individual massage therapist is to ask the therapist. I know, this strategy is stunningly simple, but it works. If she doesn't know anything about licensing, you may have an unprofessional person on your hands. On the other hand, if she knows her stuff, she can tell you exactly who to call or where to look to verify local licensing requirements in general, and hers in particular.

Because this whole licensing issue is so confusing in many areas, you're wise to consider certification as an equally, if not more, important factor in determining who to choose as your massage therapist.

Original sin?

Some massage therapists think that requiring licensing for massage is almost sinful, because they perceive what they do as art. They figure that licensing massage is like licensing a painter to paint, or a writer to write. Ridiculous! These people thoroughly oppose any attempts at control or regulation. They often live in cabins in rugged-individualist states such as Vermont, which, as an interesting side-note that has absolutely nothing to do with massage, is the only state that has managed to keep out Wal-Mart stores.

If a massage therapist has graduated from a bona-fide massage school, he has received a certificate of completion, and this certificate often notes the number of hours completed, specialties studied, and other relevant information. This certification may be the single most substantial piece of evidence of a massage therapist's dedication to his craft, especially in those areas where licensing is not required.

Another type of certification is awarded to those massage therapists who complete a test given by a certification board, such as the National Certification Board for Therapeutic Massage and Bodywork (NCBTMB). This certification is another way of determining competency.

Remember, in massage, just as in a marriage, it's not the actual piece of paper, but the level of commitment on the participants' part that is most vital to the success of the relationship. A fancy, gold-embossed massage license hanging on the wall in a frame is no guarantee that you're going to like a given massage therapist's technique. And, on the other hand, someone with no certificate or license at all may be one of the most highly skilled massage therapists you'll ever meet. When it comes down to choosing a pro, go with your heart and your intuition.

Chapter 7

The Rules for Receiving Massage

In This Chapter

▶ Following guidelines for receiving a massage

▶ Getting in tune and staying in touch

*F*rom the day you were born, your body has been hanging around you like a shadow. It never leaves you alone. You wake up in the morning, and there your body is, faithful as a puppy, thumping its little tail against your freshly washed bedspread. At first, having a body is a novelty, a fact that you can see reflected in the faces of babies and small children. Even the most mundane details about their bodies fill them with delight. "Oh boy, there's my hand again!"

As you mature, however, you become more accustomed to having a body, and it begins to bore you. This boredom usually occurs as young people enter their teenage years. "Oh boy, my hand again, big deal." At this point, they begin to pierce their bodies in various locations and cover them with decorative tattoos. By the time people are full-fledged adults, though, most of them have begun to concentrate on other things, leaving their bodies far behind. The only time they really get connected to their bodies is when they're learning a new skill of some kind, like soccer, or neurosurgery.

The result? Most people take their bodies for granted. One of massage's main objectives is to get you back "into" your body again. A good massage should rekindle your childlike enthusiasm for life.

In order for massage to help you achieve the lofty goal of getting back in touch with yourself, you need to follow certain guidelines, which I just happen to outline in this chapter. At first, some of these "rules" may seem a little simplistic to you. Others may appear irrelevant. However, I give you my personal guarantee that if you try them out when you're on the receiving end of a massage, you're going to get much more out of the experience.

So, approach these guidelines with an open mind, apply them when you feel that doing so is appropriate during your own massage exchanges, and watch your enjoyment of massage soar to levels beyond your expectations.

The rules for receiving massage are, in fact, quite similar to the Ancient Secrets of Life as passed down by Big Important Spiritual Leaders for thousands of years. Yes, it's true; you can learn every really important thing in life by lying down and getting rubbed.

Honing your skills at receiving massage is more than simply a way to feel better. It's also a way to improve your life. Read through these rules, practice them, and you'll see what I mean.

Rule #1: Keep Breathing

When you receive a massage from a professional, she may remind you several times in a soft, soothing voice to breathe. And you may be tempted to say right back to her in a not-so-soothing voice, "I'm already breathing, in case you haven't noticed."

Don't be offended. The massage therapist's comments aren't meant to imply that she thinks you're deceased, and she's not trying to insult you for your poor breathing skills. In fact, many massage therapists start each and every massage with a series of deep breaths, regardless of how obviously alive you are to begin with.

A massage therapist may tell you to take deep breaths during a massage for the following reasons:

- ✔ To help you focus on the sensations you're feeling in your body rather than the internal monologue going on in your mind
- ✔ To get you to fill your lungs and thus all your cells with fresh oxygen, enlivening your entire body
- ✔ To help you become aware of muscles that you've been holding tense so you can start to relax them

Most people walk around not actually breathing much. People tend to use only a tiny percentage of their lung capacity, just like they use only a tiny percentage of their brain capacity. Proper breathing changes that.

While receiving a massage, focus your mind as fully as possible upon the very important act of breathing. Focusing your mind on your breath brings your awareness back to your body quicker than anything else.

Going with the diaphragm's flow

The *diaphragm* is a muscle in your abdomen — it looks like a soft *pizza* shaped into a double-headed dome — that is responsible for keeping you breathing (see Figure 7-1). Most of the time, your diaphragm is contracting and relaxing without conscious thought from you, but you can teach yourself to control this activity. In the section "Exercising your breathing muscle's breath," I give you an exercise that helps you use this muscle more consciously, which enables you to exert more control over your breathing, making it fuller and deeper.

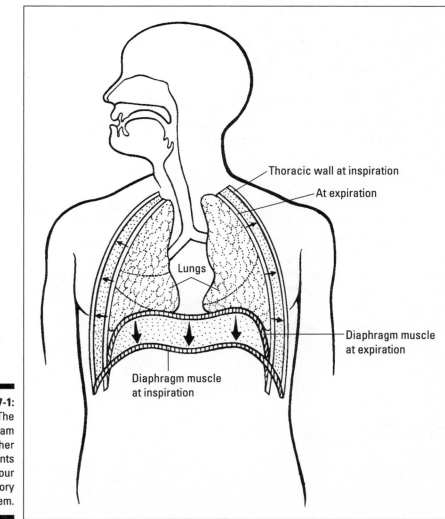

Thoracic wall at inspiration

At expiration

Lungs

Diaphragm muscle at expiration

Diaphragm muscle at inspiration

Figure 7-1: The diaphram and other elements of your respiratory system.

Exercising your breathing muscles

The next time you have the chance, spend a few minutes observing a sleeping — or at least relaxed — infant or toddler breathe. Pay close attention to the abdomen, and you can see the entire area gently lift and lower. This movement is the result of an active, uninhibited diaphragm at work.

Then look down at your own abdomen while you breathe for a few minutes. Notice a difference? Where did all the lifting and lowering go? You still have the same breathing mechanisms you always did; they're not something you grow out of. With each breath you take, you should indeed have a visibly rhythmical, moving body. Somewhere along the line, though, most people stifle themselves into taking shallow, insufficient breaths. This type of breathing is a common reaction to the act of growing older. Don't worry, you're still getting enough oxygen to survive. But, are you getting enough to thrive? By practicing deep breathing during massage, you can literally rejuvenate your body, sending extra-oxygenated blood out all the way to your toes.

The key to breathing properly while getting a massage is to take *whole breaths,* a term that basically means "breathing like a kid." Go ahead and try a whole breath now. Lie down on your back, placing your palms gently on your abdomen, and then begin this four-step process:

1. **Breathe deep and low into your lungs so that your abdomen pushes your hands upward.**

   Make sure that you're not just pushing up with your stomach muscles, but that you're actually expanding the entire abdominal area.

2. **Continue the expansion up into your ribs, allowing them to push outward toward each side.**

3. **When your ribs have expanded *out* as far as they'll go, then expand them *up* toward your head, taking the last bit of breath into the area just beneath your collar bones.**

4. **Let the whole thing collapse.**

   You don't need to try and push the air out; just let it flow. When your lungs feel empty and your abdomen is flat once again, you can restart the process.

Rule #2: Stay Loose

As you probably know, one of the main points of getting a massage is to relax. Logically, you may then think that you can just give your body to a massage therapist who will relax your body for you, like giving your car to a mechanic and expecting him to fix it.

Please release me, let me go . . .

After you receive several massages, you'll gradually become accustomed to relaxing your own muscles. Eventually you notice that you can do the same thing even when you're not receiving massage, like when you're waiting in line at the grocery store, stuck in traffic, or sitting in a meeting with your boss. "Twang," will go one of your muscle fibers, and you'll feel it beginning to tighten up. Then, silently, without anyone noticing, you send a mental message to the growing knot, telling it to go away, in the same way that your massage therapist helps you do during a massage. You can take this side benefit of massage with you wherever you go.

Expecting a massage therapist to do all your body's relaxing is called *giving up responsibility for your own relaxation,* and it's a no-no. Staying loose is your responsibility; the massage therapist can help you, but you basically have to do the relaxing yourself. So how do you do that?

You accomplish relaxation by becoming more aware of what you're feeling in your own body. During the massage, your massage therapist often reminds you to focus on "knots" or tight areas. In those moments, using the power of your own imagination, you can begin to visualize what those knots may look like in your muscles, and to let go of them.

If you're not staying loose by engaging your mind to relax your own muscles, you're missing more than half the benefits and effects of the massage.

Rule #3: Let Go

When you receive a massage, especially the first time, you may have a tendency — like just about everyone else in the world — to "help" the person working on you. You may graciously lift your limbs, hold your head up, and twist your body around, all to make things easier for the other person. Although this "helping" may seem like the friendliest thing to do, you're actually hindering the massage process and making your massage therapist's job a little more difficult. Relaxing a person who is holding her own arm up in the air as stiff as a flag pole is pretty darn hard.

The technical term for this tendency during massage is *hanging on,* and you want to do exactly the opposite, which is letting go. But what, exactly, does "letting go" mean?

The limp-arm experiment

You're basically hanging onto yourself for dear life, even the parts of your body that are painful, stiff, or tense. This hanging on is a natural tendency, but to get the most out of a massage, you have to let go. The "limp-arm experiment" is an easy way to begin training yourself to let go. All you need is a partner and someplace comfortable to lie down.

1. **Lie down on your back and have your partner lift your arm up in the air several inches.**

2. **After a few seconds, have your partner let go of your arm without any warning to you.**

   Let your arm drop back down. (Make sure that you're lying on a soft surface.)

3. **Watch to see whether your arm plops back down, limp as a noodle, or whether you hold it right where she left it, stiff as a board.**

   What do you have to do to let your arm drop back down? What thought process do you have to go through? What mental image? What body sensation?

4. **Tell your partner to lift your arm a little higher each time.**

   Instead of dropping your arm all the way back down, tell her to catch it in her other hand.

5. **Keep repeating this exercise until your arm completely lets go and your partner can drop it from any height with absolutely no resistance.**

   This ability may come naturally to you the very first time you try to let go, but normally the exercise takes quite a bit of conscious effort. You may not be able to let go until you make several separate attempts on different days. After you master one arm, you can try the other arm, a leg, or your head.

Use this newly formed skill to let go the next time you receive a massage.

If you were to take a microscope and look deep within your muscles and joints while you're getting a massage, you'd discover some specialized nerve cells that monitor the position and relative movement of your body. These cells are called *proprioceptors* (see Chapter 4).

These cells constantly tell you where you are in space, something everybody likes to have a pretty firm control over all of the time, even while asleep. These cells keep you from just rolling right out of bed every night.

About the only time you completely let go of all your holding patterns, tensions, and proprioceptive rigidities is when you're under deep anesthesia. Under anesthesia, people sometimes release the tension they normally think of as "built-in" through age or heredity, including stooped shoulders, stiff hips, ugly grimaces, and more. When they come out of anesthesia, they reclaim these habitual patterns almost instantaneously. They can't sustain the relaxation because it's unconscious. Massage, conversely, allows people to achieve a conscious relaxation, which can last indefinitely.

One of my clients suffered for years from debilitating pain due to whiplash. Then one day she received a massage from a woman at Gurney's Inn, a spa in Montauk, New York. After that massage, the pain was almost entirely gone, and it continued to gradually fade away. My client was able to make such a drastic change by letting herself go fully into the healing hands of the massage therapist. When she did, she stopped holding onto the same painful, habitual patterns that had formed in her body since the accident.

Rule #4: Stop Thinking, Start Being

The problem with your mind is that it just works too darn well, thinking and thinking and thinking without stopping all day long from the first moment you wake up until well after your head hits the pillow. This feature is fine during most of your daily activities, but when it comes to getting a massage, too much thinking is definitely a drawback.

Many people get a massage and then ten minutes later can barely remember it because they weren't really paying attention to it while it was happening. Instead, an ongoing stream of thoughts kept them from fully experiencing the massage.

When you're getting a massage, don't think about what you should have done the day before or what you plan to do an hour later. A massage is time to Be Here Now. The sensations you're feeling offer a great opportunity to quiet your mind, focus, and think of nothing else for a little while. In this way, every massage is a potential meditation. Don't get me wrong: relaxing and joking around during a massage is perfectly okay, too, but most people, at least once in a while, can benefit from a *massage meditation*. (See the sidebar, "A massage meditation," later in this chapter.)

Rule #5: No Pain, No Gain? No Way!

You may have heard of the massage-masochists who don't believe they're receiving a real massage unless they have to grit their teeth to keep from screaming through the whole thing. They're the ones you can hear yelling from behind massage room doors, "More pressure! More pressure!"

This green-beret school of massage is an unfortunate result of the "no-pain, no-gain" mentality that military academies, full-contact sports enthusiasts, and certain daytime-television talk show hosts foster. You don't need to buy into this way of thinking, and you shouldn't let this attitude scare you away from getting a massage.

A massage meditation

Meditation, in a nutshell, is the act of focusing your entire attention on just one thing, thus stopping the constant chatter inside your head and experiencing a state of timelessness, contentment, and wholeness. People achieve this state in many ways — through sports, or silence, or prayer, for example — and massage is yet another activity that you can use to effectively shut out the rest of the world and tune into your own inner peace. The next time you receive a massage, try this meditation . . .

1. **Close your eyes and begin to get in touch with your breath, as I describe in the section "Rule #1: Keep Breathing."**

   Before you receive the first touch of the massage, spend several minutes trying to clear your mind of any other thoughts. Concentrate only on your breathing.

2. **When your massage therapist first makes contact, imagine yourself breathing in through that very spot.**

   For example, if she starts by massaging your neck, imagine a stream of fresh oxygen and energy entering through your neck, exactly where her fingers are.

3. **On the exhalation, imagine your muscles in that same area becoming softer, warmer, and looser.**

4. **Continue with this awareness — breathing relaxation into each successive point that the massage therapist is touching.**

   Eventually, you become aware that the massage therapist is tuning in to your breath as well, and the massage becomes a shared meditation.

5. **Communicate with your massage therapist, both verbally and nonverbally. Together, you can create a special massage mood that will help you focus on your experience, making the massage more like a meditation (see Chapter 9).**

6. **Keep bringing your mind back to the massage.**

   You may realize, at various points during the massage, that your mind has wandered off on some train of thought. This is completely natural and happens even to advanced meditation practitioners. Simply bring your mind gently back to the breath and the relaxation. Don't worry about how "good" you are at meditation. See *Meditation For Dummies* (IDG Books Worldwide) for more guidance and tips about meditation.

So, how much pain should you experience during a massage? In my opinion, none. Zero. However, the line is indeed thin between the pleasure you receive during massage and a certain kind of therapeutic pain. Some people like to walk that line while they're getting a massage. If you want to experiment walking this line yourself, make sure to do so with an experienced professional.

Although certain muscle knots and patterns of tension do respond well to firm, well-focused pressure, you don't necessarily need to experience it for yourself. Harder massage is not always better massage, and at times the lightest touch can achieve the most profound benefits.

Rule #6: Listen to Your Emotions

Don't be surprised if during a massage one day you suddenly, for no reason at all, feel like crying your eyes out, or laughing hysterically. Massage sometimes has that effect on people. Some of the reasons for this emotional response include:

- ✔ Certain emotional memories — usually the result of powerful experiences — can resurface when your body is massaged.
- ✔ No one has touched you with care, compassion, and gentleness for a very long time. In that case, the experience suddenly overwhelms you with gratitude, bringing forth tears.
- ✔ You're a very ticklish person.

As esoteric as the first two explanations may sound, they're entirely plausible. In fact, certain types of massage are famous for stirring up emotions. Rolfing, for instance, often triggers this type of experience. The explanation for this emotional component of massage is straightforward — your body and mind have faithfully recorded your every experience, but some of these experiences were so unpleasant that you filed them away in your unconscious and shut down certain feelings in the corresponding part of your body. Massaging the affected areas can bring your awareness back to your body, thus unlocking the memories.

If you encounter one of these emotional peaks yourself during a massage, relax, breathe, and allow it to happen. Remembering that you are safe in your present environment, let your mind drift to whatever images or memories seem to be surfacing. You may find yourself remembering all sorts of things that you hadn't thought of for years, and you can benefit from letting the attendant emotions flow freely through your body, without trying to stifle them. Professional massage therapists are accustomed to this type of emotional release and know how to make you feel comfortable while it's happening. There's no need to feel embarrassed by the experience.

If, as occasionally happens, one of these resurfacing memories is particularly traumatic, as in the case of abuse, do whatever is necessary to comfort yourself. Communicate with the person massaging you, letting her know that you need to sit up again, or get wrapped in a blanket for a feeling of safety. Have some tissues nearby to dry away tears. Later you can decide whether you want to pursue these memories further with the guidance of a psychologist or other counselor.

Rule #7: Blissing Out Is Okay

Sometimes, massage doesn't just make you feel great; it makes you feel ecstatic, rapturous, and filled with bliss. The feeling is visceral. You're lying there one minute relaxing, hopefully concentrating on your breathing, but perhaps just going over your grocery list in your head, when KABOOM!, it hits you, and suddenly you're just floating there in a syrupy sea of endorphins, not knowing what to do with yourself.

I can tell you what to do: enjoy this feeling while it lasts, because, like every other human experience, it passes.

These experiences are different for everyone, and nobody knows exactly what causes them. They've been responsible for many people changing their entire lives and heading into a career as a massage therapist. And people with spiritual inclinations, once touched in this fashion, have created entire ministries devoted to the "laying on of hands."

A minister named Zach Thomas from North Carolina once had such a powerful experience receiving a massage that he went on to become a massage therapist himself. At first, his church was opposed to his hands-on work, and Zach had to practice massage privately. Eventually, though, he took his skills and his compassionate touch out to the public, performing massage for dying people in hospices and hospitals. He helped form a group called the National Association of Bodywork in Religious Services (NABRS), which is active today with hundreds of members. Much of the work the members of this association do is for those people who wouldn't otherwise be able to afford it. The nuns and priests and other clergy involved practice the actual "laying on of hands" as written about in the Bible. For more information, you can write to the organization at 337 Tranquil Avenue, Charlotte, NC 28209.

The spiritual secret behind massage? Simple. What massage really boils down to is two people just being together fully in the present moment, which has been the essence of spiritual traditions forever, especially in the East. The mystical traditions of the West have expressed similar sentiments, as noted in the phrase, "Be still and know that I am God." These understandings are mystical in nature, not reserved for any one particular religion.

Think of it this way — massage is one sure-fire way to follow the Golden Rule that exists in almost all cultures and every religion, from the Good Samaritan to the compassionate Buddha. *Do unto others as you would have them do unto you.* Well, who doesn't want to be touched with care and compassion? Who doesn't like others to help them feel better and lighten their load?

Massage is compassion turned into action.

Rule #8: It's Cool to Be Nude (Or Not)

You are, whether you like it or not, naked all the time beneath your clothes. You were born nude, just like every other human on the planet. Nudity is natural. However, each culture develops its own peculiar attitudes about nudity, ranging from those who consider it extremely awkward, embarrassing, and inappropriate at all times to those who don't think twice about it, anytime, anywhere, for any reason.

Neither attitude is healthier than the other, they're just different. The key for massage situations is to respect the attitudes of both people at all times. If either the person receiving or giving the massage is uncomfortable with any kind of skin exposure whatsoever, you're much better off to cover that area up and keep it covered than to cause discomfort. This applies to the entire body, even the legs and arms, which most people are comfortable exposing. Although gliding an oiled palm is definitely easier over bare skin than covered skin, massage has other moves besides gliding, and you can give a very good massage to a fully clothed person (I show you how in Chapter 11).

Remember this message: When you receive a massage, you're okay the way you are — nude or totally covered up. Just be comfortable.

Rule #9: You're the Boss

Even though you're lying down with your eyes closed during most massages, you're still in charge. With the slightest word or gesture, you can change the course of the proceedings. Deeper pressure? It's up to you. Slower pace? That's your call, too. Less chit-chat? Your decision.

You have complete authority to change anything that may be making you uncomfortable. Requesting a change of music, for example, is perfectly permissible, as is turning the music off altogether. If you want to be covered more modestly, just ask. Whatever you say goes. You can say exactly what you're feeling, even ending the massage at any time, for any reason you want. Period. You always have the option of standing up and saying, "Enough!"

Of course, when you're receiving a massage from a professional massage therapist, it makes sense to listen to her suggestions. If she thinks you should quiet down and focus on the massage rather than conversation, for example, it's probably best to follow her advice. However, don't mistakenly place yourself in a submissive role just because you're lying down. Even if the other person knows more about massage than you, is older than you, or has a louder personality than you, the bottom line is, when you're receiving a massage, you're the boss.

Rule #10: Be Grateful

During the massage itself, spend some time being grateful for what you're experiencing in the moment. This course is by far the best one to take, instead of the alternatives, which consist of

- ✔ Wondering when the massage is going to end
- ✔ Plotting the next time you can get a massage
- ✔ Planning your next business trip
- ✔ Worrying about the world economy

Also, be sure to share your feelings of gratitude with the person who just gave you the massage, being especially vocal about her fantastic skills and techniques. That way, she'll look forward to giving you your next massage as much as you'll look forward to getting it.

Chapter 8

Your First Massage Appointment — Step-by-Step

*P*robably the biggest barrier that stops people from ever signing up for their first professional massage is a fear of the unknown. Let's face it: If you have never ventured into a room with a stranger to get rubbed before, you just don't know what to expect, and the thought of becoming vulnerable in any way doesn't inspire you to take the first step.

But hold on. Think back for just a minute. Do you remember any experience in your entire life that was *not* scary the first time you tried it? Go as far back as your first day at kindergarten. *That's* scary. Getting your first massage is just another step along the road of discovery in your life.

Your First Appointment with a Pro

You can use the following seven steps as a guide to help you breeze through your first appointment with confidence and poise, starting before you even arrive and lasting right up until you walk out the door.

Preparation

In order to get the most out of your massage, you have to do a little more planning and preparation than you would, say, in order to go get a haircut. When you schedule your massage, keep these points in mind:

✔ Don't eat a large meal within a couple hours before starting the massage. You don't want to be lying face down on a belly full of lasagna while somebody is pressing on your back. Light meals and snacks are okay, and a larger meal several hours earlier won't affect you.

✔ If possible, don't wear a lot of jewelry, which takes a lot to time to take off and put back on again.

✔ Refrain from consuming alcohol before your massage (unless it's a sensual massage and you're sharing a bottle of bubbly with that special someone to get in the mood). Although alcohol can help relax you, it also slows your responses and deadens some sensations. You want to be alert and responsive because massage is a two-way dance and you need to do your part.

✔ Make sure to schedule enough time before and after your massage so you're not rushing to get there and flying out the door when you leave. Hurrying tends to counteract the relaxing effects of the massage itself.

✔ Turn off pagers and cellular phones during the massage. This probably seems obvious, but it may surprise you to know that beeps, buzzes, and rings have interrupted many tranquil, soothing massages.

✔ Make sure any childcare details are completely taken care of before you begin so your mind can be at ease during your session.

No particular time of day is best to receive a massage, but most people have their own personal preference. Some like the morning so they can experience the benefits throughout the day, and others like a massage right before going to bed at night. Whichever your choice is, try to schedule far enough in advance so you get the time you prefer. Many massage therapists are busy, and their "prime times" are taken up early.

Communication

When you arrive at your massage destination, especially for the first time, you need to engage in a little communication with the person who is going to massage you. So it helps, of course, if you speak the same language as that person. And I don't mean just the same native tongue, but the same *intention*, too. If what you want out of the experience is fundamentally different than what the massage therapist intends to give, you're headed for trouble.

For example, if you came in for an hour of blissful relaxation and escape from stress, but what the massage therapist intends on giving you is a session of active, muscle-stretching sports therapy, neither one of you is going to have a good time. The best time to confirm your intentions is on the phone, before you meet face-to-face, but you need to reconfirm this understanding with some clear verbal communication after you arrive, as well.

When you finally meet your massage therapist for the first time, there may be some nonverbal communication required also, in the form of paperwork to fill out, like the actual massage therapist's intake form. "Why do I have to fill out these medical forms if all I want is a simple massage?" you may ask. Well, it's for your own good. Massage affects the entire body, and it's best if your massage therapist knows as much as possible about your health history. If a massage therapist doesn't ask you to fill out a form, however, it doesn't mean she doesn't care about your health; that's just her style, or the policy of the spa or health club where she works.

Another type of communication you share with your massage therapist is both nonverbal and non-written — body language. Your massage therapist, by profession an expert in the language of the body, may try her best not to laugh out loud while your body silently struggles with embarrassment and anxiety at the prospect of getting your first massage. Just kidding! Actually, as you may imagine, massage therapists become very adept at making their clients feel at ease in a potentially uneasy situation. It's the little things they do (and don't do) that make the difference. It could be where they point their eyes or how they manipulate sheets and towels to make you feel protected and respected. It's the way they just relax and accept you when you make yourself vulnerable by being there.

Besides, they're just as eager to make a good first impression as you are, partly because it's human nature and partly because they want you as a repeat customer!

Getting comfortable

In most massage situations, after you arrive and go through your communication rituals, the next step is undressing and lying down. This can be tricky. It's the moment many people dread, and the one that keeps them from ever getting a "real" massage. The way it works is like this:

1. The massage therapist explains how you're supposed to get up on the massage table, pointing out where your head should be, and whether you should be face up or facedown. If you ask whether you should get completely undressed or not, the stock answer is something to the effect of, "Most people take all their clothes off, but you can get undressed to the level of your comfort." Then she leaves the room. Do not feel intimidated by "most people" who all so bravely get naked for their massages. It's up to you if you want to keep your underwear or some clothes on, and it's OK either way. Refer to Rule # 8 in Chapter 7, "It's cool to be nude (or not)."

2. After the massage therapist is out of the room, remember to take your time. Don't worry about getting barged in on, cause it ain't gonna happen. She knocks before coming back in, and usually she waits much longer than necessary to make sure you have plenty of time. Take this opportunity to remove jewelry, watches, and anything else that may

entangle a finger (wedding bands are okay). Usually, there is a little table or shelf to hold your belongings, and you can find a hook for your clothes. If you have long hair, you may want to tie it back so it doesn't get in the way. Also, it's a good idea to visit the bathroom *before* you lay down on the table, even if you don't think you have to go. Getting a massage with a full bladder takes a lot of the enjoyment out of it.

3. Lie down on the table in the position you were told and pull the sheet or towel up over your body, completely covering yourself.

4. The massage therapist knocks and asks if it's okay to enter again. When you give the go-ahead, she comes in, and then usually washes her hands. She does this for three reasons:

   • To reassure you that her hands are clean

   • To wash away any dirt or germs she may have contacted since scrubbing them the last time a few minutes earlier

   • In many areas the law requires it

5. She makes sure you're comfortable, checking the room temperature, tucking the towel around your body, and adjusting the lights and music. She may also slip a little pillow or piece of foam rubber beneath your knees, ankles, or head to help support you. These cushions are called *bolsters*, and they really help you feel more comfortable. If you feel a strain or lack of support in any area of your body, just let the massage therapist know.

6. After everything's set, your massage therapist uncovers just the area that she is going to work on. If she plans to massage your neck, she pulls the sheet down to the top of your chest. Massage therapists always leave women's breasts covered, and no one's "private parts" ever get exposed.

Sometimes no matter how hard you try, all these massage rules go out the window. Like the time I was working at a spa and had the opportunity to massage Dr. Ruth Westheimer. I'll never forget the experience because, for one thing, she threw her robe off before I ever had the chance to leave the room and let her get undressed. Then, full of confidence, she strode to the massage table and tried to climb aboard. I say "tried" because, as it turns out, she was a little too short to reach. I wanted to reach down and give her a boost, but I couldn't figure out how to do it without getting a little too personal with Dr. Ruth, so I averted my eyes as best I could and offered ineffectual words of general encouragement.

Luckily, she knew what to do. "Don't worry!" she chimed. "I've had this problem before!" Then she proceeded to push a chair up next to the massage table, climb onto it, and from there crawl up onto the table, where I immediately covered her with a sheet in the proper professional fashion.

Avoiding the bathrobe dance

As a massage therapist in spas, on many occasions I've entered the massage room to begin a massage only to find my client lying there, face down, rigid with nervousness, with her bathrobe tied super-tight around her waist. Before leaving the room to let her disrobe, I'd instructed her to take her robe off and lie down under the sheet I'd provided, but some clients are too tense to hear those instructions.

And so that's when we begin the bathrobe dance.

The bathrobe dance is an awkward ordeal that usually lasts about two minutes. While the massage therapist tries to assist as best he can, the client rolls, wriggles, and writhes her way out of the bathrobe while remaining face down and completely covered at all times. The client's rump usually scoots up in the air, arms and legs splay every which way, and her face turns bright red.

Then, after the robe is finally loosened from around her body and her arms are out of the armholes, the massage therapist has to drape a sheet or towel over it before skillfully slipping the robe from underneath. This entire procedure leaves the client even more tense than when she started, and more embarrassed than she would have been if she'd simply listened to the instructions.

If you find yourself on the table still wrapped in your robe, make things easy on yourself. Don't wear yourself out before the massage by wrestling with your robe. Instead, say something like, "That was so silly of me," and ask the massage therapist to leave the room again to give you another chance. Then get off the table, slip out of your robe, and lie down beneath the sheet like you were supposed to in the first place.

If, rather than a bathrobe, you have a towel wrapped around you before the massage, make sure not to lie down directly upon the knotted part so you have to do the "rock-n-roll" to loosen it. Instead, open the towel up and lie straight on the table with the towel still covering your backside.

The first touch

The very first moment of contact between you and the massage therapist can tell you an awful lot about how the rest of the massage is going to feel. Each massage therapist has a "personality" in her hands that you quickly get to know.

When the massage therapist is closely attuned to you and your body, this moment can be almost sacred. It's an intimate joining-together of your consciousness with the consciousness of another person, which just plain doesn't happen that often in the modern world.

Take advantage of this initial contact by tuning in especially closely to what's happening in your own body. In the same way that you pick up a lot of information about the person who's touching you, she's picking up a lot of information about you. It's a good opportunity for you to concentrate on your breathing and relaxation.

During the massage

During the massage, your massage therapist continues to keep you covered at all times, only exposing those areas that she's working on at the moment. Massage therapists are experts at this technique, called *draping*, and they make you feel completely comfortable, almost as if you were fully dressed during the experience.

Yes, you are comfortable and modestly covered the whole time, but what are you supposed to actually DO while you're getting a massage? That's the biggest problem many people have, especially "type A" people. They figure that getting a massage is just plain boring and that's why they decide not to do it.

Okay, so getting a massage is not exactly the same as bungee jumping from a hot-air balloon, attending a rock concert, or brokering a multi-million dollar deal in a corporate boardroom. But if you let it, massage can become compelling, thrilling even, in a very internal kind of way. It's like taking a roller coaster ride inside your own skin.

The trick is not to try and make anything happen, but to just let whatever happens happen. You're not supposed to do anything. Your massage therapist tells you if you have to move a certain way or breathe a certain way or visualize a certain image. Besides that, the less you do the better. Think of massage as a trip to the beach. You're *supposed to* just lie there and do nothing.

"But what if I fall asleep?" you gasp. "Wouldn't that insult the massage therapist?" Not at all. In fact, some massage therapists take it as a compliment that they can get their clients to relax this deeply. However, your creative input to the massage process is just as valuable as the massage therapist's input, so it's better if you stay awake. And, if you snooze through a massage, you may be missing some of the most pleasurable moments of your life. Who wants to pay good money for a nap?

If you're the type that cannot conceive of an entire hour spent doing nothing, try this: Talk to the massage therapist about things that matter, like your health. Most massage people are pretty well versed in the art of taking-care-of-yourself, and you stand a good chance of having a conversation that goes beyond mere chitchat, offering you some real benefits.

Under pressure

So, what's the right amount of *pressure* to ask for during a massage anyway? Pressure refers to how hard or soft the massage feels, how painful or soothing. Usually, your massage therapist has a lot of experience in this area and can find just the right pressure to suit your particular body type and your level of sensitivity. But there may be times when you want her to change the pressure, and it helps if you know what to ask for.

It's silly to suffer through a massage that's too soft or too hard just because you're too bashful to say anything about it. You can use this scale from 1–10 to communicate your desired pressure level to your massage therapist:

1 **Light as a feather.** The fingertips merely skim over the surface of the skin to provide stimulation to the nerve endings, but no pressure is exerted onto the body.

2–3 **Very light to light.** Many people prefer this kind of silky, gliding touch, but it drives others crazy because they think the massage therapist isn't "getting in there and working the muscles."

4–6 **Moderate to moderately firm.** This is where most massage takes place. You can definitely feel some pressure, and you know the massage is having some definite physical effects, but never so much that it's annoying.

7–9 **Firm to very firm to deep.** At these levels, you may begin to squirm a little. And you may even say something like, "What are you trying to do, kill me?" Rest assured, the massage therapist is not trying to kill you. She's just being merciless in her attempt to root out and destroy any tightness she's found. Mercilessness can be a good quality in a massage therapist.

10 **Profoundly deep massage**. This level reaches to the core of your body's deeper structures, actually altering your posture and inner alignment. This should be reserved for masochists, people with a high pain tolerance, and those who know what they're doing.

If there is a distraction of some sort, such as a loud noise or a telephone ringing, try not to take it personally. Nobody is out to ruin your massage experience. Instead of letting an interruption spoil things for you, focus instead on the exchange of positive energy between you and the person giving you the massage.

Keep communicating. When appropriate during the massage, give feedback to your massage therapist. Words spoken about the massage help keep you focused on the massage. If at any point you want the massage therapist to change what she's doing, you have a right to let her know. After all, you're paying, and the customer is always right. Let her know what you want, which may include:

  ✔ More pressure or less pressure. This is often referred to on a scale from 1 to 10 (see the sidebar, "Under pressure" in this chapter).

> ✔ More or less time spent in a particular area. But be aware that the massage therapist may be using her knowledge to achieve a certain goal, working in the area that's most effective, even if you think it's not directly connected to your problem.
>
> ✔ A glass of water.
>
> ✔ A trip to the bathroom.
>
> ✔ A chance to express your feelings and ask for reassurance, especially if a strong emotion begins to surface during your massage.

Beware of the massage therapist who claims she can only perform "deep" work and then proceeds to pummel your body even after you request lighter pressure. It's never necessary to undergo a painful ordeal in order to experience the relaxation you seek.

Coming back slowly

Take it easy getting off the table and back into your life. There's no need to hurry. In fact, most massage therapists suggest that you just lay there and absorb the effects of the massage and the relaxation for a few minutes before getting up again. Unless you're late for something urgent, such as an international plane trip to go receive the Nobel Prize at an awards banquet being held in your honor, follow this suggestion. These few minutes can be an exquisite interlude during which your cares and concerns seem a million miles away. Relish it.

Then, when you finally decide to get up, don't be shy about asking for help if you need it, as you may feel a little wobbly at first.

There is a special way to get yourself off a massage table that helps you keep the effects intact. Instead of essentially doing a sit-up and re-tensing all your muscles in order to get upright again, simply roll onto your side and push gently against the table with both hands while you slowly roll back into a sitting position. Your feet and legs will end up hanging over the edge of the table, as you see illustrated in Figure 8-1. Then you can slide your rear-end off the table like a buttered pancake.

Afterglow

When you first step on the floor again, exercise caution because massage oil left on the soles of your feet can cause you to slip. Take your time getting dressed, making sure you're not forgetting anything. It's not necessary to take a shower, as your skin absorbs normal amounts of oil or cream, though you may want to take one if you're going out later. If the massage therapist used excess oil, you can wipe it off with a towel or some rubbing alcohol before putting clothes back on, especially silk garments.

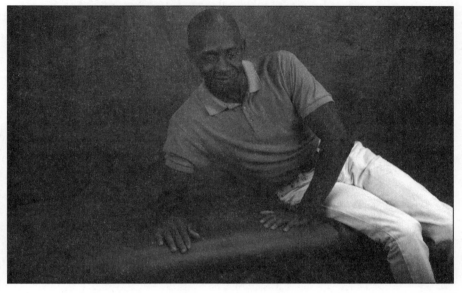

Figure 8-1:
There's a right way and a wrong way to get off a massage table. This is the right way.

Take some time to reorient yourself. Be cautious about driving your car right away as you may feel a bit "disconnected," as if your body were inside of a big box filled with cotton.

Before you leave, take the massage therapist's business card, and consider making another appointment so you don't have to worry about it later.

To tip or not to tip

You're all ready to head out the door when suddenly it occurs to you that perhaps you should tip the person who just gave you the massage. Is it appropriate? Would she be insulted if you gave her a tip? Upset if you didn't? The answer is . . . "it depends."

It depends upon where you received the massage. Was it a spa? Then a tip is almost always expected, unless the spa has a policy against it. Was it at a sports medicine clinic? Then tips are not usually part of the procedure. Did you receive the massage at home? Then a tip is definitely appreciated, as the massage therapist went out of her way to provide the service.

Overcoming the heebie jeebies

If, even after trying some of the suggestions in this chapter, you're still harboring a tiny bit of fear and loathing about massage somewhere in your subconscious mind, that's all right. I felt the same way, too, the first time I disrobed for a session as a student at the Massage School of Santa Monica many years ago.

It's perfectly natural to feel somewhat anxious at the thought of somebody you don't even know touching you for an extended period of time. And the thought of somebody you *do* know touching you for a whole hour may even be worse! In the highly sophisticated, jet-setter world of massage therapy, these feelings of anxiety are known by the technical term "heebie-jeebies." Unless you grew up in a household where massage was as common as Saturday morning cartoons, the heebie-jeebies may present a problem when you're first getting ready to climb up on a massage table and simply *receive.*

My advice? Feel the fear and do it anyway. Plunge in and get that massage. Afterwards, if you're like 99.9 percent of all people, you say to yourself, "That wasn't so bad! Why didn't I do this a long time ago?"

Some massage therapists feel tipping for a massage is inappropriate. They want their work to be considered in the same category as any other health care provider's. You wouldn't tip your chiropractor, your homeopath, or your M.D., right?

So how do you know what to do? Tipping ultimately boils down to an understanding with the massage therapist. If you're at all uncertain, simply ask, "Is tipping allowed here?" The customary tip amount in most locations is usually in the $5–$10 range, more if the massage therapist is working late, went far out of her way, or did an especially good job. And, remember, you never *have* to tip for massage. It's not like tipping a waiter, who's making the bulk of his income through gratuities. Massage therapists are usually pretty well paid for what they do. Tips are the icing on the cake for them.

Where to Go to Get Massaged

You have an array of choices when it comes to where you receive a professional massage, ranging from right in your own bedroom all the way up to super luxurious spa resorts on the island of Maui. I personally recommend Maui. Wherever you are, it helps if you know a little bit about each environment and what you can expect when you receive a massage there. That's what this section's all about.

Your own home

Getting a professional massage in your own home is great. In fact, some people think it's the crème de la crème of massage experiences. You don't have to drive anywhere. You're in safe, familiar surroundings. And, best of all, afterwards all you have to do is roll over into your own bed or onto your own couch. The massage therapist leaves, and you float off on a wave of bliss in the comfort of your own home.

What could be better?

However, there are some downsides to the in-home massage visit. For one thing, you're basically inviting a stranger to set up her business right in your own bedroom or your den, which is kind of an invasion of privacy. And another thing — when you're at home, you're surrounded by your own life. Every detail is there to remind you of your pre and post-massage existence, which may perhaps detract from the "escape" factor of your experience.

Then there are the distractions. If you have children, you can pretty much count on them wanting to crawl up on the massage table with you and "help" the nice massage person do her job. This is very endearing of the little tykes, but it's not the straight and narrow road to total relaxation.

Only sign up for an in-home massage if you're comfortable with other people in your private space and you can keep distractions to a minimum.

The massage therapist's home

Many massage therapists have a space set up in their own homes for giving massage. This can range from a dinky little corner in one end of the living room to an entire suite of offices with a separate entrance. You may like the "personalized" feeling of visiting a massage therapist in her home, where you can take advantage of the relaxing environment she has (hopefully) set up. On the other hand, if you're the type of person who prefers a more clearly defined edge between the personal and professional aspects of your transactions, the massage therapist's home may not be the best choice of location for you.

Also, you have to take into account certain practical details as well, such as whether or not the massage therapist has pets. If you're allergic to cats, and the massage therapist's house is a veritable kitty kennel, you may break out in a rash and not enjoy the massage at all.

A good massage therapist should put the rest of her life on hold while you're in her home, but some have a tendency to attend to their own business while you're there, answering the phone and the doorbell, for instance, which can greatly detract from your experience. You may need to make an extra effort to enforce rule # 9 from Chapter 7. You're the boss, even if you're in her home, and for this hour you're in charge.

Spas

Some of the most beautiful massage environments in the world can be found in spas, and you find out more about them in Chapter 15. Grand *destination spas* dot the map in every state now, and if you look in your Yellow Pages, you're likely to find a *day spa* that you can check out right in your own town.

While spas are often pleasant and luxurious, there are a couple things you should keep in mind when signing up for a massage in one:

- Massage therapists in spas only keep a (usually small) percentage of the profits, which sometimes leads them to give less than their absolute best work.

- Massage Therapists in spas are "on the clock," and you're likely to get a massage that is exactly 50 minutes long, so she has time to prepare the room for the next client. It's a rare massage therapist who can still give you a feeling of timeless bliss within that shortened hour.

- Often, the style of massage given in spas is dictated by a lowest-common-denominator mentality, and massage therapists are not allowed to use their advanced techniques for fear of alienating a clientele who wants "just a rubdown."

These warnings notwithstanding, there's no reason to believe you won't receive an incredible massage in a spa. Some of the best massage therapists work in them. Also, if you end up finding a massage therapist you really like, you can ask her whether she also takes private clients outside the spa, which may mean a better deal for her and a better massage for you. Be diplomatic when doing this though, as many spas have a policy against their massage therapists "stealing" customers in this way.

Cruise ships

Cruise ships are fun places to get massages, if you don't mind rocking back and forth a little bit while you're on the table. Almost every ship has its own spa, and you can visit for a half-hour or an hour of massage as easily as visiting the midnight buffet. A massage during your cruise may add to the exotic flavor of your trip, but there are a couple less-than-exotic points to keep in mind as well:

✔ Because floor space and portholes are at a premium on ships, massage rooms onboard are usually teeny tiny little quarters with no natural light. If you're used to ample luxurious massage spaces, you may feel a little claustrophobic in this environment.

✔ Even more so than in spas on land, shipboard massage therapists are part of a massage assembly line, and sometimes the massages are limited to half an hour. It's rough to coax the best from your massage therapist because she sees so many people come and go — none of whom are repeat customers.

✔ Make sure to sign up early — as soon as you come on board — if you're thinking about getting a massage during your cruise because the best time slots fill up fast. You may want an appointment during a "sea day," rather than in port, so you don't have to decide between getting a massage and going ashore to sightsee or shop.

Hotels

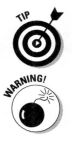

Many hotels have their own spas, so all you have to do to book a massage is call the spa desk. For those hotels without a spa, you'll want to contact the concierge to arrange your appointment.

One note about concierges: Watch out! They often take a good chunk of the massage therapist's fee for themselves, and they have a stable of ever-ready massage therapists at hand who allow them to do that. So, the quality is not always the best. You may be better off placing a call directly to a professional that you find listed under licensed practitioners in the local Yellow Pages or newspaper. That way you can avoid the fee and perhaps find higher-quality work as well.

All in all, hotel rooms are on the low end of the totem pole as far as receiving massages go. They're impersonal, they're cramped, and they often have that funny hotel-room-smell that no amount of incense or positive thinking can overcome. If you find yourself in a hotel room somewhere with nowhere else to go for your massage, and only a concierge to put your trust in, do what seasoned massage recipients the world over have done for years: enjoy it anyway. (See Chapter 17 for more info about hotel massages.)

Health clubs

Health clubs are becoming better places to receive massages. In the past, you were likely to wind up in a tiny cinder-block cubicle vibrating with the sounds of music from the aerobics room next door. These days health-club owners are more aware that their customers want a little nook of tranquility, and a well-trained massage therapist, available for massage. Depending upon the place, some of these clubs offer massage therapists a good percentage of the profits, and even a chance to run their own concession, so you may very well find some motivated individuals. The massage is often high-quality, especially if you're interested in sports-related therapy. And in a health club you can receive your massage immediately after a strenuous workout and a limb-loosening sauna.

Clinics

Many massage therapists open up their own clinics. The setup is similar to any other professional office, like a chiropractor's, a doctor's, or a dentist's. You walk in the front door into a waiting area with a potted plant, some magazines, chairs, and a reception desk. Behind the desk is a hallway with a few doors opening into rooms. The rooms behind those doors, however, can differ decidedly from other clinics. Depending upon the personality and style of the massage therapist, a massage treatment room can range from white-tiled sterility with anatomical charts on the walls to a softly glowing, plush chamber of warmth filled with the strains of celestial music.

One specialty in this area is known as the *sports massage clinic*. The massage therapists in these facilities concentrate on rehabilitating you after an injury. They often work with orthopedic physicians and physical therapists. A trip to this type of no-nonsense massage clinic may feel more like a hospital visit than a spa visit.

Student massage clinics

Because of the wide disparity between massage therapists and the environments they create in which to work, it's a good idea to go check out each environment personally, or at least get a detailed description of it from a friend, *before* you sign up for your first massage there. That way you can avoid the nasty surprises that can surface, such as when you make an appointment at your local day spa for a relaxing hour of escape only to find the massage room is directly adjacent to a bank of two dozen noisy hair-drying machines.

Part III
The Art of Giving Massage

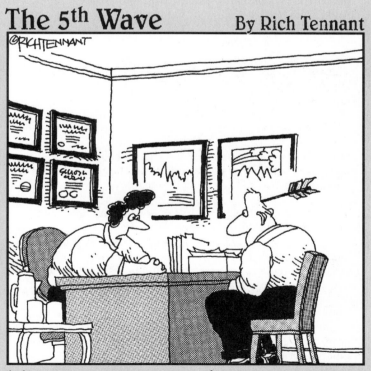

The 5th Wave   By Rich Tennant

"I really don't think a simple neck massage is going to get rid of your headaches."

In this part . . .

You're no doubt familiar with the famous expression, "It's better to give than to receive." And if you're like most people, every time you've heard someone utter that wonderful phrase, filled as it is with such a beautiful philanthropic message, you've thought to yourself, "Yeah, right. I'll take receiving any day."

But you have to admit, there's a certain gratification that comes from giving which quite often actually makes it feel better than receiving — more meaningful, more fulfilling. And the secret to achieving that kind of fulfillment is that you have to give with your whole heart. It won't work if you're just going through the motions.

This is especially true for massage. Sure, you can rub some warmed almond oil on your partner's back for 20 minutes while watching the clock out with one eye and the football game on TV with the other, but that's not what massage is all about.

Massage is about cultivating the right attitude — the *giver's* attitude — not just applying mechanical maneuvers, which any massage text can teach you.

But don't worry: In this part of the book, you're going to discover how to actually give a massage, too! And as you'll see, it's not that difficult. Just follow the simple instructions, and in no time, you'll be reproducing the very same techniques you see being performed by the highly trained models in the photographs. No problem.

That's right. *You* can become one of those people about whom everyone else exclaims, "What great hands you've got!" Just remember to focus on your "giver's attitude" as much as your manual skills, and you'll do just fine.

Chapter 9

Massage Moods: Getting the Setting Right

- -

In This Chapter

▶ Making sure that everything looks, sounds, smells, and feels right

▶ Trading places

- -

Say your husband or wife or roommate sees you reading this book for hours on end and eventually says something to you like, "Hey, how about giving ME a massage? Right now!"

Your immediate response should be:

    A. Sure, lie down on the linoleum here and we'll get started.

    B. No way, I'm too nervous about ever actually doing this stuff.

    C. I haven't finished the book yet.

    D. Okay, but give me a few minutes to set the right mood.

Yes, oh intelligent massage student, you've once again chosen correctly. The answer is D. It's definitely true that your partner appreciates it if you take a little time to set up a special environment or "massage mood" before you begin the actual massage. And, even if you're in a less-than-ideal environment, don't worry. You can materialize a magical massage mood just about anywhere if you use some of the ideas in this chapter to create your own "inner chamber."

Creating the Inner Chamber

One of the big secrets to giving a good massage has very little to do with the massage itself. It has to do, rather, with where the massage is happening. And I'm not talking about exotic locales like Bali or Atlantic City. I'm referring to more accessible locations, like your bedroom or the couch in your den.

So how do you turn these everyday places into someplace special? It's easy; the trick is to involve all the senses.

Massage, of course, relies heavily upon the senses for its effects. Your sense of touch, especially, is being bombarded the entire time you're giving or receiving a massage. But it would be a mistake to neglect the other senses; they can add greatly to your massage experience, too.

The sense of taste doesn't usually play a big part in massage, unless of course you like to use edible massage oils like strawberry, almond, and mint that are . . . whoops, I think we're straying a little beyond the scope of this chapter. Check out Chapter 19 for more information on sensual massage, including the use of all kinds of flavored oils.

Anyway, for now let's concentrate on the three remaining senses that come into play during a massage experience, also known as the 3 S's of your inner chamber:

- ✔ Scents
- ✔ Sights
- ✔ Sounds

Scents

Professional massage therapists often coach their clients through some deep-breathing techniques as part of the massage. And, as you may suspect, all that breathing includes quite a bit of smelling, too. That's part of the reason why massage pros have so much concern about the way that their work-rooms smell. In addition, they also know how powerful the sense of smell can be for healing and relaxation.

Just sniffing a whiff of corn muffins like the ones your Aunt Betty used to bake when you visited her on weekends as a kid is enough to send you reel-ing back through the years, right? Why is that so? Aromas trigger a mighty emotional response because the molecules that enter your nose don't mess around. They do not pass GO; they do not collect $200. Instead, they take a direct route straight into the midbrain area, which is the seat of your emo-tions and memories. This fact is a key to the power of *aromatherapy.*

Aromatherapy

If you use advanced grammatical techniques to break down the word aro-matherapy, you discover that it means "therapy with aromas." Aha! So, does that mean therapy with just any aroma, such as the aroma of sautéed onions, for example, or the aroma of diesel fuel at dawn?

Hardly. Aromatherapy is the use of highly concentrated *essential oils* from certain plants to stimulate the brain. This stimulation causes a positive effect on the nervous and glandular systems and thus the entire body. During a massage, you can utilize aromatherapy in several ways. In Chapter 11, you find out how to mix up an aromatherapy massage oil, but for now let's focus on three other aromatherapy tips that can help you scent your massage space.

- **Diffusers:** As the name suggests, a diffuser diffuses aroma into the air. Several inexpensive models ($10–$15) are available that use a miniature fan. Simply place a few drops of your favorite oil on a cotton pad, turn on the fan, and the scent of essential oils fills the room.

- **Candles:** Many commercially available candles have essential oils worked right into the wax, and burning one during a massage is a great way to combine effects in two of the three S's, sight and scent. Until recently, you had to visit a specialty shop to purchase aromatherapy candles, but now they're even available at your local grocery store. S.C. Johnson, for example, makers of Glade air fresheners, is now in the aromatherapy market with candles and sprays.

- **Bulb rings:** These little doo-dads were popular in the 1970s when they were used to cover up even more exotic aromas floating around the room at parties. Now they're making a comeback as aromatherapy aids. Basically, they're floppy little rings that you place over a light bulb. When you sprinkle several drops of essential oil into the ring and turn on the bulb, Presto! — instant aromatherapy.

If aromatherapy is something you're keenly interested in, I would recommend *Aromatherapy For Dummies* by Kathi Keville, published by IDG Books Worldwide, a book that promises to answer that age-old question, "How can I smell better and feel better at the same time?"

Incense

The musky, natural scents that burning incense creates can turn your inner chamber into a mystical and exotic environment, even if in reality it's just your guest bedroom. The problem is, many people overdo it with incense, fumigating the room with enough mystical and exotic smoke to choke themselves, their partner, and any unsuspecting insects living in the walls. This is not good.

When it comes to incense, a little goes a long way. Use it with moderation, and you can create just the right mood. If you're using one of those long thick sticks of incense, snap it off ⅔ of the way down and burn just the last bit. Also, you can crack a window open, weather permitting, to circulate a little fresh air with the smoke.

An altar to the massage gods

Some people go so far as to create a special altar in the area where they give their massages. This is going a bit out into Shirley MacLaine land, I realize, but when you think about it, it makes sense. A massage can be a kind of shared spiritual experience (See Rule # 7 in Chapter 7), and an altar is a way to commemorate that.

So what should be on a massage altar, you ask? You can place the objects mentioned elsewhere in this chapter, such as water fountains, candles, incense burners, and flowers on your altar.

Then you can go a step further and add a photograph or two as well. Pick a subject that reminds you of spiritual things, such as a photo of the Dalai Lama, Saint Francis, or whales cavorting in the waves.

If you spend time meditating or simply sitting quietly at your altar, you can embue the space with a quiet energy. People who join you there may notice the difference. I don't know if this is due to an actual exchange of peaceful molecules, an increase in negative ions, or what, but it can definitely be felt.

There are thousands of brands and "flavors" of incense. My favorite is the Nag Champa scent, which, although I've never been there, reminds me of a sacred meditation cave in the Himalayas.

Flowers

Nothing beats the scent of fresh flowers in your massage area. You don't need a big vase and a big budget to make it happen either. All that's necessary is a small bowl, a cup, or a mug from the kitchen cabinet that you fill with water, and a single flower. Roses or gardenias work especially well. Snip the flower off the stem and float it on the water. This fills the air with scent for hours or even days.

If you want to get really romantic, spread some fresh petals on the bed or other massage surface to set the mood. Cleopatra had her love chamber filled a foot deep with rose petals before Anthony made his big entrance.

Sights

It may sound funny to focus on the sights of a massage space because, after all, the person receiving the massage will probably have her eyes closed most of the time anyway. But during those few minutes when she first enters, and whenever she opens her eyes, she'll soak in her surroundings. There are a few simple things that you can use to add to the relaxing ambience:

  ✔ **Candles:** Candles cast an enchanting glow over any massage experience, and they can add to the scent as well, as I mention earlier.

- **Flowers:** Even a small bunch of silk flowers placed with care near the massage area shows this is someplace special.

- **Lighting:** You can do some simple things with lighting to make your space massage-friendly.

    - Turn the lights down low. This helps the person on the receiving end concentrate more on the massage, perhaps because she won't feel like you are scrutinizing her body under a microscope.

    - Throw a silk scarf over a lampshade to create instant mood lighting during a massage.

- **Color:** Drape the area with soft colorful fabrics.

Sounds

Carefully selected sounds serve two main purposes during a massage:

- They add to the mood.
- They mask other, distracting, sounds like traffic noises and TVs.

There are a number of really interesting ways to make sound a part of your massage, and you may find that some massage pros carry an entire arsenal of sound makers to add to their clients' experience. Some of my favorites include:

- **Tibetan meditation bowls:** These look like simple brass bowls, but when you glide a wooden instrument along the rim, they sing out beautifully with rich vibrant tones.

- *Ting shaks:* Another Tibetan invention, you strike these heavy brass bells together to form a clear, long-lasting tone that sets a meditative mood for a massage.

- **Gongs:** Yes, miniature versions, complete with a little gong hammer, are available.

- **Wind chimes:** A classic in the relaxing-sounds category, there are literally thousands of types available. If you can't be near an open window to hear the chimes, place them indoors near an oscillating fan to simulate blowing breezes.

And, if all else fails . . . earplugs work wonders. You can get them at your local drugstore.

Water

You know those cute little burbling pots filled with rocks and miniature waterfalls? You can find them in a lot of gift shops these days, and while they are a tad overpriced, they definitely add a lot to the ambience of a massage. If you're the industrious type, you can overcome the price problem by building a little indoor fountain for yourself. All it takes is a container, some rocks, and a small submersible water pump.

Of course, being outside near a source of natural flowing water is a great choice, too, but then you have to consider other details, such as temperature, rain, insects, and privacy.

One thing to remember — the sound of running water seems to have a powerful effect on the bladder. Make extra sure your partner visits the bathroom before receiving a massage with a waterfall nearby.

Music

Music, of course, is the most popular type of sound used to complement massage. In most big spas, for example, they pump music directly into the massage rooms from a central sound system, putting the guests in the right mood to relax and unwind.

One massage manufacturing company built stereo speakers right into the bed of a massage table so that when you lie down on it, the music literally vibrates you. While this may be going a bit far, music is still the best and easiest way for you to include the element of sound in your massage.

An entire industry has sprung up to provide music appropriate for massage. If you want to experience some of the most popular massage music, try putting one of the following tapes or CDs on the next time you exchange a massage:

- George Winston's *December*
- Pachabel's *Cannon*
- Deuter Ecstasy
- Anything by Stephen Halpern
- Brian Eno, *Music for Airports*
- Ray Lynch, *Music to Disappear Into*
- Enya, especially her *Orinoco Flow* CD
- The Cowboy Junkies, *Trinity Session* (a personal, offbeat favorite)
- Yanni, especially his *In My Time*
- Any relaxing classical music

Don't get the wrong idea here, though. Massage music doesn't necessarily have to be flutes or harps or Yanni 'til you yawn. You can be creative in your choices, and sometimes the best massages are given to the most unlikely accompaniment. See the sidebar "Reggae massage."

Reggae massage

One day when I was in charge of the massage crew at a large spa in Florida, I suddenly was completely fed up with the droning of flutes, harps, and syrupy synthesizer music that poured endlessly out of the stereo speakers in each of the 24 massage rooms. Heading to the sound control room, I secretly exchanged the well-worn New Age CDs for some reggae discs with distinctively upbeat sounds.

It was the middle of a lazy, rainy afternoon. The massage rooms were filled with customers who were all paying upwards of $5,000 per week to be there, and I wasn't sure exactly what the reaction would be. Would the customers complain? Would I be fired?

After just two hours, the verdict came in, and someone passed me the message . . . "Steve, the spa director wants to see you in her office."

Gulp.

When I arrived, the director had an expression of profound curiosity on her face. "Do you know what was going on with the music in the massage rooms this afternoon?" she asked.

"I . . . um, well . . ."

"Because whatever it was, the customers loved it. Two of them even wanted to know where they could purchase a copy for themselves! Nobody has ever asked that before."

I was glad to be off the hook, and I was happy to know that most people seemed to agree with me on the subject of massage music. It doesn't always have to be so . . . well, tranquilizing.

As a final note about music, remember that the person receiving the massage is always right. This includes being right about the choice of music, even if that choice makes absolutely no sense to you. I had one client who always insisted on receiving his massages to the accompaniment of the local rock & roll radio station. Go figure.

Location location location

Once, in a typically cramped New York City apartment, I had to give a massage on the only available large flat surface, which turned out to be a wooden dining room table. We lay a few blankets and pillows down on it, and I scurried from side to side dodging walls and other furniture, but in the end my client reported feeling quite comfortable, and he loved his massage. I wouldn't recommend this, but it just goes to show that you definitely don't need a fancy expensive massage table or a special peaceful room in your house in order to give a good massage.

You can comfortably give massages in any room, including living rooms, bedrooms, family rooms, and as the story above points out, even the dining room. There are a few issues you want to keep in mind, though, when deciding where to give a massage:

- **Privacy:** It's important to respect the level of privacy the person receiving the massage desires. If possible, choose a room where you can close the doors to keep other people out. On the other hand, some people actually prefer to be less private, and they are more comfortable in an area with some activity.

- **Warmth:** Avoid areas with a draft or air conditioning vent directly overhead.

- **Intentions:** It may be a good idea to avoid giving massage in a bedroom if the person receiving is not your romantic partner. That way you avoid possibly giving the wrong message.

- **Space:** You need some space to maneuver around in — perhaps more than you realize. Before you begin, make sure you have enough room on all sides to move without disturbing your partner.

Privacy, please

When someone's receiving a massage, she wants to pretend that she's on a secluded tropical isle, with no one else around for miles. She's a Polynesian princess, the center of attention, and the person giving the massage is focused on her and her alone. Exotic birds are floating overhead, and one lone white sail puffs out on the aquamarine horizon . . . then, suddenly, she hears a voice: "Bart just threw up on my homework!"

Yes, it's difficult for your partner to achieve her ultimate romantic illusion if, in real life, she's receiving her massage on the couch in your den, with *The Simpsons* turned up full blast on the TV.

Do your partner a favor — indulge her in her illusions. While it's not always possible to take a trip to Fiji to give your massage, you can avoid some of the more obvious distractions quite easily:

- Turn off the TV.
- Put up a little "Do Not Disturb" sign.
- Try to schedule the massage for a time when there are few interruptions.
- Turn off the ringer on the phone and turn down the volume on the answering machine.

The "massage mood"

What I've included in this chapter so far are the external aspects of the inner chamber. But, of course, when it comes to inner chambers, it's the inside that counts, and that's what this section is about. Even if you find yourself in a less-than-ideal situation to give massage, with distractions abounding, no music to listen to, and not a candle in sight, you can still create the most important aspect of that inner chamber, the "massage mood."

When you first lay your hands upon someone else to give them a massage, what do you have in your mind? Chances are, you're a little nervous, a little uncertain of how the other person is going to receive you. And that's all right. It means you care. But how about how *she's* feeling? You, as the giver, are in charge of creating the optimal mood for her experience.

In order to create an appropriate mood for the other person, what you have to do first is get into that mood yourself. By imagining yourself in one of the following four personas as you begin a massage — saint, doctor, mother, buddy — you can quickly adopt the mood that goes with it. Then, you can give your partner something that comes from deep inside, creating the true inner chamber.

Saint

Part of giving a good massage is having some simple compassion for the person you're touching. We are, after all, in the same boat, each one of us anchored to a fragile body in an uncertain world. You can reach out to others when you massage them, crossing the barriers of separation, sending the message that you understand how they feel. This is the golden rule of most religions; touch others as you would have them touch you.

Doctor

If you're just a beginner, you shouldn't be out there trying to "fix" your Aunt Jeanne's sciatica with your massage techniques. However, it helps to think in terms of helping the person feel better, not just rubbing oil on. As you begin a massage, imagine your hands filled with healing energy, communicating the intention to soothe and make whole.

Mother

Who ever cared about us more than good ole Mom? She had a level of acceptance for our quirks and our shortcomings that was just plain astounding. You can aim that same kind of unconditional love toward your massage partner (at least for that one hour), making him feel perfect just the way he is.

Touching José

(While volunteering at the University of Miami Medical Center AIDS ward, I discovered that you can create a caring compassionate "massage mood" anywhere, even in a sterile hospital room. This is the story of José, whom I met there.)

On the bright Christmas Eve morning that we entered his room, Jose's body was wracked with pain, and he was curled into a fetal position on his hospital bed. His family stood at the foot of the bed arranged like a choir — mother, father, aunts, uncles, siblings, and friends. All of them with their hands at their sides, standing several feet away.

Jackson Memorial Hospital did not employ Rob Boyte, a nurse, and me, a massage therapist. We were volunteers with the P.A.L.M.S. foundation, and we were there to touch José.

You see, nobody else would touch José because these were the early days of AIDS and everyone was still afraid, even the doctors and the other nurses. Even the family members of the victims were afraid. Everyone kept his distance.

José had received a spinal tap the night before. Convulsions ran through his body, up to his head and back down. He could only speak in broken, grunted syllables. His family translated for us.

"He says he wants the massage," said one relative.

"He thinks it would feel good," said another. "Go ahead, try."

We approached the bed. Both of us stood on the same side, facing José's exposed back. Rob gently placed one large hand on the back of José's neck, not moving it at all. I touched him, too. José didn't relax into the touch; he couldn't because of the convulsions. He moaned, but not with pleasure either like many massage clients do. Instead, he moaned with something deeper, almost like pain itself, and I knew immediately what it was. All of the family members knew what it was, too.

José was letting out the primal moan of someone who had not been touched for a long time, at the point in his life when he most desperately needed to be touched.

Subtly, José pressed his back up into my hands. I watched the family members lean forward, lifting their hands slightly, as if they too were touching José, although they were too terrified to do so themselves.

Slowly, I stroked down José's back, then back up again. His skin was cold, then hot in turns. The family members stared hard at our hands. We were not wearing rubber gloves because we knew AIDS was not transmitted by skin-to-skin contact. Everyone should have known it, but they didn't.

Slowly, José responded. His convulsions subsided. He became quiet. For a few minutes, everyone there could see that he was all wrapped up in the sensation of two other humans, four other hands, touching him, soothing him, being with him in the way that only CONTACT can provide.

Then it was time to go. The ward was filled with other patients on that Christmas Eve day. Rob and I moved to the sink where we washed our hands with red disinfectant soap. We smiled at the family, and they smiled back at the two strangers who had just shared such an intimate moment.

We left the room and moved on. Then, a few minutes later, we heard a gasp, a cry, then a high female wail come echoing down the white tiled hospital corridor. The family came flowing out of José's room one by one, their eyes wild with pain, filled with tears. One of the women looked straight into my soul then in that hallway for one brief second. What I saw in her eyes, behind the pain, was gratitude. For a brief time,

I had become her hands and allowed her to do something she would never be able to do herself. Because now, it was too late.

Nobody could touch José anymore.

Buddy

Don't let all this serious stuff about saints and doctors scare you away from giving a massage. There's another, more lighthearted, giver's personality, too, that of the buddy. You can just hang out together and have some fun while you're exchanging massage, and that's perfectly acceptable. Go ahead, put a little reggae on the CD player. Tell a few jokes to break the ice. Relax and have an easy conversation during the massage. Sometimes this is the best choice when your partner is apprehensive about receiving the massage.

The story in the sidebar "Touching Jose" is an example of how, when it comes time to actually touch a human being, the buddy blends with the saint, and the mother and doctor become two sides of the same coin.

Trading Places

It's not that difficult to find a professional massage therapist with whom you can trade money for massage. Money seems to be a great motivational tool when it comes to getting people to massage you. It can be very tricky, however, to find an amateur. By definition, you are not going to pay the amateur, and therefore you must offer some other form of incentive to get him to give the massage. Most frequently, this incentive comes in the form of a reciprocal massage. But what if that is not enough to motivate your partner?

I'm trying not to be sexist here, but statistical evidence suggests that one gender in particular has motivational problems when it comes to *giving* massage. Yes, I'm talking about males, 95% of whom, when asked by their loving partners to give a massage, develop an instantaneous and very debilitating case of temporary-fatigue-syndrome (TFS). Even the thought of moving just a pinkie finger suddenly makes them feel very tiried. As soon as the request for massage is withdrawn, however, they bounce back incredibly fast and can often be observed playing touch football just moments later.

Here are some ways to motivate a partner who is the unfortunate victim of TFS:

- Suggest to him that his love life might suffer dire consequences unless he gives you a massage.

- Suggest to him that his love life could be greatly enhanced were he to be so kind as to give you a full hour massage.

- In exchange for the massage, offer to let him go shopping at his favorite store (camping store, hardware store, computer store, or whatever his cute little male fixation may be) and don't bug him about spending money there.

- If he agrees to massage you at least three times, let him pick the destination for your next vacation (yes, even if it's bass fishing on Lake Okeechobee).

Your mate is not the only person with whom you can form a massage-trade relationship. Other potential partners include:

- Somebody who practices massage professionally (it may surprise you how many pros don't receive massage nearly as often as they'd like — your offer to trade, although you're less experienced, is likely to be met with considerable enthusiasm).

- Members of your church

- Members of your family

- Friends of the family

- Members of a sports team you're on

It may be challenging at first to find a way to be comfortable trading massages. It's an admittedly intimate form of sharing, and not everyone takes to it right away. One good alternative to jumping straight into a full body massage is to try some seated massage with the clothes still on. You may find plenty of non-threatening options in the chapters to come.

Chapter 10

All The Right Moves

*Y*es, this is the chapter where you'll find all those massage moves that you can use to turn your everyday, ordinary hands into instruments of irresistible pleasure. Your fingertips and palms will be sought after by friends, family, co-workers, and complete strangers alike. Everybody will say, "Use some of those moves on me! Me me me me me!"

Then, inflated by your newfound abilities and the quick expertise you acquire in these pages, you may find yourself thinking, like many of us did in the beginning, that these neat new massage moves you've learned actually are the massage itself. But you'd be wrong! Oh yes, very wrong.

Massage moves are not the massage; they're just the medium.

Let me give you an analogy to help explain this:

Learning massage is like learning to play a musical instrument. The moves in this chapter are the notes on the scale, plus some basic chords and combinations. They're great ways to warm up your fingers and make some rudimentary noises, but if you continue to play them over and over again, you're going to drive the people close to you crazy.

In massage, you have to go beyond the moves pretty quickly. You need to develop a "moveless movement," or "flow," in which you're concentrating not on your own technique, but on your partner's feelings, her sensations, and her reactions, just like a musician who forgets all about notes and scales, sharps and flats, and even the instrument itself. Your movements are the technique, the body you massage is the instrument, and it's the interaction between the two that makes the music.

Massage is the music, the communication, the thing that you create, NOT the movements required to produce the sensations.

Whoa! Getting a little deep here, aren't we? Sorry about that. Don't worry — the rest of this chapter's going to be very practical and concrete. After all, you still have to learn your scales before you can play Carnegie Hall.

Don't Do It, Mon!

Just like the Jamaican bobsled team, you may be all fired up to go out and practice your new moves. Before you jump off the cliff and begin massaging away recklessly on anybody who lets you near them, however, stop for a moment to consider some sage words of advice about:

- Conditions that you should NOT treat
- Places you should AVOID touching
- Moves you should NOT make

Contraindications

As innocuous as massage may seem, there are still times when you should refrain from giving one because it may adversely affect a health condition of the person who receives it. *Contraindications* is the medical term for these conditions, a word which, when you look at it closely, obviously means "Nicaraguan rebel indications." No, really, "contra" means against, as in contrary, and indications are things that tell you what to do one way or the other. So contraindications are things that are telling you not to do something.

The list of contraindications for massage may be longer than you expect, and it includes some conditions that at first glance don't seem like massage would affect at all. Take a look:

- **Fever:** When you have a fever, your body is trying to isolate and expel an invader of some kind. Massage increases overall circulation and could therefore work against your body's natural defenses.

- **Inflammation:** Massage can further irritate an area of inflammation, so you should not administer it. Inflamed conditions include anything that ends in *-itis*, such as phlebitis (inflammation of a vein), dermatitis (inflammation of the skin), arthritis (inflammation of the joints), and so on. In the case of localized problems, you can still massage around them, however, avoiding the inflammation itself.

✔ **High blood pressure:** High blood pressure means excessive pressure against blood vessel walls. Massage affects the blood vessels, and so people with high blood pressure or a heart condition should receive light, sedating massages, if at all.

✔ **Infectious diseases:** Massage is not a good idea for someone coming down with the flu or diphtheria, for example, and to make matters worse, you expose yourself to the virus as well.

✔ **Hernia:** Hernias are protrusions of part of an organ (such as the intestines) through a muscular wall. It's not a good idea to try and push these organs back inside. Surgery works better.

✔ **Osteoporosis:** Elderly people with a severe stoop to the shoulders often have this condition, in which bones become porous, brittle, and fragile. Massage may be too intense for this condition.

✔ **Varicose veins:** Massage directly over varicose veins can worsen the problem. However, if you apply a very light massage next to the problem, always in a direction toward the heart, it can be very beneficial.

✔ **Broken bones:** Stay away from an area of mending bones. A little light massage to the surrounding areas, though, can improve circulation and be quite helpful.

✔ **Skin problems:** You should avoid anything that looks like it shouldn't be there, such as rashes, wounds, bruises, burns, boils, and blisters, for example. Usually these problems are local, so you can still massage in other areas.

✔ **Cancer:** Cancer can spread through the lymphatic system, and because massage increases lymphatic circulation, it may potentially spread the disease as well. Simple, caring touch is fine, but massage strokes that stimulate circulation are not. Always check with a doctor first.

✔ **Other conditions and diseases:** Diabetes, asthma, and other serious conditions each have their own precautions, and you should get a doctor's OK before administering massage.

✔ **HIV infection:** Some people still think of AIDS as something that can be "caught" through simple skin-to-skin contact, but most of us know that's not the case. If there is no exchange of bodily fluids (blood, semen, vaginal fluids, or mother's milk), HIV can't be transmitted during massage. So, HIV infection is not contraindicated for this reason. However, some of the infections that people suffering from the later stages of AIDS experience are contraindicated, and you should avoid those infections. Loving, soothing contact is extremely important for people at any stage of infection, but in the case of any visible rashes, sores, lesions, or swelling, massage is best left to a professional. If you have any cuts or scrapes or scratches on your hands, it's an especially good idea to wear thin surgical gloves while massaging an HIV-infected person with any signs of open lesions.

✔ **Pregnancy:** Most women love to receive massage during pregnancy, and it's perfectly fine to give them one, but there are a few precautions to observe. See the sidebar about pregnancy later in this chapter.

Just a minute here! All this makes it sound like you practically have to get a medical checkup and an OK from the doctor before giving someone a massage, doesn't it? Well, in many cases, that's exactly what it means. Always err on the side of caution when you're considering giving a massage to a person with any health concerns. Check it out with his or her physician first.

The first and foremost rule here is, "Do no harm." If you're not sure about a particular condition, don't give the massage.

Bad moves

Ever watch an infant pet a cat? They often have the best of intentions, but they just can't seem to get it right. Wham! Wham! goes the beefy little hand on top of the cat's head, and the poor feline scurries away before the infant does any serious damage. Similarly, there are moves that you should not make during a massage, no matter how good your intentions are. They all cause discomfort, and some of them may even cause harm.

Pregnancy — a contraindication?

There are some people who believe that pregnant women should not receive massage. Most of these people, needless to say, are not pregnant women, whose backs and legs are often quite sore, and who love massage. There's a section in Chapter 18 on this topic, but for now I want to put your mind at ease and say that it's perfectly okay to massage a pregnant woman, as long as you observe a few simple precautions:

✔ Always make sure her legs and head are supported with pillows.

✔ Never put her in a face-down position to massage her. In her last trimester, she should lie only on her side.

✔ Only light gliding strokes should be used directly on the abdomen. Don't press directly onto or knead in this area.

✔ Always give soothing, relaxing massage moves, never heavy or deep.

✔ Avoid the ankles and heels because, according to the theory of reflexology, the heels contain special points that may stimulate labor. Going into labor during a massage is not recommended. Chapter 14 has more info and a diagram showing the location of these reflexology points.

- **Neck pulling:** Do not grasp the head firmly and pull upward, attempting to lengthen the neck (some people say this is what happened to Audrey Hepburn).

- **Neck twisting:** Only a very gentle and slow turning of the neck to one side or the other is appropriate during massage. No sudden movements!

- **Neck pulling and twisting together:** Never ever, for any reason, pull and twist the neck at the same time. This can be very dangerous.

- **Bone cracking:** Never ever try to do a chiropractic-type adjustment if you haven't been trained as a . . . duh . . . chiropractor.

- **Bone pushing:** Don't press directly on bones, especially the spine. Instead, glide lightly over these areas.

- **Hyperextension:** Basic stretches are okay, and I explain several in Chapters 11 and 16. However, don't try to *hyperextend* any joint past its normal *range-of-motion* unless you receive some serious schooling in massage. This is hard to do with the knee or elbow, which resist such maneuvers, but you can easily hyperextend the neck, for example, so you need to use caution.

Danger zones

"Endangerment sites" are super-sensitive areas on the body. These areas contain important pieces of your anatomy, like nerves and blood supply, for example, in exposed and vulnerable positions. Highly trained massage therapists can sometimes work in these areas, but if you're not a professional massage ace yourself, it's better to stay away from the following spots:

- **Front of the neck/throat:** You've heard of the expression, "Go for the jugular," right? Well, this is where you find it. Unless you're trying to choke someone, it's a good idea to stay away from this area that also contains the carotid artery and major nerves.

- **Side of the neck:** Not quite as sensitive as the front of the neck, you should still treat it delicately.

- **The *"ear notch":*** Just behind your jawbone and beneath your ear you find a little notch. It's not a good idea to jam a finger into this notch, unless you're trying to extort money or favors from the person receiving the massage, because it contains a sensitive facial nerve.

- **The eyeball:** Unless you're trying to do a Three Stooges massage (popular amongst college males), don't poke your fingers directly into the person's eyes.

- **The axilla:** This is a fancy term for the armpit which, as you know, is a sensitive area, filled with nerves, arteries, and lymph glands. Not to mention, most people are very ticklish there.

- ✔ **The upper inner arm:** Just down from the armpit, along the inside of the upper arm, is a sensitive, nerve-filled area along the length of the arm bone. Pressing here too firmly gives you that yucky-nervy feeling.

- ✔ **The ulnar notch of the elbow:** Otherwise known as the "funny bone," this spot contains the ulnar nerve which, if you touch it too hard, causes normally discreet people to curse in several languages.

- ✔ **The abdomen:** Houdini was killed by an unsuspected punch to this area, which is filled with many squishy important bits known as organs. Be especially gentle around the upper abdomen along the ribs, where you find the liver, gall bladder, and spleen.

- ✔ **The lower back:** Just to both sides of the spine, and below the ribs, is where you find the kidneys. Don't press too hard here or pound on them. Kidneys don't like it when you do that.

- ✔ **The femoral triangle:** Not to be confused with the Bermuda triangle, this area is often referred to as the "groin." It's the inner part of the line in front where your leg meets your body. If you press too hard here, you can actually cut off circulation to the leg.

- ✔ **Popliteal area:** Popularly known as the back of the knee, you should always treat this spot gingerly. It's very sensitive to pressure.

Please don't do that

The ultimate contraindication is a request from the person receiving the massage that you stop doing what you're doing. Immediately. Quit it. No more!

When a person says, "Please don't do that," then don't do that. This is especially true for well-meaning beginners, who have a tendency to press ever forward with their newfound massage skills, in spite of the complaints issuing forth from the poor soul beneath their fingers.

The following is NOT proper etiquette:

Massage partner: "It really hurts!"

You: "Oh no, it doesn't. That's just your tension melting away. Visualize your muscles as butter . . . ."

In massage, more than any other business, the customer is always right. But there are times when the person receiving the massage either doesn't know or won't tell you he's uncomfortable. How do you know what to do then? That's where body language clues come in.

Body language clues

Some people think that when they're getting a massage they have to "grin and bear it" when something hurts. They figure massage is like a form of torture, and they're prisoners of war. They certainly aren't going to display any signs of weakness or let you know you're hurting them. Other people may not even know they're uncomfortable, because their discomfort is unconscious, and so they can't communicate it to you.

In these cases, wise massage givers have figured out certain non-verbal clues that they can use to determine when their massage is too strong. These include:

✔ Curling of the toes

✔ Arching the back

✔ Inability to speak in a normal tone

✔ Facial grimaces and contortions

✔ Excess sweating, especially in a cool room

So, what should you do when your partner starts showing signs of discomfort? The answer is simple — talk about it. Simple, straightforward communication clears up most situations immediately. Some people just won't be able to believe that you honestly want them to tell you how they feel. Go ahead, surprise them.

The one word never to say when you're giving a massage

You can get away with almost any kind of amateur commentary while giving a massage to friends and family because, after all, they understand that you're an amateur. Thus, when you say, "Geez, am I pressing too hard there?" they're likely to respond with some positive criticism. However, there is one particular word that neither amateurs nor professionals should ever utter while in the middle of giving a massage. Hearing it strikes fear into the poor vulnerable person lying there receiving. And that word is . . .

"Oops."

Like a surgeon saying "oops" in the middle of an operation, or a pilot saying "oops" while making the approach for landing, your saying "oops" in the middle of a massage, although hopefully not life-threatening, simply doesn't inspire confidence. It may lead some people to imagine horrible scenarios — injured muscles, crushed arteries, or indelible marks left on the skin.

The person receiving doesn't know what kind of massage move you're attempting to perform at any given moment. So, if you don't get the move exactly right each time, don't worry; she's not going to know the difference. Not unless you say "oops," that is.

Building Your Massage Muscles

Massage requires the sustained dexterous use of certain muscles in your hands, forearms, shoulders, and in fact your entire body. You may not be using these muscles for any particular purpose right now. Like any other muscles that come suddenly into use, they may get sore when you begin using them. Don't be alarmed, as this is natural.

Here's a list of a few exercises and devices that massage pros sometimes use to help build massage muscles:

- ✔ **"Walking" a quarter:** Balance a quarter on your thumb. By using only the one hand, try to turn it over onto the top of your index finger. If you succeed, then try to flip it over onto your middle finger, and so on. When you get good, you can walk the quarter over all four fingers and catch it with the thumb again from below.

- ✔ **Finger dancing:** First, hold your hand in front of your face, with your palm facing away from you. Keeping your thumb out of the way, hold all four fingers loosely together. This is the starting position. Next, separate your fingers down the middle, two on each side. This position is shown in Figure 10-1. Finally, bring those fingers back together again, and then take just the pinkie finger and index finger away from the center. This position is also shown in Figure 10-1. Practice until you can repeat these steps over and over in a continuous loop.

- ✔ **Fingertip pushups:** For you fitness fanatics, try doing some fingertip pushups; these not only strengthen your fingers for massage, but you receive the added benefit of some powerful exercise. Be careful not to overdo it, and always check with a physician before starting a new exercise regime.

- ✔ **Grape squeezing:** In order to sensitize your fingers for delicate massage moves, you can practice squishing grapes. Simply place a grape between your thumb and your first two fingers and squeeze till you burst the skin. Practice squeezing new grapes until they're just about to burst, maintaining a constant sensitive level of pressure.

- ✔ **Lunges:** Lunges strengthen your legs and hips, making it easier for you to stand and bend and squat when you're giving a massage.

- ✔ **Dance:** Any kind of dance class is great to prepare you for using your whole body to do massage.

- ✔ **Yoga:** You won't believe how quickly you get tight and tired just from giving a simple massage. Doing yoga may help keep you limber.

- ✔ **Fist squeezing:** You can pick up a little stress-relief squeeze ball just about anywhere these days, even at the checkout counter in most drugstores. These are great not only for relieving stress, but for building hand muscles, too. There's even a special compound made just for this purpose, called "power putty," that is sold in massage stores.

- **Dumbbells:** Lighter weight dumbbells (5–12 pounds) are great for building muscles in the forearms and wrists. Simply sit on a bench with the dumbbell in one hand, support your forearm across the top of your leg, palm up, then curl and extend the forearm.

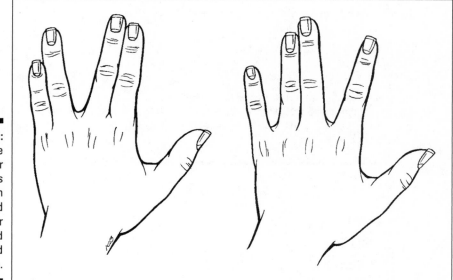

Figure 10-1: This simple finger exercise is harder than it looks, and it's great for building hand strength and coordination.

You Got 'da Moves

So, what do you actually do when you place your hands on a body and start giving a massage? Well, the first thing many people do is panic. They stand there with their hands motionless on an arm or a leg or a back, and they think to themselves, "Oh my gosh, what do I do now?"

This is where the seven types of massage moves you find in this section come in handy. After practicing them, you can rest easy that you won't draw a blank when it comes time to give a massage.

Feeling versus doing

Massage is as much (or more) about feeling as it is about doing. In fact, without really doing anything, you can still give a good massage. Through simple touch alone, you can have a profound effect on somebody else.

When I was in massage school, during the very first day in class, the instructor had us do a little experiment, which you can try for yourself.

Have your partner sit barefoot in front of you. Gently grasp one of her feet in your hands, and then DON'T DO ANYTHING. Just feel. Feel her foot, the weight of it in your hands, the contours of it against your fingers and palms, its warmth, the pulse of the blood. Resist any temptation to squeeze or press or knead.

After just five or ten minutes, slowly pull your hands away and ask your partner to note the feeling in both of her feet. Almost everyone notices a large difference; the touched foot feels as though it's been vigorously massaged. It's tingling and alive.

All you had to do to achieve that effect was to feel. No need to do anything at all.

The seven basic categories of movements are:

- ✔ **Gliding**
- ✔ **Pressing**
- ✔ **Kneading**
- ✔ **Rubbing**
- ✔ **Shaking**
- ✔ **Tapping**
- ✔ **Stretching**

Slip-sliding away: The pleasures of gliding

Usually the first move you make on any particular part of the body is gliding. Why glide first, you say? Why not just get right to the pressing and muscle-squeezing part of the massage? Three reasons:

- ✔ Gliding is a great way to warm up the skin and underlying muscles while simultaneously spreading your oil or massage cream.
- ✔ You cover a lot of territory during a glide, too, so it's perfect for "introducing" your hands to your partner.
- ✔ You'll get a feel for your partner's body and discover which areas may need the most attention during the rest of the massage.

Depending upon the amount of pressure you use, a glide can be light and ethereal or downright intense. Usually, at the beginning of a massage, you want to start with lighter gliding and then progress to the more heavy-duty stuff later, after your partner trusts your touch.

Take a look at Figure 10-2. These pictures make gliding look easy, right? What could be simpler than just running your hands along someone's skin? It's a little trickier than that, though. Good gliding is something you learn over time, with practice.

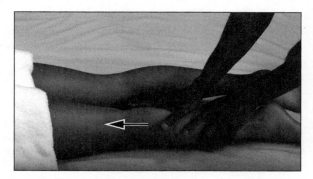

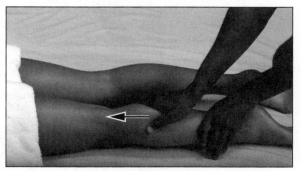

Figure 10-2: Long, soft, light gliding (top); sliding-down-the-banister gliding (middle); squeezing-toothpaste-through-a-tube gliding (bottom).

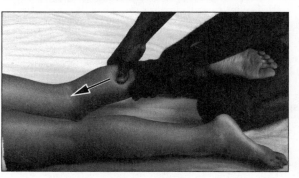

Here are three basic types of gliding:

- ✔ **Long, soft, light:** You can create the lightest type of gliding by just barely brushing the fingertips or palms across the skin in a feather-light fashion. This type of movement is also known as a *nerve-stroke* because it calms the nerves.

- ✔ **Sliding down the banister:** This movement follows the contours of the body more closely. As you glide, you mold your hands to fit the body, just like a little kid who molds himself to fit over the banister as he slides down it into the foyer. This is typical gliding, the type you use to spread oil, warm the body, and so on.

- ✔ **Squeezing toothpaste through a tube:** This is intense gliding or gliding with an attitude. When you try it on your partner for the first time, you may get a stunned reaction. You achieve this by wrapping your hands around a leg or an arm and squeezing firmly while you glide, as if you were trying to squeeze toothpaste from a giant tube. The most typical places for this maneuver are on the calf and the forearm.

Start out slowly, and always, always make the motions toward the heart because you actually move blood through the veins with this move. Watch out for the contraindications of varicose veins and phlebitis.

Good places to glide

You can glide just about anywhere there's an expanse of skin to move over. Tight little nooks and crannies, like between the toes for example, are not good places to glide because there's not enough open territory. However, you can still glide on smaller surfaces, even over the eyelids (provided your partner is not wearing contact lenses). Simply adjust your hands to the area you are touching. Thus, a forehead glide would include just your fingertips, while a glide to the leg would include your whole palm.

For all types of gliding, you need to turn your hands into super-sensitive, micro-adjusting instruments that constantly change to conform to each and every little hill and valley on your partner's body. Imagine yourself trying to smooth out a sheet of plastic-wrap around an irregularly shaped piece of fruit, allowing no air-pockets or wrinkles. Got it?

"X" marks the spot: Pressing

"Out, damned spot!" — *Shakespeare*

Great poets throughout the ages have understood the value of getting rid of spots. And it's no wonder. If you've ever received a back rub from someone and suddenly felt them press exactly the right spot, you know the sensation is swift and unmistakable. Immediately, you say something like, "Yes, there it is. That's the spot!"

So, what is the "spot" anyway? Massage pros have all kinds of fancy names for it, like "trigger points," or muscle spasms, or adhesions. Whatever you call them, these points of tension or pain are what we're trying to get rid of in massage, and pressing on them skillfully can help achieve that.

I envision these spots as tenacious little criminals who invade our bodies and take some of our muscles hostage. They're tough, resourceful, and they thrive best when we don't know exactly where to find them. Massage helps us locate where our tension spots are hiding so we can ferret them out. Just the right amount of pressure can send them this message:

"It's no use. We know you're in there. Come out with your hands up. Let the hostages go, and you'll get off easy."

Of course, if the "spots" don't leave your muscles alone, you have to go in with some heavy firepower. That's where pressing comes in. Here are a few steps you can follow to find spots and press them into submission:

- **Zeroing in:** First, while you're warming the tissues up during your pre-liminary gliding strokes, feel for areas that are unusually tight, hard, or sensitive. (See the "Under pressure" sidebar in Chapter 8.) After you're done gliding over a certain area, come back to these targeted spots one at a time and zero in on them by using just your fingertips or thumbs.

- **Pushing the walk button:** You know those little rubberized buttons that you push to change the light to green at intersections? They give a little at first, but then you get the feeling that you have to push harder. You can't quite tell if you're holding it down or not, so you hold it in firmly for a few seconds, much longer than you'd hold, say, the on/off switch on a desk lamp. Well, that's the same kind of pressing you can use in your massage — good, firm, sustained pressure is what makes pressing work, as shown in Figure 10-3.

- **Pinpoint pressure:** You not only need the right spot; you need the EXACT right spot. This can mean an itty-bitty micro-difference in the location of your fingers or thumb. Keep feeling around until you can tell you're directly on "top" of the spot. Usually this feels like you could easily slip off of it on either side.

- **Keep adjusting:** As you feel your partner's body respond, you can adjust your pressure accordingly, lightening your pressure as the tension dissipates.

Good places to press

Finding the right spots to press may sometimes feel a little tricky to you. After all, the body has about a million different points on it. How do you tell where's a good place to apply pressure and where's not a good place? There are two answers:

✔ You have to practice feeling for these points (this is the art of palpation, which you find out about in Chapter 4).

✔ Certain points are common to most people. After you practice on several willing massage partners, you'll build your skill in locating them.

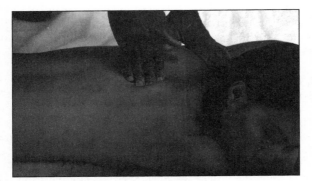

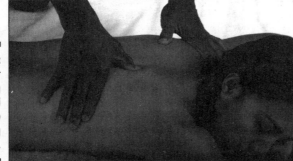

Figure 10-3: Finger pressing (top) and thumb pressing (bottom).

The spots we are talking about in this section are not *shiatsu points* or *acupressure points,* which are spots along energy pathways in the body. You get to know a few shiatsu points in Chapter 11; the spots we're talking about here are occasionally found in the same areas, but they're a different animal altogether.

Let's do the twist: Kneading

After you master the art of kneading, you may be in great demand because kneading, in my opinion, produces the most pleasurable sensations of all the maneuvers. It gets in deep to flush out tension while at the same time stimulating a large surface area on the skin.

Your kneading technique can make or break you as a massage giver, so I recommend practicing quite a bit on this one. If you practice building your massage muscles, as suggested earlier in this chapter, you can be a better kneader because this particular maneuver requires a lot of strength in the hands.

In order to knead effectively, you must banish fear! The biggest mistake novice kneaders make is kneading too tentatively. As a massage teacher, I've spent hundreds of hours hunched over students guiding their hands into bigger movements. "Get more flesh between those fingers!" I cajole them. "Twist your arms around some more. Use your whole body to make the movement."

This is good advice for you, too. A wimpy knead is much worse than no knead at all. Here are some ways to make your kneading big, bold, and beloved by all who encounter it:

- **Come on everybody, let's do the Twist:** Chubby Checker would have been disappointed if he looked out on the dance floor to find dozens of people just standing there and sort of half-heartedly bending a little at the waist. When he said twist, he meant Twist!, as in twist-tie and twist-off-top and wow-look-at-that-twister-about-to-destroy-the-barn! The number one rule for kneading is to use your whole body to create a twisting movement around the area you're working on. See Figure 10-4, which shows how your hands can move around a thigh in a circular wringing motion.

- **Baker making bread:** Of course, when we think of kneading, the image of a baker often comes to mind, with his hands wrist-deep in pliable flour, constantly squeezing, rolling, and pushing. In fact, those are the three components of a successful knead. After you have twisting down, add these steps to complete the picture:

  - **Squeezing:** During your twist, the hand that's furthest away (the right hand as shown in Figure 10-5a) is *squeezing* in as much flesh as possible between the fingers and palms.

  - **Rolling:** The right hand *rolls* the squeezed flesh back toward you while the near hand begins its journey away from you, pushing more flesh into the fold, as shown in Figure 10-5b.

  - **Pushing:** Finally, you're in the position shown in Figure 10-5c, and your right hand starts *pushing* while your left hand takes over the squeezing and rolling.

- **Pinching and rolling:** This final type of kneading is often called skin rolling. It's reserved for areas that normally don't respond too well to bigger twisting, squeezing, and rolling maneuvers. It's a little tricky to do, but most people love the way it feels. First, pinch a roll of flesh between your thumb and the first two fingers. Then, keeping your thumb locked in position, glide your whole hand over the skin while "walking" your first two fingers forward so that they push a constant roll of skin back against your thumb as shown in Figure 10-5d.

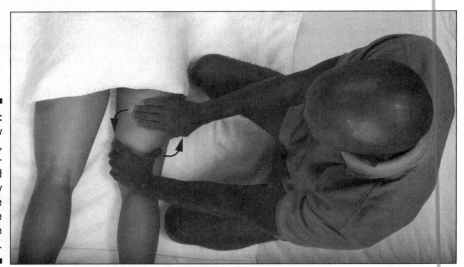

Figure 10-4:
Notice how your hands, arms, shoulders, and entire body move around the area you are kneading.

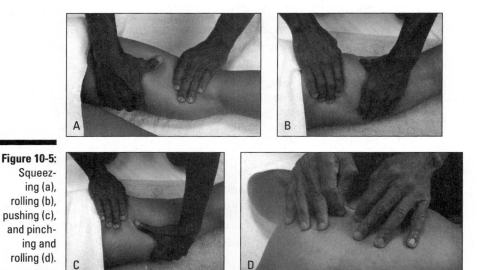

Figure 10-5:
Squeezing (a), rolling (b), pushing (c), and pinching and rolling (d).

Good places to knead

By definition, to knead something means you have to grasp it between your fingers or palms. Therefore, areas of the body that you can't grasp, you can't knead. It's simple: no flesh, no knead. That's why it's trickier to knead skinny people than to knead fleshy people. That's why it's trickier to knead a knee than to knead a thigh. That doesn't mean you need to knead a whole handful of flesh to get the job done, though. You can perform the last type of knead-ing, skin rolling, even on areas with almost no fat, like a supermodel's upper back, for instance.

Wax on, wax off: Rubbing

The secret to successful rubbing, or *friction* as massage pros call it, is to make the pressure from your fingers or palms strong enough to stay station-ary on the surface of the skin while moving the layers below. In other words, your fingers don't glide while they rub, although they can definitely move around quite a bit. Take, for example, the maneuvers you receive on your head when you get a shampoo at a salon. A good shampoo person employs friction techniques, holding her fingers steady on a certain part of your scalp while manipulating your head beneath it. If she simply glides her fingers across your scalp, the sensation is disturbingly inadequate.

Another analogy for rubbing is waxing your car. You take a buffing pad in one hand and you rub the wax on. Then with a rag in the other hand, you rub the wax off. Your fingers are never in contact with the car itself, but the car receives the effects, not the buffing pad or rags. So it is with massage. Your fingers are in contact with the skin, but you're affecting the layers below.

Here are a few rubbing techniques that work well for various parts of the body:

- ✔ **Miser's rub:** Especially good for the fingers and toes, the miser's rub will remind you of someone rubbing a gold coin between their fingers, as shown in Figure 10-6a.

- ✔ **Circular:** Making sure your fingers are planted securely, move the skin over the tissues below it in small circles, as shown in Figure 10-6b. You can move your hand gradually along the skin's surface, creating a series of circles over an entire area.

- ✔ **Cross fiber:** In any given area of the body, the muscle fibers are running predominantly in one direction or another. On the inside of your upper arm, for instance, the biceps muscle runs from your shoulder to your elbow, up and down. If you rub in a cross-wise direction over these fibers, from the inside of your arm to the outside, you're making a *cross-fiber* movement, as shown in Figure 10-6c. This action is especially good for people who exercise a lot or are in the later stages of recovering from an injury because it promotes the repair of scar tissues.

Good places to rub

You can rub most everywhere, but you have to be careful in sensitive areas because rubbing can be a little annoying if it's done, say, on the eyelids.

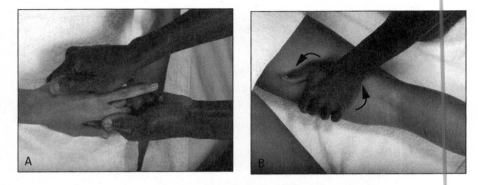

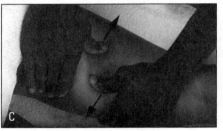

Figure 10-6:
The miser's
rub (a), the
circular rub
(b), and the
cross-fiber
rub (c).

Shake, rattle, and roll: Shaking

Some people are afraid to get too "physical" when they give a massage, which doesn't make much sense when you think about it. They incorrectly assume that every massage move has to be as smooth and soothing as the next CD from Enya. But this is not true. Some of the best moves actually jostle you around quite a bit.

You have to imagine what the shaking is actually doing internally to the muscles, tendons, and bones where they attach to each other inside the body. It's like loosening fruit from a tree. Imagine that you're standing on the ground in front of an apple tree, and one big perfect juicy apple is still left just barely clinging to a high branch. Grasping a lower limb, you *shake with the intention of loosening something at a distance from you*. This is the essence of shaking in massage, too.

Of course, you don't want to literally loosen muscles from bone so that they fall off, but you do want to help ease the muscles' tight grip of chronic tension, especially in the joints. Shaking is great for this, and there's a fine art to it. Here are three different versions that you can practice:

Vibration

No other massage move feels quite as dramatic as vibration. It's a show biz move, a move with pizzazz. But first of all, you have to figure out how to do it, which isn't that easy for most of us. Here are the steps (and see Figure 10-7):

- Placing just your fingertips on the area to be vibrated (try the back, which is easiest to start with), stiffen all of your joints from your fingers all the way up to your shoulders.

- Try making your entire arm tremble as one unit, as if you were extremely cold and shivering uncontrollably.

- Pressing firmly, concentrate all of that trembling down into your fingertips.

- Simultaneously, drag your fingertips slowly down over your partner's back, remembering to imagine your movements loosening muscles all along the way.

Be careful not to vibrate a fingertip directly on top of the spine as you may cause some discomfort or bruising.

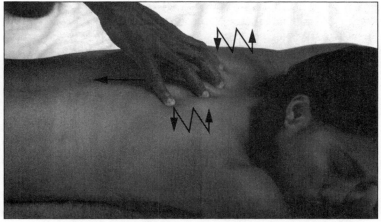

Figure 10-7:
Creating high speed vibration takes concentration and a willingness to look spastic.

Shaking

In this move, you grasp one part of your partner's body (usually a limb) and then recreate the same kind of rigid trembling you did for vibration. It can be a slower trembling, though, even languid, but the intent is still to loosen deep muscles. See Figure 10-8.

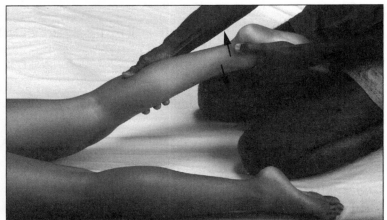

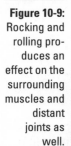

Figure 10-8:
Shaking is similar to vibration, but you grasp instead of press.

Rocking & rolling

A doctor named Milton Trager developed a kind of massage called, appropriately, *Trager*, which includes an awful lot of rocking and rolling, as shown in Figure 10-9. One of the results of a really good Trager massage is a deep release of tension from areas that you wouldn't be able to get to with your fingers, like deep inside joints. You can recreate some of the effects of this type of massage by doing some very gentle rocking and rolling of your own. You find out more about how to apply this to specific areas in the next chapter.

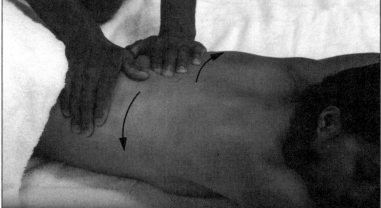

Figure 10-9:
Rocking and rolling produces an effect on the surrounding muscles and distant joints as well.

Good places to shake

The limbs respond exceptionally well to shaking. However, if you shake the head, you're coming dangerously close to a chiropractic maneuver, which is a definite no-no.

Larger areas such as the back and thighs respond well to vibration, and you can rock the whole body, especially when your partner is lying face down.

Get into the rhythm: Tapping

This is the type of movement that you see movie actors performing when they think they're doing some really authentic massage on-screen. It also seems to be the preferred move for overweight Russian men giving massages in bathhouses. Yes, I'm talking about the famous karate-chop family of massage maneuvers, otherwise known as tapping.

This family of moves is based upon one major concept: getting pounded on feels surprisingly good. This is true, as long as you tap judiciously, with the right amount of pressure. To achieve seasoned tapping prowess, practice with the three basic hand-shapes for tapping: the open fingertip, the karate hack, and the loose fist. All of them are done with "soft" hands because, after all, your intention is not to attack ninja-style but to increase circulation and soothe sore muscles.

The secret to all good tapping is the rhythm. If you're not a natural born drummer, try slowing your tapping down until you reach a rhythm that you can sustain easily. It's not speed that counts, but consistency.

- ✔ **Fingertip tapping:** This is the lightest tap, excellent for faces and the top of your head. A lot of cosmetologists use this move to bring extra circulation to the cheeks, creating that "rosy glow" look. Tapping is shown in Figure 10-10a.

- ✔ **Karate hacking:** Make sure to keep the hands limp and not treat your partner's body like a board you're trying to break. Don't hack directly on bony areas, of course. Keep your wrists loose and let the edges of your flopping fingers do a lot of the hacking for you, as shown in Figure 10-10b.

- ✔ **Loose fist pounding:** You have to be extra careful when using your fists for tapping, but they definitely come in handy if your partner is one of those NFL linebacker types who doesn't seem to respond to normal massage manipulations. Don't tighten your fists completely when tapping, and resist the temptation to do a Rocky-Balboa-side-of-beef-in-the-freezer move. See Figure 10-10c.

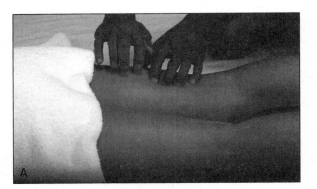

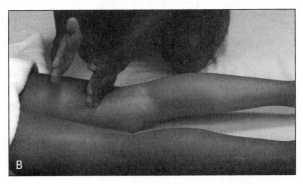

Figure 10-10:
Fingertip
tapping (a),
karate hack-
ing (b), and
loose fist
pounding (c).

Good places to tap

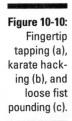

Tapping feels good just about anywhere, but if you tap someone too hard on the top of his head, he's likely to think you have something against him. The usual rule is: the more flesh in an area, the more force you can tap with, progressing up the scale from fingertips to hacking hands to loose fists. Bony areas like the knees need light tapping with just the fingertips. Also, go feather-light on the kidney area on either side of the spine in the lower back. Certain spots you may not think of, like the bottom of the feet for example, are great places to hack. And of course the ever-popular back, buttocks, and thighs are great places to practice "getting into the rhythm."

Keep it loose: Stretching

Stretching is really good for you, and a lot of people don't stretch as much as they should in order to stay limber and youthful. You can help solve this problem by incorporating a few stretching moves right into your massage.

Stretching feels really good as long as you follow three easy guidelines:

- ✔ Ease your partner into it.
- ✔ Easy does it while you're doing it.
- ✔ Ease your partner out of it.

Remember that each joint has a limit as to how far it will stretch in any and all possible directions, and this limit is called its *range of motion*.

Don't try stretching any part of the body past its normal range of motion because, if you do, it will hurt. A lot. Stop long before you think you reach the maximum stretch. Always ask your partner for feedback about how the stretch feels. Some people are super limber and you can twist them like pretzels while others can take very little stretching before it becomes uncomfortable.

Be especially careful when stretching your partner's neck, moving it slowly and in only one plane at a time: left to right, up and down, or ear to shoulder. And don't *hyperextend* the neck, or any joint for that matter. (See the *contraindications* section earlier in this chapter.)

There are three basic types of stretches you can apply during a massage:

- ✔ **Passive stretching:** Passive stretching doesn't mean you should have a ho-hum attitude about the stretch. It means your partner just lies there passively and doesn't assist you at all while you stretch him, as shown in Figure 10-11.

- ✔ **Active assisted stretching:** This type of stretching, shown in Figure 10-12, requires your partner to move through the stretch while you help her stretch a little further. It's not recommended for lazy partners who just want to lie back and have you do all the work during the massage.

✔ **Active resisted stretching:** In this one, your partner resists the movement of the stretch that you're giving him. When he stops resisting, you are able to stretch him even further. This one's good for strengthening muscles and can be considered a kind of mini-workout.

Figure 10-11:
In this passive stretch of the knee and thigh, you press the person's ankle toward her buttock while she just lies there letting it happen.

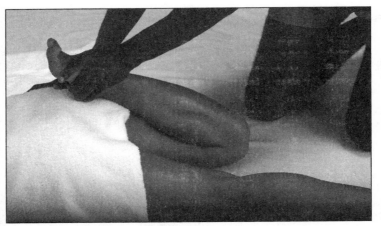

Figure 10-12:
In active assisted stretching, you help your partner stretch a little further.

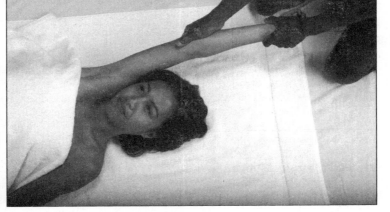

Good places to stretch

The multitude of joints in the body make it possible to do a large variety of joint manipulations and stretches in many areas such as the toes, ankles, knees, hips, shoulders, elbows, wrists, and hands. You find out about a few all-time favorite stretches in the chapters to come.

Massage moves in a nutshell

Here are some simple general guidelines that you can apply to all the preceding maneuvers and use in every massage you give:

- ✔ **Follow the contour:** When in doubt about what particular move to make, just trace the body's outlines with your fingers for a few moments, applying pressure according to what you feel. It's better to keep moving in a constant flow rather than stop and say something like, "Now, what was that next maneuver again?" This can be annoying to your partner.

- ✔ **Do no harm:** Don't press too hard or work on areas that may be too delicate, such as sprains, strains, or scar tissues soon after injuries. Of course, avoid all contraindicated areas and conditions. Ask for a physician's advice if there is anything that gives you concern.

- ✔ **Stay in the moment:** The easiest way to look at a massage is piece by piece. Concentrate on one movement at a time, and one area. Work on just that leg first, and worry about what you're going to do on the arm later. One move at a time, one after another, creates a whole massage.

A ticklish situation

Some people out there will flat-out refuse to even consider the possibility of getting a massage because they're afraid they would giggle so hard they would fall right off the table. These folks consider themselves "ticklish," but what is a ticklish person anyway? Most of us are sensitive when we get poked in the ribs or stroked lightly on the bottom of the feet, but some people claim any kind of touch at all elicits the "tickle response."

When someone complains of being overly ticklish, you can follow these steps to help them get over it:

1. **First, explain that surface tension in the muscles causes excessive ticklishness.**

2. **Explain that you are going to get "underneath" this layer by applying firm pressure that affects tissues below.**

3. **Gradually apply pressure with as broad a surface as possible, for example, your entire palm instead of your fingers.**

4. **After you "sink down" to a depth that is not ticklish anymore, make your movements slow and steady, gently rocking back and forth, pulsing up and down. Avoid kneading, pressing, and vibration.**

5. **Move slowly from one area to another, staying away from the areas your partner reports as most seriously ticklish.**

6. **If your partner shows any signs of discomfort, discontinue movement and simply apply steady firm pressure.**

The Massage Dance

So, you may be asking yourself, what am I supposed to be doing with the rest of my body while my hands are massaging someone? Good question. Can you guess the right answer?

A. It doesn't matter, as long as you remain in a generally upright position and don't fall asleep.

B. Something constructive, such as learning a foreign language with audio-cassettes, because otherwise you're just wasting your time.

C. Absolutely nothing; stay as stiff and still as possible so you don't distract the person you are massaging.

D. Make every move a "whole body move" by engaging your entire self in what you're doing, turning the massage into a dance.

The answer, of course, is "D." In fact, it's so important to use your entire body properly while giving a massage that massage pros have given this practice a name — *body mechanics*.

It may seem like a lot of extra effort at first, but in the long run it's easier if you use proper body mechanics and engage your entire body while giving a massage rather than relying on the strength of your arms and shoulders alone. Actually, using your arms and shoulders alone is guaranteed to burn you out really quickly. You may end up saying something like "This is WAY too difficult." Then you may quit, offering muscle-fatigue as an excuse to your partner after just ten minutes.

Here are a few guidelines to help you fine-tune your body mechanics:

✔ **Root yourself:** Your movements should feel like they're coming from the place where your body is rooted to the earth. Don't get off balance and lose your center of power. You need to ground yourself enough so that it's difficult to knock you over when you're giving a massage.

✔ **Move from below:** Whether you're standing or kneeling down next to your partner to give the massage, generate your movements from your legs and hips, not just your upper body, as shown in Figure 10-13.

✔ **Maintain straight lines:** When you apply pressure, do it in a straight line from your shoulders down to your fingertips. Bending your joints and then applying pressure puts extra pressure on your thumbs, wrists, and elbows, and should be avoided. Figure 10-14 shows you what I'm talking about.

Figure 10-13:
If you're standing, keep your knees soft and move from your hips. If you're kneeling, still move from your hips.

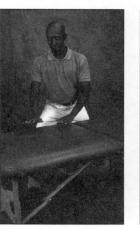
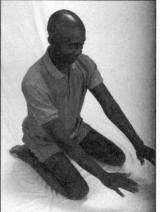

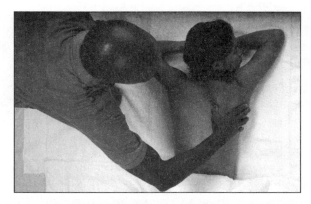

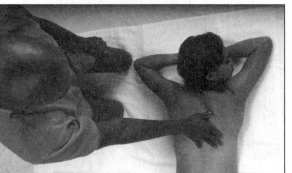

Figure 10-14:
The wrong way (top) and the right way (bottom) to apply pressure.

  ✔ **Be kind to your thumbs and wrists:** Thumbs take the biggest beating when giving a massage, and wrists come in a close second. Be extra careful not to rely only on these delicate instruments to do your heavy-duty massage work. Give them a break every once in a while by using your knuckles and forearms.

  ✔ **Lean a lot:** Instead of straining your muscles to get the job done, use your body weight. Simply LEAN on the person you're massaging by placing your center of gravity several inches away from her, then falling forward and supporting yourself on her body. This takes a little practice because our civilized instincts tell us not to use other people's bodies as counter tops. Go ahead and try it, though. It saves you a lot of work.

Massage Gizmos

Ever wander around inside one of those expensive gadget gift shops like the Sharper Image and suddenly realize that about a quarter of the inventory is massage gizmos of one kind or another? They have vibrating chairs, tables with rollers built in, and devices to buzz you, press you, knead you, jab you, and squeeze you. Seeing all this, you can definitely come to a couple very important conclusions:

  ✔ Massage gizmos are a great way for manufacturers and retailers to make lots of money.

  ✔ Massage gizmos are a great way for you to spend lots of money.

So, naturally, the question comes to mind — are they worth it? In my opinion, most of them are. And, fortunately, they don't all cost tons of money either. You can get a nifty little massage device at your local pharmacy for $12.95.

There are three main reasons why people use massage gizmos:

  1. They're fun and kind of neat looking.

  2. They can help save your hands a lot of work.

  3. They actually make you feel better.

Often, people overlook reason number 3. This is strange, because that's the whole point of using them, right? The little gizmos can really make you feel better, but you should also exercise the same cautions and observe the same contraindications when using them as you do when using your fingers.

Before you go out and purchase your own massage tool, I have a little secret for you, and you have to promise not to tell anyone else. Ready? Here it is:

JUST ABOUT EVERYTHING FEELS GOOD WHEN IT'S RUBBED AGAINST YOUR BODY! THE SECRET IS NOT THE TOOL, BUT THE TOUCH.

Whoops, I said that kind of loudly, didn't I? Maybe even some of the gizmo makers heard. But it's true. Don't take my word for it. Go out in the backyard and grab a smooth, palm-sized rock. Wash it off, of course. Then have someone take a rounded end and gently rub it against your back muscles. Wow! Feels fantastic, doesn't it?

The truth is that you don't really need these custom-made massage doohickeys, but all sorts of neat designs are out there, and some of them, admittedly, feel quite a bit better than rocks from your backyard. The ones that apply vibration and pressure are especially effective. Everybody should have at least one such gizmo in his or her home. But which one are you going to choose when there are so many shapes and sizes available, as shown in Figure 10-15? This section attempts to make a little sense of the whole massage device market for you by breaking it down into three categories: gravity-assisted gizmos, pressure tools, and mechanical devices.

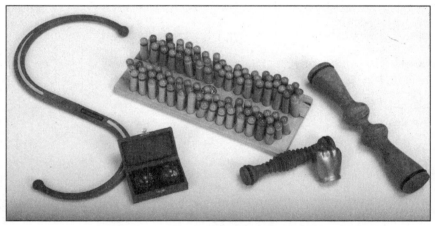

Figure 10-15:
The choice of massage gizmos continues to grow.

Gravity-assisted gizmos

These tools utilize your own weight to massage various parts of your body:

- **Foot rollers:** There are many of these, and most of them look basically like wooden cigars: stubby, brown, and round. Some have grooves etched into their surface, and others have a series of interconnected rolling balls. By running your feet over them, you stimulate nerve endings and *reflexology* points (see Chapter 14 for more on this). You can even buy sandals with hundreds of tiny knobs on the soles that massage your feet as you walk.

✔ **Back rollers:** Several versions are available. They look similar to the rolling pin your mom used to use to make pie crusts. The most famous is the Ma Roller, which has two bumps in the center that are placed on either side of your spine. The instructions say not to roll your back down over the knobs, but that's what everyone does, because that's what feels the best and has the most profound effect. Be careful when using these not to accidentally roll hard wood onto your spine itself.

✔ **Stretchers:** We all need to stretch, and sometimes we could use a little help from devices like the "body bridge" which is basically a curved table that you bend over backwards on, letting gravity do the stretching.

✔ **Body Balancer:** A massage pro named Grace Apfel in California, trying to recreate the support and flexibility she offered clients with her own hands, created the device shown in Figure 10-16. You fill the holes with pegs of different heights that you adjust to your particular needs, then lie down upon them and just relax. It's a good way to let gravity do the work in easing some of your back pains for you.

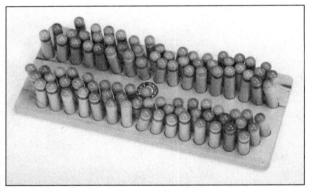

Figure 10-16:
Massage gizmos have become more and more elaborate in recent years.

Pressure tools

All sorts of devices are available now that you rub on the body with varying degrees of pressure. You can get them in specialty shops, but they're increasingly available in more common outlets such as drug stores. Basically, they stimulate *acupressure* points and trigger points. You can use them to exert pressure on tough knots and sore spots. But be careful: The materials used in these tools are usually hard, like stone or wood. Just a little pressure goes a long way.

- ✔ **Little knobby things:** Many little odd-shaped items are now sold that you're supposed to rub across your body (or somebody else's body) for fun, pleasure, and relief from stress. Some of them even have names and personalities, like the Happy Massager from the Tender Loving Things Company, Inc. or the Dolphin Massager. You can even order a Handy massage tool from the back of this book, designed by yours truly. It's a hand-shaped instrument with a perky personality that you can use when your own hands are too tired or not in the mood to give a massage. All of these utilize the same simple concept: Pressing on people makes them feel better. Try them, you'll like them.

- ✔ **"Captain Hook" devices:** Ever wish you could rubberize your arms and reach around to massage a knot in the middle of your back? That, in essence, is what these curved devices allow you to do. You can use them to hook onto otherwise unreachable tight spots on your posterior surface. Popular brands include the Backnobber and the Thera Cane.

- ✔ **Professional pressure tools:** There are certain tools that you can only get in massage clinics that are meant for professional use. One particular device looks like a sharpened pencil eraser stuck into the side of a wooden peg. Neuromuscular therapists use them to work on deep tissues. If you find professional tools somewhere, you're better off not buying them. They can cause harm if not used by skilled hands.

- ✔ **Rubbing gloves:** Several brands of textured gloves are now available. You slip them on and then apply pressure and friction over the skin. The gloves both *exfoliate* the skin and stimulate nerve endings. They feel great, too.

Mechanical devices

There are many mechanical devices on the market that utilize electricity to create vibration and kneading actions. They range in price from just a few bucks to major capital investments.

- ✔ **Thumper:** This is probably the best-known in its class, and its name says it all. It gives a heavy thumping action that simulates a pair of "chopping" hands. Great for after workouts or to combat chronic tension, but it ain't cheap.

- ✔ **Vibrating doohickeys:** Dozens of these line the shelves, and there's always one that has batteries and is available to test. That's because the manufacturers know that they feel great and that you may want to take one home when you feel it for yourself. That's a good tactic. However, after you get home, these items tend to see more use as conversation starters than therapeutic devices.

- ✔ **Shiatsu massager:** This type of unit has kneading "fingers" built into it. You put it behind you in a chair and lean back against it. According to many reports, they can work wonders. Greg, a journalist friend of mine, swears by his. He has a back problem that is exacerbated by long hours sitting at the computer, and he credits his Shiatsu massager for saving his career.

- ✔ **Massage furniture:** Panasonic and other well-known manufacturers have gotten in on the massage game with electronic chairs and tables that give you a massage while you recline on them. These are fun items to have around the house, but the novelty often wears off pretty quickly, and before too long you're left with a slightly odd lumpy piece of expensive furniture.

The best gizmo of all

When it comes to any of these gadgets, the bottom line is this — they are fun, helpful, and neat, but no amount of technology or ingenuity can create a tool more adaptable, powerful, or sensitive than the human hand. Even the device makers themselves know this. Living Earth Crafts, one of the largest massage manufacturers in the world, has a slogan: "There is no substitute for the human touch."

Tom Myers, a famed anatomy teacher and structural massage expert, agrees. Holding his own hand up for inspection, he often comments, "Twenty-five-million years in the making. Hard to beat that kind of engineering."

Chapter 11

Putting the Moves Together

● ●

● ●

I was recently watching an episode of the sitcom *Friends* on TV, and one of the main themes of the show concerned the effects of massage on friendships and relationships. The Monica character thought she gave a great backrub, but her boyfriend Chandler thought otherwise. The whole show centered on how he should break the bad news to her.

We humans are sensitive creatures, and when we give something as personal as a massage to someone else, we're making ourselves vulnerable to his or her judgement. What if they don't like our technique? What if they don't like *us?*

When you give of yourself through massage, it's natural to be afraid of what people may think and to wonder, secretly, if you're doing it *right* or if you're *good enough.*

I think you should forget all about that stuff. Your massage abilities are not something to be proud of, or ashamed of. Your abilities are something you should share.

As long as you tune in and become sensitive to your partner, you can give a good massage. The idea is not to focus on *being* good, but to focus on *doing* good.

If Monica had not been so proud in the beginning, she wouldn't have forced her own concept of what she thought was good onto her boyfriend, which set the stage for her to feel rejected and ashamed later.

Be sensitive. Tune in. Do good. If you do these things, you never have time to worry about whether you're good or not. As long as your heart is into what you're doing, you're guaranteed to do it the *right* way.

Setting Up

First, you need to go over just a few preliminaries to make sure you're set up and ready to go. I assume that you've created a suitable *inner chamber* for your massage experience and that you've practiced a few moves from Chapter 10. You know what to do and what not to do, and now you just have to get yourself ready and do it.

Table for one?

One thing you may notice is that the massage in this chapter is being given on the floor. It's pretty much guaranteed that you have a floor available someplace to work on, right? But there's a good chance you don't have a massage table like the ones the pros use. For those of you not familiar with them, massage tables are oblong, folding, padded tables. Most of them have legs of adjustable height, like the one in Figure 11-1. These tables are great tools, and if you get serious about massage at some point, you may want to consider investing in one. New ones cost a few hundred dollars.

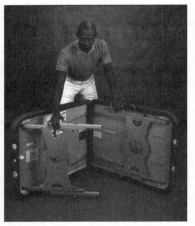

Figure 11-1:
Massage tables look like folding, adjustable-height, oblong, upholstered card tables.

The floor can be quite a comfortable place to get a massage, especially if you add a few pillows, a sofa cushion or two, plus a sheet and towels, as you can see in Figure 11-2.

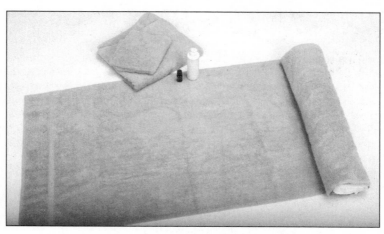

Figure 11-2:
You can create a perfectly comfortable massage space on the floor.

Many massages have been given on beds, but in those cases the massage often leads to other activities — like sleeping! That's right, it's very tempting for the giver to just roll over and lounge around instead of working like he should. When you do give a massage on a bed, arrange some towels near the foot or along one edge, so that you don't have to be up on the bed yourself the whole time you're giving the massage.

Sheets, towels, and so on

Don't use your best sheets and towels to do a massage on because the oils and creams can leave stains and a musty oil smell behind. Also, the color white seems to show off oil stains the most. Many spas use darker colored linens, like green or blue, for this reason.

Other things you may want to have around include heating pads, blankets, bottle warmers, and other such comfort-creating devices. Nothing's worse than getting a massage and not being able to concentrate on how good it feels because you're shivering the whole time.

It's also a good idea to have some extra pillows to use as *bolsters* for support beneath your partner. Massage pros use specially made bolsters, as mentioned in Chapter 8, but you can use normal pillows just as effectively. If you use one of your nice pillows, it's a good idea to cover it with a towel to keep it from getting stained by oil.

Oil's Well That Ends Well

Yes, it's true. Massage can be an oily endeavor. In fact, in some countries, such as India, oil plays a major part in the whole procedure, and about half way through a massage people in Delhi end up glistening with a layer of lubricant. This is okay (as long as you have lots of towels around to sop up the extra oil afterwards). In fact, the Indian system prescribes large amounts of oil — usually sesame oil — on purpose for its lubricating and detoxifying effects. The common wisdom in most other countries, however, is that you should use just enough lubricant to, well, lubricate.

This is how you best use oil during a massage:

1. **First, choose the oil (see the sidebar later in this chapter).**

2. **Second, make sure the oil is not cold.**

   When you apply cold oil to your partner's skin, it may cause her to hit you or kick you, which is not desirable. The best way to warm the oil is to place the bottle in hot running water for a few minutes, or use a baby bottle warmer, until the oil is warm to the touch. Don't microwave the oil, which can potentially overheat it, causing an equally adverse reaction from your partner.

3. **Cup one palm and pour a small amount of oil into it.**

   Ideally, you want to keep the back of your cupped palm in contact with your partner so that you maintain a constant connection. The amount of oil depends on the size of the area you are massaging, the amount of body hair in the area, and the maneuvers you plan to use. You may have to experiment a few times to get the amount right.

4. **Rub your palms together for a few seconds to further warm the oil and then glide your hands over the skin, spreading a smooth layer of oil over the whole surface you are massaging.**

   The correct amount is the amount that leaves the skin lubricated, but no puddles of oil or "greasy" spots.

Getting creamed

Skin creams and lotions are a good alternative to oil, and in fact many professional massage therapists would not be caught using anything else. Cream absorbs more quickly into the skin than oil, so you don't slide around so much. Good ones leave a lubricating layer that makes it easy to work. A lot of pros choose a brand called Biotone.

Bottle placement

There is an age-old feud that has gone on between massage therapists for decades over where to place the oil bottle during the massage. I know that this may seem silly to you, but you can rest assured that it's a debate taken very seriously by otherwise intelligent adults. There are basically two camps — those that propose placing the bottle next to the person, where it's handy but liable to get knocked over; and those that propose keeping the bottle out of harm's way, on the floor for example, where it's harder to reach but less likely to get kicked or spilled. Some people go as far as to keep their oil bottles in a specially made holster strung around their waist like a six-gun. This gives the average massage therapist a Wyatt Earp kind of look that is perhaps not ideal for inducing relaxation.

Where should you put the bottle of oil during a massage? In my professional opinion, speaking as a massage therapist who's been working in the field for almost 20 years, it doesn't really matter. Whatever's most comfortable for you is best.

The type of bottle (and especially the cap) does matter, though. You can make things much easier for yourself if you choose a squeeze-top type cap that pours a tiny bit of oil at a time. Pump tops work well, too. If you use a wide-mouth opening, chances are you may end up with oil all over the place, especially if you have your massage area dimly lit with candles.

Your own oil blends

You can incorporate the concepts of aromatherapy into your massage by adding a few drops of *essential oil* to the oil you're already using, which is then called the *carrier oil*. Typical carrier oils include grapeseed, sweet almond, jojoba, avocado, and sesame, which are all good as a base for the essential oils. To make your own aromatherapy oil, blend two dozen drops of essential oil with 2 ounces of carrier oil. For added aromatherapy benefits, place a few drops in a *diffuser* to fill the room you're in with the same scent you're using for the massage, as I suggest in Chapter 9.

Table 11-1 lists the essential oils I use in my spa therapy workshops and a description of their basic effects:

Table 11-1	Essential oils
Oil	*Properties*
Cedar	Reduces fluids in body tissues, diuretic. Warming in baths.
Clary sage	Balances female hormones. Good for scalp problems.

(continued)

Table 11-1 *(continued)*

Oil	Properties
Eucalyptus radiata	Excellent for lungs, respiratory system. Muscle tonic.
Geranium rose	Balances the skin by affecting sebum. Balances emotions, too.
Juniper	Calming and purifying.
Lavender	Anti-bacterial (first-aid kit in a bottle), calming, good for skin.
Lemon grass	Stimulates digestion. Antiseptic, detoxifies lymph. Uplifting.
Orange	Mood elevator.
Peppermint	Stimulates alertness. Good for headaches, colds.
Pine	Pain killer. Natural deodorant.
Rose	Excellent for the skin.
Rosemary	Hair tonic. Astringent. Good for oily skin.
Sandalwood	Grounding and relaxing. Spiritually uplifting. Aids aging skin.
Tea tree	Antiseptic, antifungal, antibacterial. Good for the skin.
Vetiver	Grounding and calming.
Ylang ylang	Aphrodisiac. Relieves tension/stress. Balances dry skin.

The Rules for Giving Massage

Just as there were some rules for receiving, there are rules for giving, too. For the most part, these are things I've mentioned all along throughout the previous chapters, but it helps if you review them here, right before you actually begin giving a massage.

1. **Do no harm.** This is the number one rule for giving a massage. Refer to Chapter 10 and make sure you're aware of the moves that you shouldn't make, the places that you shouldn't press, and the conditions you shouldn't treat.

2. **Think 3-D.** Refer to Chapter 4 and try to visualize the physical structures beneath the skin that you're affecting with your hands during the massage.

3. **Use your whole body.** Remember to use correct *body mechanics* (see Chapter 10) in order to save your own body from overexertion while applying just the right amount of pressure for your partner.

So many oils, so little time

Walk into any bath and body shop or health food store and you see at least a dozen choices in massage oils. Which is the best one, you ask? Is it the special formula designed by the spiritual healer Edgar Cayce who "received" the recipe while in a trance? Or is it the "mango tango" scented blend that your favorite boutique down the street recently released?

Several oils available straight from the shelf in your local grocery store are usable, if not ideal, for massage. Almond oil is used in spas around the world, and you can use sesame oil and olive oil, too. But the special oils formulated just for massage really are better. They have more nutrients for the skin, and they create just the right amount of lubrication. In my opinion, it's worth the extra money you spend to get a high-quality massage oil.

There are a few things you want to look for when choosing an oil:

- **Ingredients:** Check the ingredients. A common addition to several oil blends, for example, is lanolin, which comes from an animal source and turns some people off.

- **Scent:** Make sure the scent is not overpowering or synthetic.

- **Viscosity:** Everyone has his or her own preference as far as the right viscosity goes. "Thin" oils, such as mineral oil, feel a little watery and spread unevenly. This is not recommended. "Thick" oils like coconut leave a "greasy" feeling. Test a little on your palm before buying to find an oil somewhere in the middle of this spectrum that works for you.

4. **Focus on the other.** This is no time to be thinking about politics, sports, the weather, or your upcoming turn to receive. As fully as you can, focus on your partner, what she's feeling, and how you can make her feel better.

5. **Go out of your mind.** After you figure out the moves, practice the technique, and focus on your partner with all your concentration, then you can stop thinking. That's right. Let go of your extraneous thoughts, and even your thoughts about doing a good job.

6. **Get creative.** Go ahead, go crazy; just let yourself feel whatever you're feeling and go with your intuition. Want to leave one palm on your partner's forehead and the other on her stomach completely motionless for ten minutes? That's probably exactly what she needs. As long as what you're doing is generated from caring and commitment to your partner, it is going to be the right thing.

7. **Let love flow.** Certain people develop an ability to send a very distinct and palpable sensation of love into their fingers and palms. You can feel it when they touch you. Everyone else has the potential to develop that ability. Why not use massage as an opportunity to explore your own innate abilities to send a powerful message of caring to others through your touch and presence? There are worse ways you could spend your time.

The Massage

Okay, here it is, the moment you've all been waiting for. You can only talk about it for so long without realizing that massage is not really about talking, it's about feeling. And as Bob Marley once said, "He who feels it, knows it."

Soon, you are going to be sailing away toward hours of massage bliss. All you have to do to get started is follow these five easy steps:

- ✔ Cleanliness first
- ✔ Take your positions
- ✔ Invocation
- ✔ The force, Luke, remember the force
- ✔ The first touch

Cleanliness first

You're all set up, the mood is right, the lights are low, and now, before you do anything else, there's one critical procedure you must follow before starting the massage — wash your hands!

Good hands

What does it mean to have "good hands?" It's the one quality that millions of massage lovers around the world use to describe the essence of an excellent massage therapist. As in, "Oh, that was the best massage I ever had. You have got great hands." But, because that quality is so vague, it's a little difficult to reproduce or teach to someone else. Good hands? What does that mean?

Having good hands, as it turns out, is not really about your hands. It's about *YOU*. It's the way you focus on your partner, the way you become sensitive to her, and the way you care. It's also about following some very simple guidelines, which I call the "rules for giving massage." You can find those rules right here in this chapter.

Follow these simple principles, and you may even go beyond having good hands to having "great hands" one day.

But do I have to cut my nails?

Once I was hired to present a massage workshop at a huge annual convention of nail technicians (manicurists) in Detroit. I never knew so many manicurists existed before. Demonstrating some basic massage moves on the feet of one class member, I then told them to exchange similar moves. Soon, the room was filled with sounds of pain and discomfort.

These women had nails an inch and a half long. Sharp nails. Some of them had holes drilled in the ends of their nails, and miniature charm bracelets dangled through them. It was impossible for them to practice massage.

If you have long nails, it's going to be awfully hard for you to give a good massage. One of the first things people are told when they sign up for massage school is to cut their nails, and you can often tell a massage pro by her extremely short and neatly trimmed nails.

Does this mean you have to lop off your own dearly beloved nails in order to give a massage? Not necessarily. If your husband is the only person you're going to be massaging, and he likes it when you run your long nails down his back, don't worry about cutting them. You can improvise massage moves by using your palms and the bottoms of your fingers, keeping your nails lifted up out of the way. However, if your nails are long and your intention is to get better at massage and perform all the moves described here to their fullest, you have some serious clipping to do in your near future.

Washing cleanses away dirt and grime, and it also protects you and your partner from nasty bacteria. It's a good habit to get into.

Take your positions

To begin the massage, you and your partner both have to be in the right positions. In the routine shown in this chapter, you start with your partner lying on her back, and you sit up near her head.

Some people are sticklers about this whole positioning issue, but I don't believe in starting every massage in the same position every time. In fact, starting over and over again in the same position can lead to complacency and a boring massage. It's better to begin each massage where you are drawn to begin by your intuition, your partner's suggestion, and your observation. Is she all hunched over by tight back muscles? Then by all means start the massage with her facedown, working on her back. The sequence of the massage shown in this chapter is not the only way.

Invocation

You may recall that in Chapter 5, I describe a massage I received from Wesley, who's a native Hawaiian massage therapist and healer on the Big Island. What I didn't describe was the prayer Wesley used to begin the massage, sitting humbly on the floor beside me, melodiously intoning some words in Hawaiian: *"Kou makou makua iloko okalani."*

This invocation was meant to make both Wesley and me at one with the source of life. He learned it from his teacher, Auntie Margaret, and she in turn was taught it by her elders.

Although you may feel a little funny at first, it may be appropriate for you to say a couple of words of invocation as you're about to start your massage. They don't have to be in Hawaiian; something simple is fine, such as, "I summon the powers of healing and wholeness to be with us during this massage." Just say them from your heart, and you get your message across.

The Force, Luke, remember the Force

Remember, you're not just dealing with a pile of flesh and bones here. Your partner is more than a series of points to be pushed and muscles to be kneaded. She has a magical inner spark, too. According to many massage philosophies, especially those from the East like *Shiatsu*, the body is filled with invisible pathways that are pulsing with this inner energy, variously known as *chi*, *ki*, *prana*, *universal-life-force-energy*, and *the-force-Luke-remember-the-force*.

You can give a better massage if you simply stop for a moment at the beginning of the massage and focus on that force that exists within you and your partner. Remember the scenes from *Star Wars* when Luke was zeroing in on the Death Star using nothing but his intuition? The voice of his mentor was there in his head all along urging him to "remember the force." Tune into your own inner guidance as you begin the massage, and you may surprise yourself with how well you do.

The first touch

This is the crucial moment, when all of your preparation and practice is put to the test. Ninety-five percent of what your partner needs to know about your massage is completely obvious in the first split second, with the very first touch. At this juncture, you go forward into the realm of being and doing rather than thinking, and a new thing is created, the massage.

Reaching both hands down, place them gently and consciously on your partner's back, as if you were touching a sleeping child and trying not to wake her. Put one up on the top of the spine near the head, and the other down by the base of the spine. Then just touch for a moment, with no need to move. You can actually summon the "force, Luke," and say your invocation at this time, too. (See Figure 11-3.)

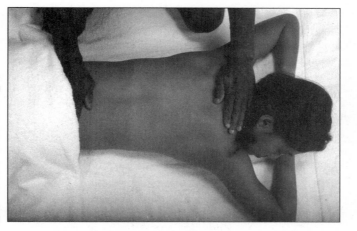

Figure 11-3:
After you summon the forces within, reach out and touch someone.

Hold this position for a minute, with your hands on your partner's spine, simply communicating your presence and loving intentions.

Then you can begin.

Note: You may notice that I haven't included any stretches in this chapter. That's because I explain stretches in the sports massage section of Chapter 16. This doesn't mean you can't use them during your full body massage, too, though. In fact, I highly recommend stretches. After you master some of the stretches, sprinkle them liberally throughout your massage for optimum effect.

The back

The back is a great place to begin a massage because many people equate massage with a "back rub." Although it looks large and solid, the back is actually prone to lots of little aches and pains, and much of the tension and everyday complaints people have can be found there. Thus the famous phrase, "Oh, my aching back." And finally, the back is the least vulnerable area to touch someone, psychologically speaking, so people are more likely to relax and "let you in" when you begin there.

1. Without moving your hands from the position they're in, simply begin to rock your partner gently from side to side, by using the tailbone as a kind of handle for the heel of your hand. When you get good at it, you can extend your rocking maneuvers further up the back and down onto the buttocks and even the legs. The idea is to get a wave-like motion going through your partner's body so that she starts to melt into the floor.

    When you want to get someone out of the mood they were just in, and into the mood of getting a massage, nothing beats rocking.

2. People either love skin rolling, or they really don't like it at all, so you have to experiment a little and ask your partner how it feels. Start by getting a grasp on the skin at the base of the neck between your thumb and your first two fingers, then "walk" this roll down the back, keeping it between your fingers the whole time. This takes some practice, so start with a partner who doesn't mind playing guinea pig.

3. Use your fingertips to "hook" into the muscles alongside the spine near the tailbone. Then start vibrating your hand while dragging it with medium pressure back up toward your partner's head, as in Figure 11-4a. Repeat this three times.

4. This long gliding movement spreads oil and further warms up the entire area. See the section on oil earlier in this chapter for the proper oil-spreading technique. Glide down with both hands on the muscles on either side of the spine, with your fingers pointed in toward the middle. When you reach the base of the spine, swivel your fingers toward the outside and glide back up as shown in Figure 11-4b. Repeat this gliding four or five times, using light pressure at first and then slightly firmer pressure.

5. When you reach the base of the spine on the fourth or fifth glide, stop and apply circular rubbing all over the sacrum, or tail bone, as shown in Figure 11-4c. You may notice that when your partner is lying down this bone is tilted in such a way that it presents a relatively flat surface, so you can lean your weight forward from your partner's head and apply pressure to it.

6. For this next move, start with your thumbs at the top of your partner's back, one thumb on either side of the spine. Then push your thumbs down along the "ridge" of the erector spinae muscles *very slowly,* with medium to firm pressure, as in Figure 11-4d. This should take 30 seconds or more. When you get to a tight "spot," slow down and let your thumbs sink into it even more slowly, making a mental note to revisit this area later. Remember to use proper *body mechanics* so you don't overstrain your joints while pushing. After you reach the base of the spine, glide your way back to the top.

7. With your thumbs atop the shoulders and your fingers up on your partner's back, knead the tops of the shoulders, also called the trapezius muscles, as shown in Figure 11-4e. While you're doing this, you can feel for tight spots and then stop for a moment to apply pressure with your thumbs directly on those areas.

8. Switch your position to your partner's side. Then, using medium pressure, glide your hands up the back, separating them at your partner's shoulders and gliding back down with lighter pressure. Do this two or three times, being careful not to press too hard directly over the spine.

9. Reaching across your partner's back, drape your fingers over her side, then pull back slowly, actually lifting her body up a tiny bit as you engage in a nifty "reverse glide," as shown in Figure 11-4f.

10. With "small" kneading movements, using mostly just the fingers, reach down and pull up the muscles along the back of the neck, alternating one hand after the other, as shown in Figure 11-4g. You can be firm, but be careful not to pinch your partner. Also, make sure not to pull her hair when you're doing this maneuver. You should also avoid reaching around too far with your fingertips because you may end up in an *endangerment site* on the throat.

11. Now is the time for you to really focus in on the tight spots you discovered during your thumb glide down alongside the spine. Start at the base of the spine and place your thumbs in the little groove that's formed between the spine itself and the *erector spinae* muscles that run up alongside the far side of the spine. Then press out toward the opposite side of the back, moving your thumbs in a little reverse "J" motion over the muscle, as shown in Figure 11-4h.

Never press directly on the spine itself while you're doing this move. Instead, keep your thumbs pressing away from the spine at all times.

The main difference between a good massage and a mediocre one is that a good massage is always custom-made for each person every time. So, customize this maneuver and apply it exactly where your partner needs it this time, seeking out the tight spots you find during your earlier gliding, and then concentrating on them.

12. With your partner's hand lifted onto her lower back, it's easy to see the shoulder blade, which automatically lifts up and reveals itself. A great way to release tension in this area is to run your fingers along the lifted inner edge of the shoulder blade, pressing in and down while you do so, as shown in Figure 11-5a. Sometimes you can feel the shoulder blade lifting even further from the back as you relax the muscles.

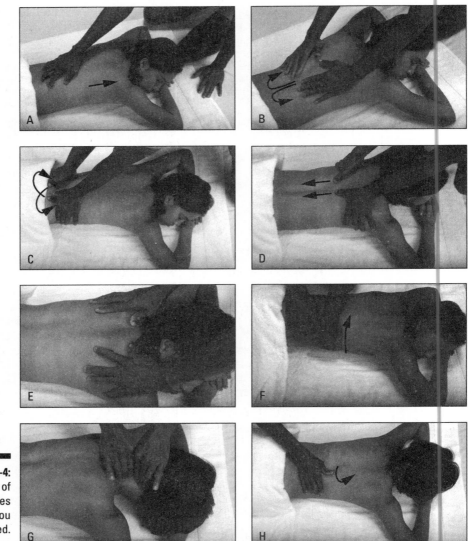

Figure 11-4:
A series of
back moves
to get you
started.

13. Use your thumbs to zero in on the spot that lies about midway out from the spine at the level of the armpit. It's right at the base of the inner edge of the shoulder blade, and is usually tight on almost everyone. If you can find this spot and do a thumb press with firm pressure for 10 seconds or longer, you may feel the entire shoulder "fall" away from the back in relaxation.

Knots, and what to do with them

As you get used to gliding over people's bodies with your hands, you may quickly realize that no two bodies are the same and that, in fact, the same body can even feel different on different days. Eventually, you'll know how to distinguish a "knot" from an area of normal muscle tone. Then you can apply the techniques you find in this chapter and Chapter 10 to start relaxing those tight places.

You could easily spend an entire hour just dealing with your partner's knots, so you have to

decide when enough is enough, and move onto the next area. This is a tough call, because your partner's knots and sore spots are the areas that need the most attention.

In general, during a full body massage, spend no more than 5 minutes on any particular tight spot. If you want to focus on it more later, schedule a special session just for that purpose.

14. Tap all across the upper and lower back, being careful to avoid the spine, as shown in Figure 11-5b. This is a typical way to finish massaging the back, and every body part for that matter. It feels good, but I find it sometimes disrupts the calming, soothing effect of the massage. Only use tapping if your partner wants it, or if he's about to jump off the table to engage in some activity, in which case some serious karate chops and loose fist pounding are called for. Otherwise, stick to some soft fingertip tapping at this point, or leave it out altogether.

15. After you press and rub on all the major spots, it's time to bail out of the back area, but you don't want to make your exit too obvious, lest you shock your partner and cause sudden back-massage withdrawal symptoms. So make your departure from the back a gradual one and use gliding *connective strokes*. See the sidebar, "Creating wholeness" later in this chapter.

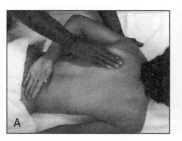 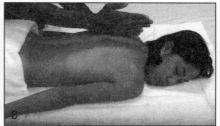

Figure 11-5: More moves for the back.

Creating wholeness

You can create a better experience for your partner if you never really "finish" one part of the body. Because, if you finish, that means the clock is ticking, and the massage is slowly dripping away. It's better to create the illusion of timelessness by connecting all the pieces of the massage together into one whole.

So, after you "finish" the back, that doesn't mean you shouldn't allow your hands to move there again. In fact, it's a good idea to add some "connective strokes" throughout the massage so that it feels as though you never completely finish with any particular part of the body. You can even connect the front of the body to the back by reaching beneath your partner during certain moves, as you see later in this chapter.

Back of the legs and buttocks

The buttocks contain the largest muscle in the human body, and they do a large percentage of the work. Without them, you couldn't walk, sit, or dance the "Bump." Buttocks really deserve a lot of respect, but often they've been disparaged and have unfortunately become the "butt" of many off-color jokes. Don't let this flippant attitude about buttocks keep you from spending some serious time there during your massage.

1. After you glide your way down from your partner's back and reposition yourself by your partner's legs, apply some oil to the entire back surface of one leg with firm gliding strokes, circling your outer hand around at the buttock and gliding more lightly back down.

2. Lift your partner's foot, supporting it with both of your hands while applying circular rubbing all around the ankle bone with your thumbs and fingertips of both hands, as shown in Figure 11-6a.

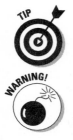

   It helps your partner relax if you can get her to "let go" of her lower leg and allow you to take the full weight of her limb in your hands. Take a look at the "Limp arm experiment" in Chapter 7 for a reminder on how to do this.

   Be careful not to press too hard directly on the upper ridges of the heel bone right behind the anklebones, because it is a sensitive area and may be uncomfortable for your partner.

3. Before you put your partner's foot back down, do some gentle shaking movements, using the foot as a "handle" to move the leg, as shown in Figure 11-6b. This can help relax the muscles of the entire limb, right up

into the joints, in this case the knee and hip. Practice until just using a gentle shaking at the foot can produce a rhythmical movement throughout the body up to the head.

4. The largest muscle in the calf is actually separated into two "bellies." It feels great to run your thumbs or the tips of your fingers up the middle of the calf, separating the two sides, as shown in Figure 11-6c. You can also make a straight line up on either side of the middle.

5. While you knead the calf muscle with a back and forth motion, move your hands up and down also, so you cover the entire muscle, as shown in Figure 11-6d. Stop about ⅔ of the way down from the knee because the calf tapers down to the Achilles tendon there and becomes too thin to knead. At that point, you can continue by squeezing the tendon between your thumb and fingers down to the ankle.

6. Grasping the leg just above the ankle with both hands, use the webbing between your thumbs and forefingers to create a tight seal. Then squeeze in and push up at the same time, moving slowly, as shown in Figure 11-6e. Stop when you reach the back of the knee. With this maneuver, you can actually help move stagnant blood out of the limb, improving circulation. If you do it correctly, this move may incite your partner to say something like, "Whoa, that's intense!" Take this as a sign that you're doing things right, but also make sure that you're not squeezing too hard. There's a fine line between intense and painful.

Remember to apply only very slight pressure over the back of the knee! And be careful to avoid any varicose veins.

7. Making your hands into fists, apply pressure with the knuckles into the back of the upper legs, called the hamstrings, as shown in Figure 11-6f. Knuckling is a form of gliding that is especially appropriate to this area because each knuckle slides between the long bands of muscles here.

8. This move feels like an ice cream sundae for the leg muscles. Knead from the top of the leg down to the knee, moving up and down three to four times. To make this move most effective, try keeping as much of your hand in contact with the skin as possible as you squeeze, roll, and push.

9. Depending upon how big any particular buttock is, you have a variety of choices of where to press, but to be most effective you have to find just the right spot. In order to do that, palpate the outer upper edge of the tailbone (sacrum), and then go straight down toward the leg half way across the buttock. This should be right in the middle. Press directly in here with thumbs, as shown in Figure 11-6g. Use your fingers, fist, or elbow at an angle perpendicular to the surface. Hold this move for 5 to 10 seconds. This move is particularly beneficial for sciatica pain.

Turning over

In my opinion, not enough is said about the art of turning over during massages. Often, this turn is the only physical effort a massage recipient has to make for over an hour. And, as it comes right in the middle of the experience, there's a potential for it to be disruptive and a little jarring. For these reasons, most massage pros are quite gentle with their clients when it comes time for them to turn. In a soft, soothing voice, they say something like, "All right, Mr. Smith, I'm going to ask you to gently roll over onto your back now. Take your time."

You have to watch your wording carefully because there are those who take what you say too literally. I have one client who is a world-class athlete, and once when I asked him to "flip

over," he literally flipped, springing a foot off the table and twisting over in midair to come crashing back down on the table, splintering one of its wooden legs.

When it comes time for your own partner to turn over, follow the example of the pros:

- ✔ Be gentle

- ✔ Speak softly

- ✔ Give them as much time as they need

- ✔ Assist them if necessary, offering support

- ✔ Use the words "roll over" or "turn gently, please" instead of "flip"

10. Knead the thick muscles of the buttocks, particularly on the upper, outside portion, which often tends to be the most sore, as shown in Figure 11-6h. You have to watch where your fingers are going while you squeeze, roll, and push here, though! It's kind of a tight area to work in.

11. Because the buttocks include the largest muscles in the body, they can withstand some heavy percussion movements. Use loose fists and firm pressure, but be sure not to pound with your fists on the tailbone, which is much more delicate. Then move the tapping down the leg, opening your fists so that you're doing karate-chop moves. Remember to lighten up over the back of the knee!

12. Apply light fingertip brushing up the back of the leg and onto the back, then back down again. After pummeling, pressing, squeezing, and kneading your way across your partner's back, fingertip brushing is a really good way to remind your partner how nice you are. You can extend the move from the feet all the way to the head.

After you finish the first leg, switch to the other leg and repeat. Remember, because you already connected the back with the first leg, you want to do some connecting strokes when you begin the second leg as well. So, make your initial gliding on the second leg go up and over the buttocks and onto the lower back.

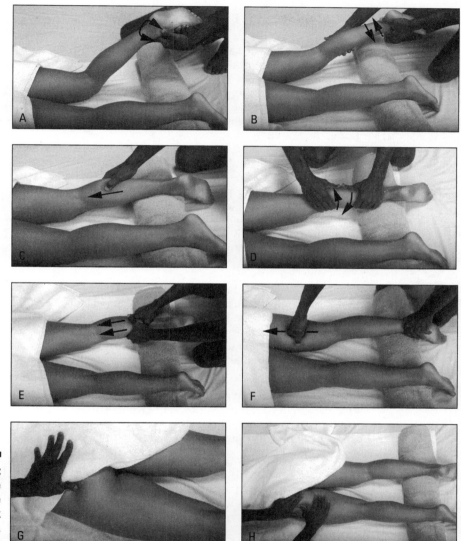

Figure 11-6:
Giving the back of the legs a kick in the pants.

Face and scalp

After your partner has turned over, you are presented with entirely different terrain to massage. The front of the body is a little more perplexing. There are more intricate surfaces to deal with, as well as more private, vulnerable, and delicate areas. Therefore, you need to be more of a diplomat while massaging the front of someone's body. Most people allow just about anyone to give them a backrub, but when it comes time for you to touch the front of their body, they have to trust you.

The face, for example, is quite a private area. Although it's exposed to the world for all to see, it's not there for all to touch. You have to be sensitive as you begin to massage your partner's face. Avoid large gestures, or quick movements. All of your maneuvers here, including those you make before you even touch your partner, should be smooth, deliberate, and slow.

You probably don't need any extra oil for the face. The oil left over on your hands from massaging the back is sufficient.

1. Start by placing your hands gently on the side of your partner's head, thumbs resting on the forehead. This is the perfect position from which to start massaging the forehead with some thumb gliding and firm circular rubbing. First, glide your thumbs out from the middle toward the sides, starting low by the brow, making three to four lines progressively higher. Then begin making circles with your thumbs, as shown in Figure 11-7a, all across the forehead.

2. Leaving your hands in about the same position, begin using the fingertips instead of the thumbs. Circle your fingertips into the side of the head around the spot where sideburns would start if your partner had some, as shown in Figure 11-7b.

3. Using the tips of your first two fingers, trace around the edges of the bones that surround the eye — across the brow, down along the nose, and around the top of the cheek bones, as shown in Figure 11-7c. You may try a little mini-kneading along the same path with your thumbs and fingertips.

   If you apply pressure very near the eyes or directly on the eyelids, make sure your partner isn't wearing contact lenses.

4. Glide your fingertips lightly across the top and down along the sides of the nose, being careful not to block your partner's breathing passages. At the base of the nose, near the outside edge of the nostrils, is a good place to apply light to moderate pressure and small circular rubbing, as shown in Figure 11-7d, which helps open sinuses in the area.

5. Use your thumbs in an "opening" gesture to fan out across the cheeks from just under the inside corner of the eye down toward the jawbone. The pressure you apply should be light to medium.

6. At the corner of the jawbone, slightly in front of and below the ear, you find the chewing muscles. In order to palpate them, ask your partner to clench her teeth, which makes these muscles bulge slightly out to the side. Then apply circular rubbing with the fingertips, as shown in Figure 11-7e, all around this area. Locate the highest point on this muscle, directly in the center, and use some pinpoint pressure directly inward for 5 to 10 seconds while suggesting to your partner, "relax your jaw, let your mouth open slightly, and just breathe."

7. Use some pinch and roll kneading to walk your fingers and thumbs from the jaw muscles out onto the chin, as shown in Figure 11-7f. Glide back softly and repeat twice more.

8. Most people love for you to massage their ears. Use your fingers and thumbs to pinch and roll the ear from the lobe up around the edges to the top, as shown in Figure 11-7g. Repeat this twice and then tug gently for a second on the top, back, and bottom of the ear.

9. The scalp is often mistaken for a thin flap of skin without much potential for massage moves, but actually it's a great place to use medium to deep circular rubbing with the fingertips, as shown in Figure 11-7h. Keep lifting your fingers up slightly, moving them a half-inch or so, then placing them firmly on the scalp again. During the rubbing, keep your fingers glued to the scalp and move the muscles below it over the cranium. Be careful not to pull your partner's hair while doing this move.

TIP

Favorite places

Everyone has his or her own particular favorites when it comes to getting a massage. Some swoon over an ear massage, while others go into ecstasy as soon as you lay a finger on their forehead. Oftentimes, you can find these "favorite places" somewhere on the head, neck, or face, although other areas like the hands and feet are popular, too.

Encourage your partner to communicate with you about any areas that feel particularly therapeutic or pleasurable. Then, during her next massage, spend more time focusing on the area she likes the most. She'll enjoy the sensation and appreciate you for remembering.

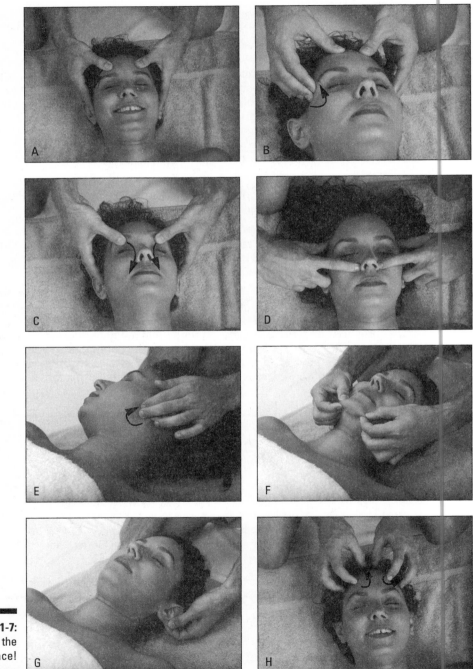

Figure 11-7:
Face the
face!

Neck and shoulders

We refer to just about anything that bothers us as a "pain in the neck." Perhaps this is because the neck is particularly vulnerable to feeling pain. Filled with delicate nerves, vertebrae, and vessels, your neck can give you pain if you simply turn your head too quickly. Massage is a great way to soothe some of the minor complaints that people experience in this area, many of which are a reaction to stress. Be especially sensitive when massaging here, "tuning in" to your partner's muscles and letting what you find guide your movements. Sometimes, simply by adding your awareness to the equation, you can help your partner get rid of that pain in the neck she's been complaining about.

1. The "shoulder swoop" move may be a little tricky at first, but after you master it you have a great tool under your massage belt. Pouring a small amount of oil into one palm, rub your hands together, then place them on your partner's upper chest, with your fingers pointing inward, as shown in Figure 11-8a. Slide your hands outward, pivoting your palms on top of the shoulder so that your fingers end up beneath your partner's upper back, as shown in Figure 11-8b. Finally, glide your hands in and up the back of your partner's neck to the base of her head, lifting slightly while you do so, as shown in Figure 11-8c.

2. Slip your fingers beneath your partner's neck, cradling her head in your hands. Then lift very gently just until you can turn her head to one side, supporting it in your bottom hand. Rock her head back and forth slightly until your partner no longer tries to hold onto her own neck muscles. You can then use the other hand to apply circular rubbing to the muscles in the back of the neck, as shown in Figure 11-8d. Move your circles up and down, and when you find a tense spot, apply some pinpoint pressure. By using both hands for different purposes (one massaging, the other cradling the head), you have extra-effectiveness with this move.

3. Still supporting your partner's head in one hand, use the other to knead up and down the back of the neck. Practice switching the position of your hands during this maneuver until you can create a fluid sensation for your partner — left, right, left, right. This feels darn good.

4. Supporting your partner's head with both hands, lift up and forward, bringing her chin toward the chest, as shown in Figure 11-8e. Hold this position for about 5 seconds, being careful not to twist your partner's neck. Then slowly lower her head back down. I believe this is the only stretch you should try with the neck until you receive further training.

5. Pushing down with your palms, glide across the tops of your partner's shoulders, also known as the trapezius muscles. As a more intense alternative to this move, you may try using the knuckles to glide in this area, too.

6. Take the muscles on top of your partner's shoulders between your thumbs and fingers, kneading with a good amount of pressure, as shown in Figure 11-8f. As your fingertips reach down beneath your partner's back, curl them up so you're applying pressure in that area at the same time.

7. Now that the neck and shoulders are warmed up and relaxed, use some pinpoint pressure with your thumbs to zero in on the tight spots you find, as shown in Figure 11-8g. Remember to keep a straight line from your elbows and shoulders to your thumb so you don't stress your joints.

To create a smooth transition, finish the neck and shoulder area with another shoulder swoop. Then move down onto your partner's left shoulder and arm with a long flowing glide, which leaves you in position to begin massaging the hand.

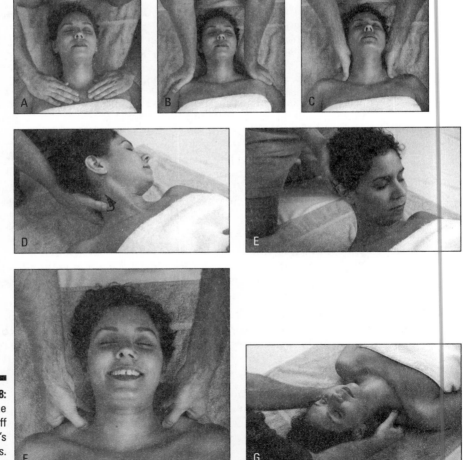

Figure 11-8:
Taking the burden off someone's shoulders.

Arms and hands

Arms and hands are some of the most active parts of most people's bodies. Think about it. Even couch potatoes use their arms and hands to reach for the potato chips and open cans of beer. In fact, just about everybody is so used to doing things with their arms and hands that, at first, you may find it challenging to get your partner to "let go" in this area (see the "Limp arm experiment" in Chapter 7 for help in getting your partner to "let go"). However, this doesn't mean that you can't perform some spectacularly beneficial and pleasurable massage moves here.

The secret of good arm and hand massage is to make your moves smaller and to focus on the little details. Every pinkie finger counts!

A typical reaction you may get when you begin massaging in this area is, "I didn't know my arms were so sore until you started doing that!" Good massage techniques can put vitality back into this active, expressive part of your partner's anatomy.

1. Your initial gliding in this area spreads the oil, of course, but it also does much more. At this time, you help your partner "let go" and loosen up. You accomplish this by offering some support to the limb at the wrist and elbow while you're gliding. This means you're actually picking the arm up and supporting it with one hand while gliding with the other. Practice switching hands with this lift-support-glide maneuver until you get fluid with it.

2. Begin kneading the palm. You've already picked up your partner's hand, so you're in the perfect position for this move. You can flip your partner's hand up and down to work at different angles, spreading open and squeezing between the bones of the palm.

3. You have to build up a little dexterity in your fingers in order to get this knuckle rolling technique down. One at a time, curl your fingers closed into a fist then open them back up again over your partner's palm, as shown in Figure 11-9a.

4. Squeeze each finger as you pull slightly at the same time, moving up from the base of the finger to the tip, as shown in Figure 11-9b. Make sure to rub the sides of the fingers as well as the tops and bottoms.

5. The pressure point in the webbing between one's thumb and index finger is especially good for helping to relieve headache pain. The best way to massage it is with direct pressure from your thumb, as shown in Figure 11-9c. Hold this pressure point, pushing in toward the bones of the hand, for approximately 5 seconds.

6. This little move feels surprisingly good. While holding your partner's hand palm-down, you apply circular rubbing over the top of the wrists, as shown in Figure 11-9d. For serious wrist problems such as *carpal tunnel syndrome* (CST), see Chapter 13.

7. The forearms are jam-packed with muscles all crying out for attention. In this move, you use your thumbs to trace lines straight up the forearms from the wrists to the elbows, as shown in Figure 11-9e. This is a deep gliding that is meant to sink down between the bands of muscle in this area.

There are special massage moves for the forearm that are effective on tennis elbow, and you can find out about them in Chapter 16.

8. Your kneading movements on the forearms are basically a smaller version of the ones you used on the legs, but this doesn't mean they aren't just as effective. Try to get as much of the muscle tissue between your thumb and fingers as possible, and remember to involve your whole body in the movement, all the way down to your hips, as shown in Figure 11-9f.

9. With your partner's elbow bent and resting on the ground for support, encircle the arm at the wrist with both of your hands, creating a tight seal around the entire circumference. Then begin pushing up the arm *very slowly* until you reach the elbow, maintaining firm pressure the whole time. This "squeezing toothpaste through a tube" glide is great for tired, achy arms that need some renewal.

10. In order to massage the entire upper arm from one simple position, lift your partner's arm up, supporting it at the elbow, allowing her hand to fall back toward the floor near her head. Then use your free hand to massage the upper arm. For example, in Figure 11-9g the left arm is supported by your left hand, allowing the right hand to massage the biceps. In Figure 11-9h, your right hand supports the elbow, leaving the left hand free to massage the triceps.

As you're doing this move, make sure to keep track of where your partner's hand is. If you're banging it against the side of her head, it detracts from the pleasure of the experience.

This is a perfect position for stretching the upper arm and chest, too, and you find instructions on how to do just that in Chapter 16.

11. Grasping your partner's hand near the wrist, shake the whole arm gently until you can see some movement way up at the shoulders, neck, and head. Try positioning her arm at three different angles to achieve a different stretch on the shoulder joint: down by her side, out at a 90-degree angle, and up by her head.

12. Finish the arm with a light fingertip glide that floats up over the shoulder to the chest, where you're going to massage next.

    Repeat this sequence on the opposite arm.

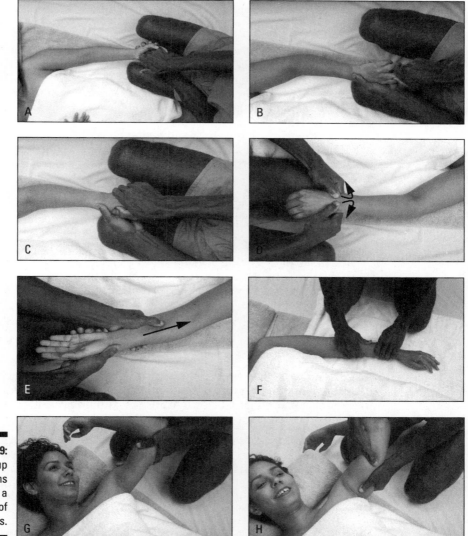

Figure 11-9: Taking up arms against a sea of troubles.

Torso

As a species, we've taken a big collective risk by standing erect on two feet and exposing our defenseless underbellies to the world. The front of your body, especially the abdomen, can be a very vulnerable area, and you have to be extra sensitive when applying massage moves here.

Your abdomen is the physical home of many emotional realities such as fear, anger, and intuition. That's why we say we have a "gut instinct" about something. You're not just massaging a stomach when you place your hands on your partner's belly. You're massaging her soul. This fact has been recognized by many Asian cultures, such as the Japanese, for example, who have even given this soul-in-the-belly a name: the *hara*.

Make your movements on the chest and abdomen gentle at first, until your partner relaxes a little and allows you to massage more deeply. Keep in mind that your touch here penetrates to the deepest layers, both physically and psychologically.

1. Place your thumbs across your partner's upper chest muscles below the collar bone, with your fingers reaching down toward his sides, as shown in Figure 11-10a. Begin some kneading, which, as you soon discover, is a tricky maneuver to perform without causing your partner to squirm and writhe in fits of hysterical giggling. Yes, this area can be quite ticklish. Start out gingerly, like a kitten pawing a pillow, then gradually intensify, always staying within your partner's comfort level.

    This area can be extremely sensitive, especially on people who exercise a lot or who are overly ticklish. Be careful not to poke your fingers into your partner's ribs or armpits. And make sure to use extra oil if your partner has a lot of chest hair.

2. Lifting your hands off the chest just slightly, begin pressing back down by using pinpoint pressure of the thumbs along a line about two inches below the collar bone, as shown in Figure 11-10b. This can have a beneficial effect on your partner's breathing, "opening" the upper ribcage.

3. Placing your fingertips near the top of the breastbone, push in gently and then begin circular rubbing as you move slowly down toward the abdomen, as shown in Figure 11-10c. As your fingers skim over the edges of the breastbone on either side, you find ridges and valleys where the ribs attach. Make a small circle in each one of these valleys, too, as you move down.

4. Gliding on the abdomen not only spreads oil and relaxes muscles; it also aids digestion. Your large intestine runs clockwise starting on the lower right-hand portion down by your hip bone, up along your side, across

the base of your ribs, and down your left side. When you massage in this same direction (clockwise), you're helping the digestive organs do their job. Press in with firm but sensitive pressure so your movements affect these organs as well as the muscles on top of them, as shown in Figure 11-10d.

When you get really good at circling your hands over the belly, try speeding up your movements a little by letting your left hand glide right over the top of the right each time they cross paths, without pausing to lift the left hand up. This creates a smoother flow for you and a neat sensation for your partner.

5. Right around the navel, in the pit of the belly, is where people often store pent-up emotions. By gently touching several points here, applying just the softest pressure inward, as shown in Figure 11-10e, you can help coax the emotions out. It's possible that your partner may sigh with relief or even begin to cry when you press here with sensitivity and compassion. This is a good time to offer nonjudgmental support and perhaps even suggest a positive image, or visualization, your partner can focus on. See the sidebar, "Visualize whirled peas," later in this chapter.

6. This move offers a chance to massage the lower back while your partner is lying face up, and it's a nice stretch, too. Slide both hands over the waist until the fingertips slip down all the way to meet at your partner's spine. Then curl the fingertips up to apply a little pressure as you simultaneously lift the whole lower back a fraction of an inch upwards and glide your hands back toward the abdomen, as shown in Figure 11-10f. Repeat this move three times.

During this move, make sure you're not putting too much strain on your own back. Position yourself close to your partner's side, and use your legs and hips to do the lifting.

7. Finish the abdomen with a glide that swoops around your partner's side at the hipbone, onto the front of the legs, and then down to the feet.

Front of the legs and feet

Think of how many miles your feet and legs have put in for you, selflessly hanging around beneath the rest of your body, taking you everywhere you want to go, seldom asking for anything in return. The average person doesn't realize how great a good leg and foot massage feels, and so you can surprise your partner with the simple, effective techniques in this section.

You finish the full body massage on the legs and feet because this is where we stand, literally. Ending here leaves your partner feeling more grounded and "down to earth."

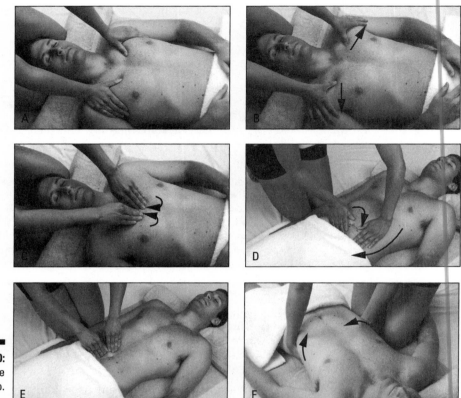

Figure 11-10:
Torquing the
torso.

Feel free to spend some extra time on the feet. Although the full foot massage isn't described until Chapter 14, you can incorporate many of those moves here as well.

1. Begin by pushing in with both thumbs on the bottoms of your partner's foot and then "spread" the sole open as you move your thumbs out toward the side, as shown in Figure 11-11a. Use firm pressure and repeat this move three times.

2. By using the thumb on the sole and forefinger on top of your partner's foot, rub between the long bones of the foot, as shown in Figure 11-11b. You should find a "groove" between the bones that you can easily slip your finger into.

Make sure to press sideways, as well as inwards, against the foot bones.

3. Holding the top of your partner's foot in one hand, use the knuckles of the other hand to "rake" into the arch of the foot in a continuous one-knuckle-at-a-time movement, starting with the pinkie finger, ring finger,

middle, then index, over and over, as shown in Figure 11-11c. Done correctly, this move feels exquisite, but you have to build up considerable finger dexterity to achieve that.

4. As if you were squeezing a coin, rub each toe between your index finger and thumb, as shown in Figure 11-11d. Start with the little toe and progress toward the big toe, making sure to rub on the sides of the toes as well as the tops and bottoms.

5. Then, find the exact location of your partner's shin bone, also called the tibia, and then apply firm pressure with both of your thumbs together along the outside (lateral) edge of this bone as you glide your way slowly up toward the knee, as shown in Figure 11-11e.

6. You have to use mostly the tips of your thumbs and fingertips to knead effectively on the front of the lower leg because, as you may notice, the front of the lower leg is mostly bone. Contain your kneading/squeezing movements to the fleshy areas on either side of this bone as you move up and down from near the ankle up to the knee, as shown in Figure 11-11f.

Visualize whirled peas

At many points during the massage, you can offer a visualization to help your partner relax and melt more fully into the experience. These visualizations usually incorporate three ingredients:

- ✔ A reminder about how important it is to breathe during the experience.

- ✔ Some guidance about what specifics to think about during the visualization.

- ✔ A positive message meant to uplift your partner's state of mind.

I cover breathing pretty extensively in Chapter 7. After you have your partner breathing evenly and deeply, then it's time to suggest an image to visualize, and when it comes to visualizations, concrete is better than vague. Make the images you suggest extremely specific, including textures, colors, sounds, and even aromas.

An example of something vague to visualize is World Peace. Plenty of people may tell you to visualize it, but how do you do that? What does

world peace look like? What color is it? How big is it? How would it taste? Does it need any salt?

I personally find it much easier to imagine smushed vegetables, which perhaps explains the existence of a well-known bumper sticker that urges us to "visualize whirled peas." It may sound silly at first, but can't you just see them there, swirling around topsy-turvy inside the blender, eventually turning to green mush as the blades increase from chop to blend to puree?

Of course, the image of pureed peas itself is not enough for a fully effective visualization. You have to include the ever-important uplifting New Age message, which in this case may well be, "See the color green as a vast see of tranquility. Imagine each pea as a grain of green sand on an unending beach of bliss."

Or something like that.

7. Reaching around behind your partner's knee with your fingertips, lift slightly while making circles over the sides of the knees with your thumbs, as shown in Figure 11-11g. Use moderate pressure inward against the knee while making this move, and monitor your partner's response closely; some people are ticklish in this area.

8. Continuing up over the knees, use your palms to glide with firm pressure in an upward direction on the front of the thigh, also known as the quadriceps muscles. Slide back down the thigh with light pressure and repeat four to five times.

9. Apply kneading to the front of the thighs. This is where you can use some really big movements, sliding your hands all the way from the inside of the thigh to the outside in a constant motion. Remember to use your whole body to create the kneading motion, not just your arms and hands. And don't be surprised if you work up a sweat during this move.

10. Imagine a line running along the outside of your partner's thigh from knee to hip (right where the stripe is on many warm-up suits). Starting at the knee, apply pinpoint pressure with your thumbs to a series of points along this line, as shown in Figure 11-11h. Hold each point for 3–5 seconds, then release and move up to the next point. When you reach the hip, slide back down and repeat one more time.

This area is often very sensitive on many people, so you have to be careful when pressing here. Start out softly and increase pressure gradually. You can tell if you push too hard by noticing that your partner tenses his leg. If this happens, lighten your pressure.

11. This is an advanced move that requires quite a bit of trust on your partner's part. You are putting him in a vulnerable position, one leg bent at the knee, with the hip open to the side. By using your palms, press down firmly just above the knee, then glide slowly up toward the hip, as shown in Figure11-12a. For even more intensity, use your knuckles instead of your palms. Glide your hands back down to the knee with light pressure then repeat twice more.

Lighten your pressure as you approach the upper thigh, which contains many delicate nerves and vessels.

12. Lay your partner's leg flat again, and then glide your hands upwards over the thigh. When you reach the hip, swivel your outside hand around and slip your fingers toward your partner's lower back, as shown in Figure 11-12b. Glide up as far as you can alongside the spine, then press your fingers up into the muscles there as you slowly pull back down toward the hip again, letting some of your partner's weight do the work of pressing. When you reach your partner's leg again, continue gliding down by using both hands on the back of the leg, lifting slightly to get your hands underneath. Finish your glide down at the foot.

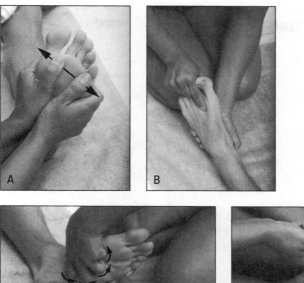

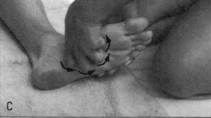

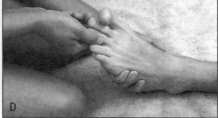

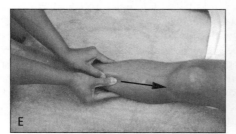

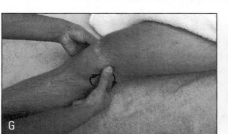

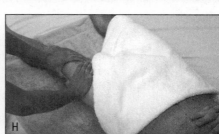

Figure 11-11:
Fleet moves
for the feet
and legs.

13. Cupping the heel in your palm, lift your partner's leg just an inch or so, reminding him to "let go" if he tries to lift the leg for you. Shake back and forth with a vibrating motion.

14. Your last move on the leg is a light fingertip brushing down from the hips toward the feet to leave your partner feeling "grounded."

Repeat this entire sequence on the other leg.

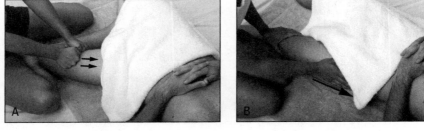

Figure 11-12:
Finishing up
the feet and
legs.

The grand finale

As with so many things in life, like fireworks and circus acts, in massage it's the grand finale that really counts. Sure, you can apply superlative techniques all throughout the massage; flowing from one bliss-inducing maneuver to the next in seamless perfection; but if you finish with a ho-hum squeeze of the toes and then rush off to grab a cold one from the fridge, you're going to leave a slightly disgruntled partner behind. It's like watching a good movie with a bad ending: All anyone can talk about is how bad the ending was, not how good the rest of the movie was.

The way you end the massage leaves a lasting impression. To make your finish the best it can be, follow these steps:

1. Use long gliding strokes that flow over the entire body, starting at the feet and moving up onto the torso then down the arms, as shown in Figure 11-13. This is the lightest kind of long-soft-light gliding, not meant to actually affect the tissues beneath the skin, but rather to send your partner a message of connection (see the sidebar, "Creating wholeness," earlier in this chapter).

You don't have to wait until the end of the massage to use *connective strokes.* In fact, you can use them throughout the entire massage to connect everything together. Starting an arm? Connect it to the neck you just finished a moment earlier. Go ahead, experiment. Connect away! The point is to make your partner feel that you're treating his body as a whole, not segmenting it into chunks.

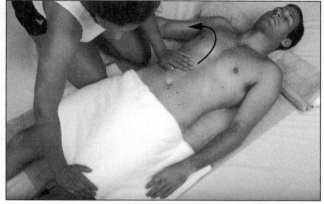

Figure 11-13:
Whole-body connective strokes create a sense of wholeness and continuity for your partner at the end of a massage.

2. To finish your massage, place one hand on your partner's forehead and the other gently upon his belly, letting them rest there in contact, but without pressure, for 30 to 60 seconds, as shown in Figure 11-14. You may begin to feel his pulse, or some warmth emanating from his body. This is good. Just tune in to whatever it is you're feeling and, for just these last few seconds, make sure your partner knows he's the center of the universe.

This type of intentional hand placement to balance your partner's inner energy is known in some quarters as *polarity*.

The last moment of the massage is as important as the first. When you finally break contact with your partner for the last time, make it a conscious, gentle letting go.

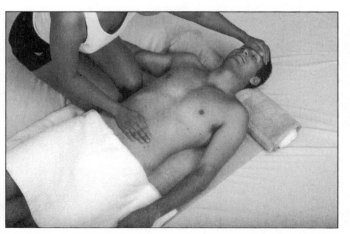

Figure 11-14:
Placing your hands softly on two areas also creates a sensation of connection.

Part IV
Massage at Work

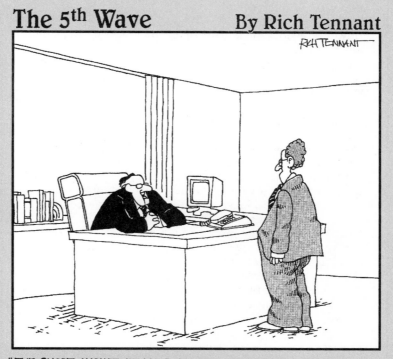

The 5th Wave   By Rich Tennant

"THE SHORT ANSWER TO YOUR REQUEST FOR A RAISE IS 'NO'. THE LONG ANSWER IS 'NO, AND GET OUT OF MY OFFICE.'"

In this part . . .

Not too long ago, work used to be a very physical activity for almost everybody on the planet. Sure, there were always a few pharaohs, high priests, and ladies-in-waiting whose main activity was flicking fingers and shouting commands, but for 99.99 percent of humanity throughout our entire history, "work" meant physical work, and we used our bodies a lot.

As you may have noticed, this is not the case anymore. In a sense, we've all become pharaohs, masters of a digital domain in which we push around bits of data as if they were slaves. Click a button, and your wish is executed. Most of us check our bodies at the door when we walk into work each morning.

However, even though many of us don't use them as much anymore, our bodies are still subject to high levels of stress and strain. Recently in the U.S. alone, absenteeism went up 25 percent in one year, and stress was the top reason sited for missing work.

Luckily, massage is here for us, ready to breathe some life back into our corporate bodies. It is now possible for massage to become a part of your life at work, where you may need it the most. I'm talking about corporate massage here, which is the subject of Chapter 12, in which you find out how to take advantage of the growing number of massage pros who specialize in on-the-job stress reduction.

Of course, a massage pro might not always be available, and you need to know how to de-stress yourself on the job too. Chapter 13 is all about self-massage and stretching that you can do right at the desk or workstation. In addition to relaxation techniques, you'll discover some basics about how to combat a very serious problem many office workers, and others, face: carpal tunnel syndrome (CTS).

The work environment also forces many of us, especially females, to wear strange, sadistic contraptions on our feet, what Steve Martin called "cruel shoes." We then walk around on hard, unnatural surfaces all day, until our feet end up needing some serious massage attention of their own. Chapter 14 explains reflexology, a type of massage that concentrates on the feet, with the added benefit of affecting the entire body through its actions as well.

Chapter 12

The New Coffee Break: Corporate Massage for a Digital Generation

- -

- -

Guess which of the following touch-gurus wrote these words: "Touch is a very powerful message. It is very honest. People know immediately when you touch them if you care about them."

A. Brian Weiss, psychiatrist and author of *Many Live, Many Masters*.

B. Deepak Chopra, proponent of Ayurveda, the ancient healing science of India, and author of books such as *Quantum Healing*.

C. Ram Dass, modern mystic and author of such classics as *Be Here Now*.

D. Ken Blanchard, corporate consultant and author of the business best-seller, *The One Minute Manager*.

Strangely enough, the answer is D, and Blanchard is basically talking about a pat on the back, not a massage. But his statement does point out the great need for people in the work environment to use the right kind of touch with each other.

Appropriate, stress-relieving touch in the workplace is so important that an entirely new category of massage has been invented in the past several years to specifically address this issue. This category is called *corporate massage*, and it has become quite popular in offices and workplaces around the world. With corporate massage, a professional massage therapist comes to your office with a specially designed chair that you sit on to receive a massage with your clothes still on. This saves time and makes the whole massage procedure easy, safe, and acceptable.

You've probably heard more than you want to about sexual harassment, abuse of power, and ruined careers, but the wrong kind of touch in the workplace can get you in a lot of trouble. Corporate massage, however, can help fulfill your *touch quotient* (your natural need for touch) while in an environment that otherwise stifles much healthy contact.

Corporate Massage

Your first reaction to the thought of massage at work may be less than positive for several reasons. As you contemplate the idea, you may come up with some of the following:

✔ Can I really handle the thought of my co-workers lining up to get undressed and rubbed with almond oil in the employee lounge?

✔ What will my (wife/husband/girlfriend/boyfriend, and so on) say?

✔ Won't the boss think that this kind of massage is a waste of time? Or, if you're the boss: Won't my employees take advantage of this and turn the office into a massage parlor?

✔ Will I be in an awkward position on a table or chair and look stupid while receiving a massage at work?

✔ How much will the massage cost?

✔ Will it mess up my hair?

These concerns are all rational, and this section is meant to set you straight on what corporate massage really is so that you'll run straight out to contact your nearest practitioner and at least give it a try.

What does corporate massage look like, anyway? Well, imagine this scenario: It's late on a Friday afternoon. Your whole department has been under intense pressure to wrap up that humongous project you've been working on for months. Nerves are frayed. Happy hour is looming. No one can think about anything but escape. Then right at four o'clock, in walks a healthy-looking individual toting a strange, padded, chair-like contraption that he proceeds to unfold over in one corner. This is the "corporate massage" that your boss promised.

One brave soul offers to go first, and the rest of you watch while he sits down — fully clothed — on the device, which seems to support all of his weight easily at the knees, elbows, chest, and head. As he leans forward and relaxes, you can feel the pressure on your own limbs start to dissipate, too. The massage therapist begins with some strong kneading of the shoulders and upper back.

"Ahh, this is great!" roars your co-worker through the circular face rest. Quietly, but quickly, people start to drift over to that side of the room, and soon a line begins to form. One after another, everyone is treated to ten minutes of much-needed relief, and a funny thing starts to happen. Happy hour is no longer calling so urgently. As you stand around chatting with newly relaxed colleagues, the ideas begin to flow again, and you end up staying till after 7 p.m., coming up with a few great new concepts that will make this project even better.

Yes, scenarios like this one can actually occur. Massage in the workplace has many such benefits, including the following:

- ✔ Increases employee morale

- ✔ Lowers stress

- ✔ Decreases overuse injuries

- ✔ Provides some high-touch to counterbalance high-tech environments

- ✔ Offers employees something new and different

The benefits of this type of massage quickly outweigh the concerns I mention at the beginning of this section:

- ✔ Nobody has to undress, and if they really don't want their hair messed up, they just have ask the massage therapist not to massage their head.

- ✔ The massage is usually given in a public space and is very conservative.

- ✔ The boss realizes that happy employees are productive employees.

- ✔ Employees who receive this extra benefit are more likely to feel grateful and be more responsible.

So you're left with one last issue — who pays for all this? Normally, payment is handled in one of three ways:

- ✔ **The company pays:** This scenario, which is the most common, allows employees to forget about whether or not they can afford the massage, and it makes the boss look great.

- ✔ **Everyone contributes to a pool:** This scenario is less common, but some companies still choose it. Pulling those few dollars out of your pocket may hurt at first, but what you receive is better for you than the typical office-pool birthday cakes.

- ✔ **Everyone pays separately:** This scenario is the least common. Though it may prove quite popular, paying separately often leaves people feeling a little at loose ends. Should they pay? Should they not pay?

No matter what the scenario, the massage therapists often appreciate tips, unless everyone is aware that a service charge has been added up front.

Either way, the massage more than pays for itself almost immediately. A massage pro brought in once a week or once a month can truly upgrade the total work experience of everyone involved.

In addition to chair massage, many corporations now offer full body massage through their wellness programs, employee fitness programs, and so on. My advice? Take advantage of this benefit immediately.

Call a local corporate massage provider and ask him to come in for a free "demo-day." With the prospect of potentially gaining a new, ongoing client, he'll probably be eager for the opportunity to prove how good he is with no investment on your part. This approach is also a way to convince your boss that the expense involved is worth the improved morale and productivity. This situation is win-win-win: The massage provider wins new business. Your boss wins happier workers. And you win as the hero who introduced this great new idea to your co-workers.

Massage Chairs

Massage in the workplace goes by various names, including corporate massage, on-site massage, and chair massage. But regardless of what you call it, this type of massage is guaranteed to involve the use of a specially constructed device known as the *massage chair* (see Figure 12-1).

Massage chairs were originally developed in the U.S. by a man named David Palmer who wanted an easy way to massage his clients on the job at the Apple Computer company. Now, several models are available from a number of suppliers. The basic idea is that people can lean forward into the device, taking a load off their hips and legs and thereby position themselves perfectly to receive a back, neck, and shoulder massage. Getting into one of these things is more like lying down than sitting in a chair. Try it sometime; you'll be amazed at how supported and relaxed you feel.

Although they may look slightly intimidating at first, massage chairs are actually quite easy to get into and out of. Here's how they work:

1. **Place your knees against the pads and lean your chest forward onto the support; then wrap your hands around front and place your arms on the arm rest.**

   The chair will be adjusted for you so that the face rest is the correct height; simply lean forward into it and feel your weight shift and become distributed evenly throughout your body.

   If you're wearing a dress, you can still get on. Just swivel your legs in modestly from the side.

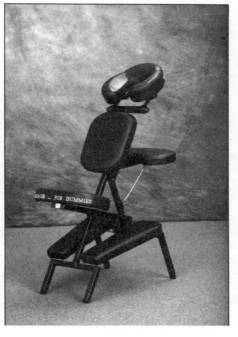

Figure 12-1:
The massage chair, a strange-looking but comfortable piece of equipment. (This one was custom made for the authors by Golden Ratio Woodworks.)

2. **Make sure that the face rest is covered with a tissue or towel, for sanitary reasons.**

   Wipe the surfaces down after each treatment to prevent body oils from building up on the material.

3. **Let the chair take your weight and the massage therapist do the rest.**

   Don't try to support yourself in any way during the massage. Just relax and enjoy!

Make a little vow to yourself right here — the next time you spy one of these strange contraptions somewhere with a massage therapist standing by ready to work, take the plunge and jump aboard. You can find them in malls, at airports, in special storefronts like The Stress Station, and even on street corners. See what happens!

Of course, not everyone has access to chair massage. Perhaps you live in a small town where no one has ever heard of this concept before. Maybe you work at a place where people would look at you like you're insane for suggesting that you pay somebody for the privilege of sitting in such a strange contraption.

Taking the chair on the road

Offices aren't the only place where massage chairs are put to good use. You also see them in the front lines at athletic events and disaster sites, among others.

For example, after Hurricane Andrew struck in south Florida, I and a crew of other massage therapists headed to the epicenter with our trusty massage chairs to provide neck, shoulder, and back relief for weary soldiers and Red Cross volunteers.

If you don't have a specially made massage chair around, you can use a normal chair to receive many of the same benefits. As shown in Figure 12-2, simply turn the chair around and sit in it backwards. Then lean forward onto a pillow while your partner works on you. The techniques pictured in this chapter are done in a professional massage chair, but you can recreate them easily at home by using this setup.

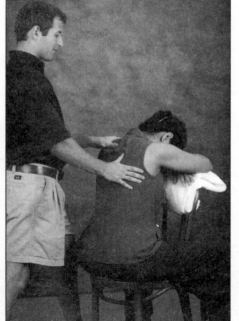

Figure 12-2:
If you don't have a custom-made, $400 massage chair, a regular chair turned backwards works pretty well, too.

The Chair Routine

Following is a simplified version of the chair massage routine that people learn in classes and workshops. You can follow it exactly or feel free to concentrate on the areas where your partner needs the most work.

You don't need any oil or cream to do this type of massage, and your partner definitely doesn't have to take his or her shirt off. Also, creating an ideal "inner chamber" (as described in Chapter 9) for this experience isn't so important either. Think of chair massage as a rough-and-ready kind of experience that you can enjoy anywhere, anytime, no matter how many distractions surround you.

The photographs in this chapter show some basic maneuvers. You're free to develop your own style based on the moves I show you in Chapter 10.

Shoulders and upper back

The shoulders — where almost everyone holds a good amount of tension — are best part of the body to begin a chair massage. After your partner is comfortably seated, start with some kneading in that area (see Figure 12-3).

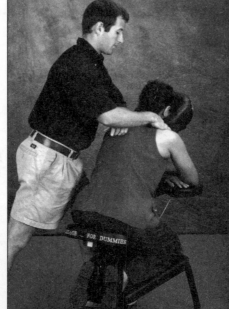

Figure 12-3:
The chair offers a perfect angle from which to work the shoulders using hands, forearms, and elbows.

1. **Grasp the tops of both shoulders firmly, with your thumbs in back and fingers in front, and then begin kneading.**

   Your kneading can be relatively firm. For variety, switch both hands to one shoulder and then the other, but return to both-shoulder kneading at the end.

2. **With your palms facing down, press the meaty underside of your forearms directly down on top of your partner's shoulders.**

   For a more intense sensation, turn your hands palm up and press the forearm bones into the shoulder.

3. **For the ultimate in pressure, bend your arm and use the point of your elbow as a finely honed instrument to zero in on tight spots atop the shoulders.**

   Use the fingers of your other hand to guide the elbow precisely into place, and then ease slowly into pressing because this move is very intense.

4. **Stepping back a couple feet, *lean* into your partner's back, supporting yourself with your thumbs against the ridge of muscles on either side of the spine.**

   Lean back, slide down, and press again, hitting several points down along the spine to mid-back.

5. **With your elbow on the muscles alongside the spine, hit roughly the same points that you did with your thumbs.**

   Be careful not to press directly against the spine with your elbows as this could be quite painful.

Arms

When a person is seated in a massage chair, her arms are easily accessible. Support the entire weight of the arm in your hands while you're working on it so your partner doesn't have to help you.

1. **Squatting or bending at your partner's side (see Figure 12-4), use both hands to encircle the arm, starting at the top near the shoulder, and then squeeze.**

   Release the squeeze, move down a couple inches, and squeeze again, repeating this process all the way to the wrist. If you want to add something to this move, try pressing with your thumbs as you're releasing pressure with your palms.

2. **Follow the hand massage routine from Chapter 11.**

   Don't languish there too long in a squatting or bending position or you'll end up with a sore back yourself.

3. **Standing up and stepping back a bit, grasp your partner's arm at the wrist and elbow then apply a little gentle shaking.**

   Afterwards, gently bring the arm back around to the front and lay it down again.

4. **Repeat the process on the other arm.**

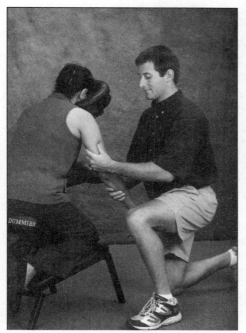

Figure 12-4:
You massage the arms from a squatting position either in front of the chair or to the side.

Lower back

The lower back is the hardest part to get to during a chair massage because it's so low. You can kneel if you want to, or squat, to make these moves more comfortable on yourself.

1. **When you finish the arms, brush lightly down the back to the lumbar area, get into a squatting or bending position again, and apply some firm pinpoint pressure (as described in Chapter 10) with the thumbs into the muscles on either side of the spine (see Figure 12-5).**

   Be careful not to press too firmly in the kidney area. (See Chapter 10 for the reasons.)

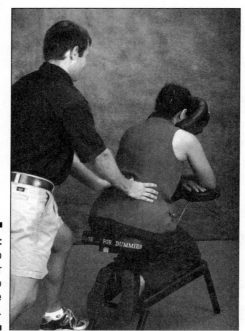

Figure 12-5:
You have to
squat or
kneel to
work the
lower back.

2. **Press in firmly with the heel of your hands against the upper portion of your partner's buttocks, and then make rapid circles with the right hand going clockwise and the left counterclockwise (see Figure 12-6).**

First made famous in the movie, *The Karate Kid*, this move incorporates a little coordination on your part, along with some good old-fashioned rubbing. I know, it's complicated, but you can do it!

Neck

As you can see in Figure 12-7, the neck is in the perfect exposed position for you to work on it to your heart's content.

1. **Standing slightly to the side, use the thumb and fingers of one hand to knead up and down the back of the neck.**

You can switch back and forth from side to side and hand to hand.

2. **Starting at the base of the skull, press in with your thumb on the muscles to one side of the spine.**

"Walk" your thumb down that muscle to the top of the shoulder, pressing in at half-inch intervals as you go. Repeat this maneuver two more times, each time slightly further away from the spine.

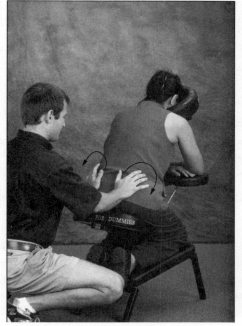

Figure 12-6:
Pressing with the heels of the palms, move the left hand counter-clockwise and the right hand clockwise.

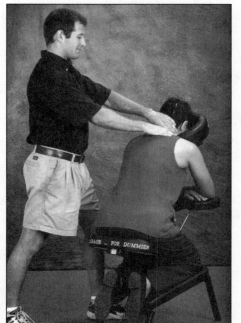

Figure 12-7:
With the head tilted slightly forward into the face rest, massaging the neck is easy.

3. **With your thumb on one side of the spine and your fingers on the other, make small firm circles on the base of the skull where it attaches to the neck.**

Head

You can modify the three steps in this section in many different ways, depending on your intentions and the situation you find yourself in. If you're giving seated massage to someone who's going out on a date ten minutes later, for example, don't mess her hair up too much because she wants to look neat when she stands up from the chair.

1. **Plant your fingertips firmly on your partner's scalp and make small circles, moving the tissue below but not sliding over the hair (see Figure 12-8).**

   Repeat in several spots. Before you start, ask your partner whether he minds having his hair messed up a bit.

2. **Reaching your fingers forward on both sides of the head, find the temples (which are partially covered by the face rest in a professional massage chair) and press in for 5 to 10 seconds.**

   This move is great for people with minor headaches.

3. **Use your fingertips and thumbs to apply mini-kneading all over the outside rims of the ears, pulling gently up on the tops and down on the lobes.**

Finish

Chair massage is usually an invigorating experience, and people often have to get back to work or another activity soon afterwards. Tapping over the entire back with moderately firm pressure of the fists or open hands is a great way to finish the experience and send them off into the world again.

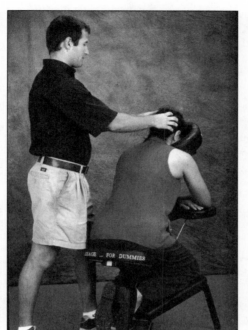

Figure 12-8:
The scalp,
temples,
and ears are
all easily
accessible
in the chair.

Chapter 13

Cubicle Maneuvers: Self-Massage for the Keyboard Jockey

*Y*ou're not always going to be able to convince somebody else to give you a massage. Like it or not, at times you'll be sore, achy, tired, emotionally needy, and just plain crying out for a massage, but the people around you will be much more interested in the football game on TV, or in going to lunch.

Don't despair. There are some simple massage techniques that you can use on yourself, without the need for anyone else's participation — or sympathy. And, coincidentally, those very techniques appear in this chapter!

These moves work equally as well at home, of course, but I'm including them here in the massage-at-work section because that's where so many people end up all stressed-out, with no outlets to relax. Sure, you can stand up in your cubicle and sing the Frank Sinatra tune, "I did it *my* way," to take a slight edge off the tension, but wouldn't quietly engaging in a few self-massage techniques be easier — and a little more discreet?

Some of these moves not only feel good, but can actually make quite a difference in your productivity level, which should make your boss happy, too. The techniques to fight carpal tunnel syndrome, for instance, can help keep you tapping away at the computer for years, and spare your company some expensive worker's comp bills at the same time.

So, limber up those fingers (use the massage-muscle building tips from Chapter 10 if you'd like) and get ready for a treatment from one of the most talented, and reliable, massage masters around — you.

Self-Massage: The Basics

Say you're sitting at your desk. Your neck is killing you, but you don't want to ask a co-worker to massage it because the other people in your office may get nervous, jealous, or both. What're you gonna do? Well, you can grab that nifty massage gizmo that you have stashed in your bottom drawer, but it makes a loud, buzzing noise. Instead, sitting right there in your chair, you can give yourself an entire mini-massage, get some good relief, and be relatively discreet.

Self-massage is as easy as following a few simple guidelines. Don't stress the rest of your body out while trying to relax one spot. Use correct *body mechanics* (see Chapter 10) while applying self-massage moves, just as you do for partner massage. Here are the basic rules for self-massage:

- **Keep breathing:** This rule holds true whether you're massaging a partner or yourself.

- **Focus on the sore spots that you find and be willing to experience a little "pleasurable pain":** At the same time, don't overdo it — self-inflicted, black-and-blue marks are hard to explain.

- **Be intuitive:** Nobody knows better than you where that tight spot is. Using the routine in this chapter as a mere template; follow your own inner guidance.

Self-Massage Mini-Routine

Keeping the points from the preceding section in mind, you can move straight into a ten-minute mini-routine right at your desk. If you're at home, you can do this on a sofa or a stool just as easily as you can on your chair at work. In fact, you can do this routine anywhere you can sit down, although you may look a little funny massaging your own feet on a city bus.

Irrigate your head

One of the biggest causes for all of your problems, whether you know it or not, is a non-irrigated head. Think about it. All day long you're walking or standing or sitting, and your head is the highest point on your body. Your heart has to pump the blood against gravity to supply your brain, which can leave you feeling foggy-headed at times. Have you ever experienced that in the middle of a long day at work? Why not help your brain stay sharp by irrigating it with extra oxygen-rich blood?

A great way to start the self-massage routine is to simply lean forward in your chair, getting your head somewhere in the vicinity of your knees. Keep your feet flat on the ground and clasp your hands behind your back, as shown in Figure 13-1. If you feel limber enough, raise your hands up toward the ceiling for a nice stretch.

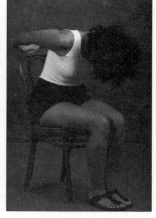

Figure 13-1:
To start the self-massage, lean forward in your chair and bring some fresh blood to your brain.

Stretch your arms and upper back

Sitting upright once again, continue your warm-up by reaching across your body with one arm and grasping it at the elbow with the opposite hand. Pull the elbow in against your chest (see Figure 13-2), which should create a stretching sensation across your shoulder. If you don't feel a stretching sensation, either you're super-limber, or you're not pulling on the elbow firmly enough.

Repeat with the other arm.

Reach around to the back of your neck this time, grasp your elbow once again and pull to the opposite side (as shown in Figure 13-3), which stretches your upper arm and further opens your shoulder joint. For an extra stretch, bend toward the side you're pulling with at the same time.

Repeat with the other arm.

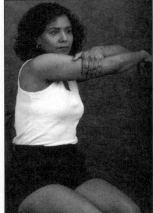

Figure 13-2: Sitting up straight again, reach across your body to stretch the shoulder and upper back.

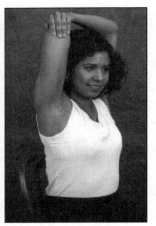

Figure 13-3: With one hand behind your head, raise the elbow, grasp it with the opposite hand, and pull for another stretch.

Massage your temples, face, and jaw

Time to start the actual massage moves. Reach up and apply circular rubbing — see Chapter 10 — to your temples, as Figure 13-4a shows. This move is a good way to combat tension headaches. Make your circles slow, deliberate, and firm, staying in contact with one area on the skin while you move over the bones below.

Sliding your fingers up on to your forehead, continue the circular rubbing until your fingers meet in the middle above the nose (see Figure 13-4b). Then push in with the fingertips and glide back toward the temples again, keeping firm pressure against the skin the whole time. Repeat two more times.

You may be surprised at how much tension gets lodged in your jaw muscles. Tension hides out there like an enemy soldier wearing camouflage gear, especially while you're sitting at your desk, straining forward to concentrate on the computer screen. With the proper pressure and sensitivity, you can flush this tension out.

Using your fingertips, press in at the angle of your jaw, and while you're pressing, open and close your mouth slightly, which allows you to find the exact point that feels like it's holding the most tension. Apply slow deep circular rubbing to that spot, plus a little pinpoint pressure (both moves are described in Chapter 10), until you feel your jaw start to relax and drop (see Figure 13-4c).

Use enough pressure with these moves to sink your fingers into the jaw muscles slightly but not so much that you feel pain. Be careful; the jaw's a sensitive area.

Using your thumbs, "hook" them in to press up against the bone just beneath your eyebrow, right next to your nose, as shown in Figure 13-4d. This is another good headache point. Hold the pressure for about 5 seconds.

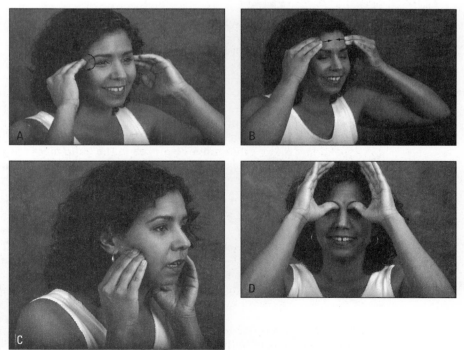

Figure 13-4:
Massaging
all around
the face.

Rub that neck

Reach around to the back of your neck with both hands and hook your thumbs up under the base of the skull (see Figure 13-5a). Press in firmly and hold for 5 to 10 seconds. This move alone should leave you feeling more alert and relaxed.

Now drop your head forward and pick a hand, any hand (probably your dominant one), to perform kneading on the back of your neck as you see in Figure 13-5b. Squeeze from the base of your neck up to your head and then back down again. Repeat twice.

Turn your head to the left and reach across with your left hand to knead atop your right shoulder and up onto your neck, using your thumb to press into any knots you find along the way (see Figure 13-5c). This move also provides a good stretch for your neck. Repeat on the opposite side.

Squeeze your arms and hands

Starting at your shoulder, begin squeezing down your arm, as shown in Figure 13-6. When you reach a tender spot, hook your thumb in and hold for a moment. Stop when you reach your wrist, glide lightly back up to your shoulder, and repeat one more time.

Repeat on the opposite arm.

Pinch the webbing between your thumb and forefinger of your opposite hand (see Figure 13-7). Hold for 5 to 7 seconds. This spot may be quite sensitive. You can also do some coin rubbing on the fingers, circular rubbing on the wrists, and any of the other moves featured in the hand massage section of Chapter 11 — modified, of course, to be performed by one hand on yourself.

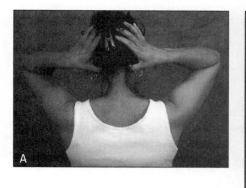
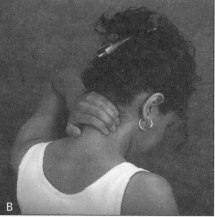
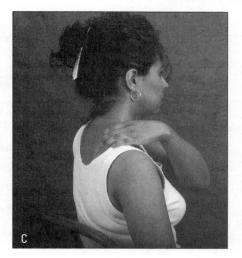

Figure 13-5:
Getting rid
of that pain
in your
neck.

Massage your lower back

Scoot forward to the front of your chair and reach around to your lower back.
Using your thumbs, press into several points along the muscles beside your
spine (see Figure 13-8). Then lift and press onto the base of your spine (the
sacrum) itself, hitting several more points. You can also use your knuckles
quite effectively in this area by balling your hand up into a fist and "rolling" it
over the area.

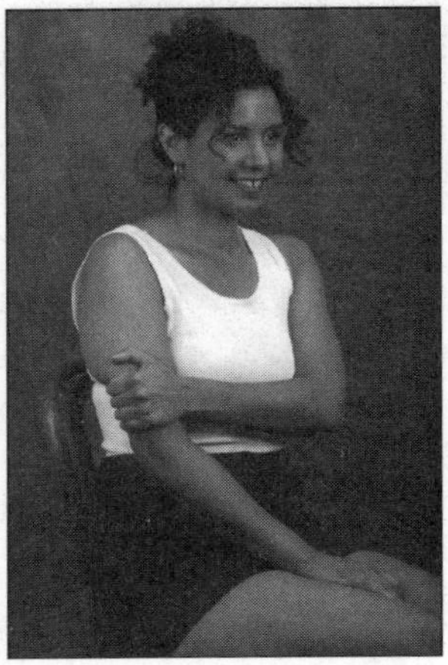

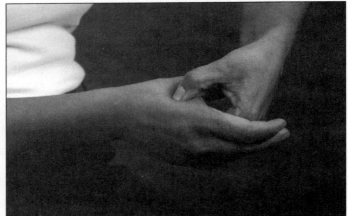

Figure 13-6:
Squeeze
down your
arm from
shoulder to
wrist.

Figure 13-7:
Press firmly
with your
thumb. This
spot some-
times helps
relieve
headaches.

Squeeze your legs

Bring one foot up onto your knee and use both hands to squeeze down all the way from your upper thigh, across the knee, and to your ankle, pressing in with your thumbs along an imaginary line down the inside of your leg. (See Figure 13-9).

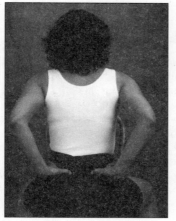

Figure 13-8:
Reach around to your lower back and use your thumbs and/or knuckles to press in.

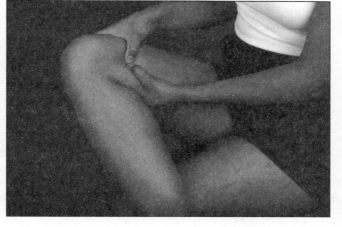

Figure 13-9:
Bend one leg and place your foot on your opposite knee to massage down your leg.

If you're in an area where you can take your shoes off, by all means do so and apply as many of the foot massage moves from Chapter 14 as you can.

When you finish the self-massage mini-routine, take a couple of deep, relaxing breaths (see the "Breathing lesson" sidebar in Chapter 7) before you dive into whatever activity you have lined up next.

Why massaging yourself feels different

You may notice that even when you apply self-massage techniques with an incredible amount of verve and enthusiasm, they still don't feel quite as good as when somebody else applies the very same moves on the very same parts of your body. But why?

The reason is simple. Massage, like tickling (you can't do that very well to yourself either), is primarily a social interaction. Studies (yes, actual tickle studies by serious researchers) have shown that preschool children couldn't be tickled when they were in a bad mood or by someone whom they didn't like. They were poked in the ribs and brushed on their feet, but the reaction was completely negative. It seems that tickling is as much about relationship and context as it is about contact. And so it is with massage. A large part of the enjoyment of a massage is the social interaction with another person, which actually causes the sensations to feel different.

Carpal Tunnel Syndrome (CTS)

You've probably heard the phrase *carpal tunnel syndrome* (CTS for short), and you know it has something to do with pain in the hand and wrist area, right? That's the "syndrome" part of the phrase. But what is the carpal tunnel anyway? An underground passage for carp? A tube running through your hand somewhere? No, the carpal tunnel is actually an area in your wrist, surrounded on three sides by the little bones of the hands (carpal bones) and on one side by the transverse carpal ligament, as shown in Figure 13-10. Several tendons pass through this "tunnel," along with the *median nerve,* a very important nerve that supplies sensation and action to most of your hand.

Inflammation or swelling of the tendons and tissues that surround the median nerve can compress it within the carpal tunnel's constricted space. This decidedly un-fun experience can cause pain, numbness, tingling, burning, and loss of hand strength, amongst other problems. Repeating the same wrist-intensive activity, such as typing on a computer keyboard, over and over and over again, triggers this inflammation.

Compression of the median nerve was recognized as a problem as far back as 1854; in 1947, Dr. George Phalen made his first diagnosis of "carpal tunnel syndrome." Today, this condition debilitates people at an alarming rate. It now affects approximately ten percent of all workers who engage in repetitive activities with their hands.

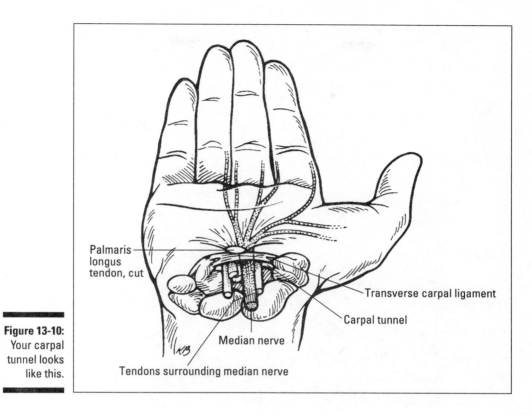

Palmaris longus tendon, cut

Transverse carpal ligament

Carpal tunnel

Median nerve

Tendons surrounding median nerve

Figure 13-10:
Your carpal tunnel looks like this.

Do you have CTS?

If you've been experiencing some funky sensations in your own hands and arms lately, don't panic. You may just have some normal aches and pains caused by overwork. A nice vacation and some well deserved wrist-rest will put you right back in shape. However, CTS is not something to take lightly. Many people end up having to undergo surgery, endure considerable pain, and lose valuable time at work because of this condition.

As with any health problem, early detection is the key to effective treatment. If you notice any of the symptoms in the following bulleted list, immediately seek medical advice, in addition to trying the exercises and massage techniques in this section:

- ✔ You wake up in the middle of the night or first thing in the morning with numbness, tingling, and an achy feeling in your hands.
- ✔ Your little finger seems to be unaffected while the rest of your fingers experience pain and numbness.

- You begin losing strength in your hands: Your grip becomes weak; you begin dropping things.
- You experience pains shooting down your forearms.
- Your hands and wrists become swollen.

One way to test yourself for CTS is to take *Phalen's test*, which is quite easy to do. Completely flex your wrists and hold the backs of your hands together — without force — for 60 seconds (see Figure 13-11). Any numbness, tingling, or pain, indicates a positive test, and you should seek a physician's opinion.

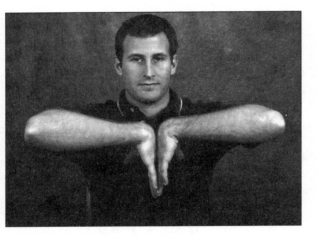

Figure 13-11: Phalen's test for CTS. The backs of your hands are together, but without pressure, for 60 seconds.

What you can do about CTS

At first, you don't have to do much to combat CTS. Simply shaking out your hands vigorously relieves the initial numbness or tingling. But the pain can progress to a point that makes your work unpleasant or even impossible. (CTS is not uncommon, by the way, in massage pros who're using their hands all day in quite intensive ways.)

The best strategy at this early stage is, of course, to stop doing what's causing the pain. However, because your pain-causing activity is often your money-making activity as well, the pain is often overruled. If you must continue the activity, you can do several things to try and improve the situation. Just one or a combination of the suggestions listed here may help you:

- **Take breaks:** Even short breaks during the work day help relieve the repetitive stresses you're putting on your hands.

- **Get ergonomic:** Make sure that your wrists are as straight as possible while working and that your back is upright. Use wrist rests for your keyboard and mouse. Don't press weight onto your wrists while working.

✔ **Immobilize it:** Use inexpensive splints and braces (available in drug and medical supply stores) to immobilize your wrist while working and even while sleeping.

✔ **Ice your wrist:** An ice pack on your wrist helps reduce the inflammation of tendons and tissues in your carpal tunnel.

✔ **Apply heat:** Heat helps soothe tightened muscles in your upper arms, shoulders, and neck that often accompany CTS.

✔ **Seek treatment**

- **Chiropractic:** Spinal adjustments may help relieve pressure on the nerves of your arm and hand, reducing pain.

- **Acupuncture:** This therapy balances the entire system and may help heal the injured nerve.

- **Ultrasound:** High-frequency sound waves may help relieve pain and inflammation.

- **Physical therapy:** Physical therapy includes many types of therapy that can help rehabilitate the wrist area after treatment.

- **Massage therapy:** Certain massage therapists are experts in CTS relief.

- **Homeopathy:** Some good anti-inflammatory ointments and creams are available that can be used alone or in conjunction with any of the other treatments. Homeopathy utilizes minute amounts of a remedy that would cause symptoms (in this case inflammation) in a healthy person.

- **Surgery:** Surgery involves cutting (and sometimes severing) the transverse carpal ligament that surrounds your wrist, which is a pretty dramatic step to take. Pressure is taken off the median nerve, and eventually scar tissue grows in to fill the gap. Sometimes, in later stages, it's the only thing that will help. But then you run the risk of re-experiencing the pain as the scar heals and the tissues tighten around the carpal tunnel once again.

✔ **Use the exercises and self-massage techniques in this section.**

Exercise and self-massage for CTS

The following are simple techniques that are meant to help, not cure, CTS. Remember, always seek the advice of a physician when treating any serious health problem.

If you want some up-to-date information on CTS, visit `www.sechrest.com/ mmg/cts/ctsintro.html`, where you can even view an animation of what CTS surgeries look like.

Chinese exercise balls

Steve Chagnon, a massage therapist who studied in China and the U.S., has developed a treatment program for CTS sufferers, and he offers a simple approach for people who want something they can do for themselves. According to him, Chinese exercise balls are an effective, consistent way to treat this situation.

Chinese exercise balls are inexpensive and widely available in department stores, specialty shops, and Chinese grocery stores. They're a little smaller than a golf ball, and they come in pairs. To use them, you put them both in one palm and rotate them around each other, using only the one hand to create the movement (see Figure 13-12).

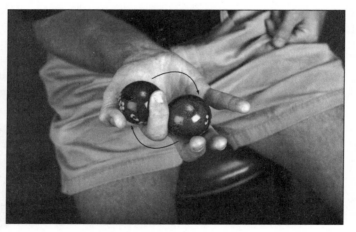

Figure 13-12:
Using the Chinese exercise balls is a quick and easy way to relieve some CTS pain.

Most squeeze-gizmos get all your muscles flexing and extending at the same time, but with the exercise balls you're only flexing one muscle at a time, in rotation, which helps to pump your lymph fluids. Traditionally, the exercise balls are said to stimulate reflex points in the palm, but this lymph-pumping action is a more important factor in addressing CTS, according to Chagnon, who believes that a build-up of lymph fluids in the wrist area is a major contributing factor to the condition (see the explanation of the lymph system in Chapter 1).

Just using the exercise balls five minutes a day will help. You may want to keep them nearby and pick them up during computer downloads or while booting up. Warming up your arm and hand muscles in this way at the beginning of a work session is especially important.

Self-massage for lymphatic drainage

"Once you realize how it works," states Chagnon, "CTS can be looked at as a plumbing problem with the lymph fluids." Since 60 percent of lymph flow is in the top ⅜ inch of your skin, all massage moves lymph. His technique, called *Specific lymphatic massage* clears superficial tissues of excess lymph fluids and in doing so reduces the volume of lymph fluids in the extremities as well.

When your hand and wrist hurt, the natural tendency is to start massaging at the site of the pain, but starting at the "lymph drain" (a point just under your right collar bone where your lymph empties back into your circulatory system) and working your way back along to the problem is actually more effective. Leave direct manipulations of your painful wrist to a massage pro instead of jabbing in there yourself, no matter how tempting it is.

Although you're working far from the painful area itself, this move helps unclog the main lymphatic drain where it all dumps out into the circulatory system at the junction of the *subclavian vein* and jugular vein. Lymph drainage massage in this area reduces hydraulic pressure on all the tissues down the arm into the wrist and carpal tunnel.

Using very light pressure (about the amount you feel when a nickel rests on your skin), lay your hand on the opposite side of your chest with your palm down and your fingers alongside the lower edge of your collar bone. Then slide your skin up over your collar bone with a very short stroke of only ¼ to ½ inch long (see Figure 13-13). Continue with this move for about 5 minutes on whichever side of your body is affected or 5 minutes on each side if you're experiencing pain in both of your hands. Then you may want to drink a glass or two of pure water to help flush your system of toxins.

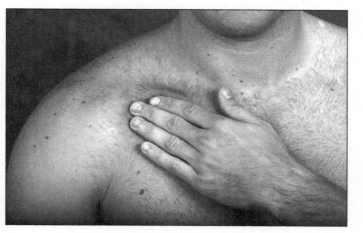

Figure 13-13: A light pressure on the skin up over your collar bone helps drain lymph from the arm, improving CTS.

Just this one move itself will offer some relief by beginning to drain lymph from the area. For more information on the technique, visit Chagnon's Web site at www.carpaltunnelmassage.com.

Another technique you can use is some self-kneading on your forearm, as shown in Figure 13-14. Overuse of the muscles in this area can be a main contributing factor to CTS, and releasing some of the tension there may help reduce pain.

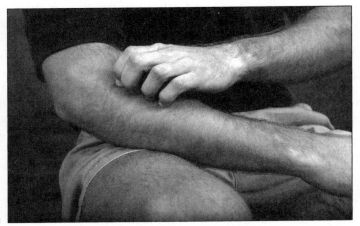

Figure 13-14:
Kneading on your forearm loosens muscles and aids circulation.

Chapter 14

Relief for the Feet with Reflexology

. . . .

In This Chapter

▶ The problem of high heels and other enemies of the feet

▶ Reflexology

▶ Foot massage routine

. . . .

*O*ne great universal truth exists outside the boundaries of any race, religion, or culture. A truth that has stood for centuries throughout human history, it is so fundamental that most of us take it for granted. That truth is this: Almost nothing beats a good foot rub.

Yes, I'm aware that some people are not big fans of foot rubs and in fact don't want their feet touched at all. In this chapter, however, I flagrantly disregard these people, because the vast majority of us absolutely love foot massage. In fact, entire civilizations have been built up and sustained for the sole purpose of giving certain people enough power, money, and influence to be able to get other people to rub their soles.

You may know a certain person in your own circle who is famous for giving "good foot." Some people seem to have a special knack for it, almost as if foot massage were a completely separate entity from body massage. Foot massage isn't really separate from the whole-body massage we discuss in Chapter 11, but feet definitely deserve a chapter of their own. After all, feet have a massage technique all their own, called *reflexology*, which we cover in this chapter.

High Heels and Other Enemies of the Feet

If you're a woman and you wear high heels, you have an especially big problem to deal with. I'll never forget the first woman I saw on my massage table with high-heelitis. She was lying down, relaxed and comfortable, but her legs and feet were still bent into the position they would have been in if her shoes had still been on — feet extended, toes pointed down, calves flexed. Extended wearing of those torture devices we know as high heels can actually change the shape of your lower body. The effects reach all the way up into your hips, lower back, and spine.

If you're a man and you wear high heels, you'll have the same problems with your calves and lower back, plus the added problem of seldom finding anything at a clothing store that truly matches your choice of footwear. What a dastardly predicament!

The common problems certain shoes cause are some of the reasons that a large number of massage pros wear Birkenstock-type sandals. We want to give our feet and bodies a little break from the pounding they take on the cruel streets of life.

Part of the reason feet get so sore is the delicate nature of their structure. They sustain your entire weight during walking, standing, running, and so on. Thousands of pounds of cumulative pressure, day in and day out, press on 26 relatively small bones. Add to that the fact that you have approximately 72,000 nerve endings in each foot, making them some of the most sensitive parts of your body, and you can see why keeping your feet happy can be a tough job.

Reflexology

The feet deserve massage, just for being feet, but another reason exists for concentrating some extra time on your feet and perhaps even devoting an entire session to foot massage. I'm talking about *reflexology*. You've probably heard this strange word somewhere before, right? Maybe on the Discovery Channel, or in a magazine with a picture of a New Age M.D. on the cover. But did you really know what the word meant? Quiz yourself by trying to complete the following sentence. Reflexology is:

    A. The practice of stimulating certain points on one area of the body (usually the feet) that have an effect on corresponding reflex areas in other parts of the body.

B. The art of developing fast reflexes for use in such real-world situations as gunfights and race car driving.

C. The act of flexing something over again after you've flexed it once already.

D. None of the above.

The answer, as you may have suspected, is A, but just knowing that doesn't do you much good, does it? Not unless you know a little of the background of reflexology and the philosophy behind this unique therapy, as well.

Zone Therapy

The origins of modern reflexology are rooted in another treatment method called *zone therapy*. In 1917, Dr. William H. Fitzgerald of Boston City Hospital published a book called *Zone Therapy, or Relieving Pain at Home*. In it, he stated that many types of health problems could be helped, or even cured, by applying pressure to various strategic points, mostly on the hands.

This whole idea did not catch on like wildfire, but one of Dr. Fitzgerald's associates, a therapist in his office named Eunice Ingham, took the idea and tweaked it a bit, experimenting with many people, mostly on their feet, which she thought were more sensitive than the hands. Eventually, she wrote her own books, *Stories the Feet Can Tell*, and that follow-up favorite, *Stories the Feet Have Told*. Ingham's work and her books heralded the birth of modern reflexology.

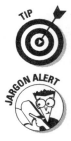

The work of Eunice Ingham is continued today at the International Institute of Reflexology, founded in 1973. You can call or write the institute to request books, charts, tools, and more.

But just what is *zone therapy* anyway? According to zone theory, your body can be divided (metaphorically, of course) into long slender pieces. Everything that's going on in any one part of a particular zone can be felt in a distant part of that same zone. You can see, then, how something happening in your abdomen can be reflected, or felt, in your foot. By stimulating a certain point in the foot, you can treat the pancreas, for example.

All of this talk about reflexes and zones may leave you feeling a little "zoned out" yourself, but don't let that worry you. The whole concept is pretty simple if you just remember that the bottoms of the two feet put together can be looked at like a miniature map of the entire body. So the head is up by the big toe, the spine goes down the middle, and so on. Figure 14-1 shows a reflexology chart.

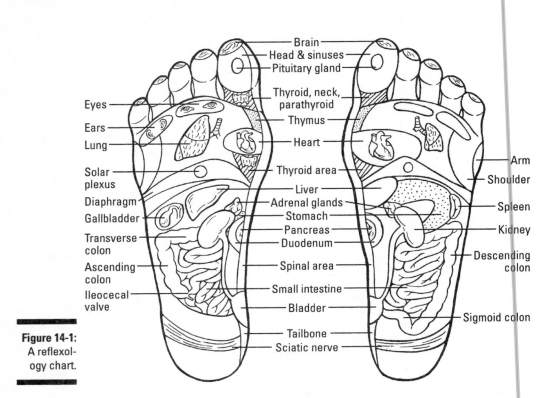

Figure 14-1:
A reflexology chart.

Some people swear by reflexology as a life-saving healing method. In fact, the woman I learned the technique from was diagnosed with a serious form of cancer and not given much chance of survival. None of the conventional treatments seemed to be helping, so as a last resort she turned to a Greek man in his nineties who specialized in reflexology. He also recommended coffee enemas. Within several months, this woman was cured and has been living a normal, productive life for over 20 years. (After the experience, however, she did develop a slight aversion to coffee shops.)

Frankly, nobody can tell you why reflexology works. But the truth is it often does. Reflexology is still a *theory,* but one with practical applications, and it certainly won't hurt you to give it a try. It may indeed help your overall health, but at the very least reflexology is guaranteed to feel darn good on your feet.

Foot Massage Routine

This section gives you a 20-minute foot massage routine based on the principles of reflexology. The routine is so easy to do that almost anyone can follow the instructions and perform the entire routine from start to finish the very first time, even members of the United States legislature. So, of course, that means you should have no problem at all.

Positioning

First, get yourself and your partner in a comfortable position. The partner-reclining position shown in Figure 14-2 is the one favored by professional foot massagers around the world, but you can also position your partner on a bed or massage table so that her feet are just at the edge. She can even lie on the floor. Also, pay attention to the way you're bending over to access your partner's soles and toes. You don't want to hurt yourself while trying to help someone else.

You can perform this routine through stockings or socks if you don't want to remove them. So far, though, no method has been devised to perform reflexology through a pair of shoes.

Points to remember

If you want to remain friends with the person you're giving the foot massage to, keep in mind a few things when you're about to dig into her soles:

- ✔ Start on the left foot. This compliments your partner's natural digestion and circulatory patterns.

- ✔ Don't use oil, because it makes the foot too slippery. Corn starch works well to absorb excess moisture, so rub some on your partner's feet before you begin.

- ✔ Always talk to your partner and ask for feedback.

- ✔ Don't diagnose any problems or treat someone for serious disorders (leave that to physicians).

- ✔ Don't use any instruments or tools to push against the feet (such as pencil erasers for example, which have been known to get lodged between toes). Use only your fingers and thumbs.

- ✔ Never push so hard that you cause pain or discomfort. If your partner is in pain, ease up your pressure a little bit.

- ✔ Finish one foot completely, and then go on to the next.

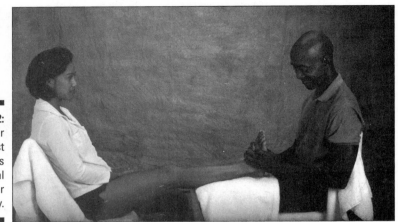

Figure 14-2:
Kick your feet up. Rest a spell. This is an optimal position for reflexology.

Basic moves

You can make certain basic, time-tested moves on the feet. These moves have been passed down by practicing reflexologists from generation to generation, and now you can use them, too. This section provides you with detailed explanations of these moves and how to use them yourself.

Cradling

Cradle your partner's foot (at either the ball of the foot or the ankle) in both palms, with your fingers pointing straight ahead. Then move your hands back and forth rapidly, just an inch or so (as shown in Figure 14-3). This move is especially good for warming up, and you can also use it in the middle of a foot massage to give your partner a little extra pleasure. Cradling feels so good it was called "dessert" by one of my colleagues who specialized in reflexology at a spa where I worked.

Thumb walking

The most basic move of all in foot reflexology is "thumb walking," which is a lot trickier than it looks. Start by placing the pad of your thumb firmly against your partner's foot (as shown in Figure 14-4a). Then bend the thumb and creep it forward like an inchworm across the surface, pressing in while you do so (as shown in Figure 14-4b). Every time you bend your thumb, move your hand forward just slightly. You may want to practice this technique a little before subjecting your partner to a spastic or weak inchworm movement.

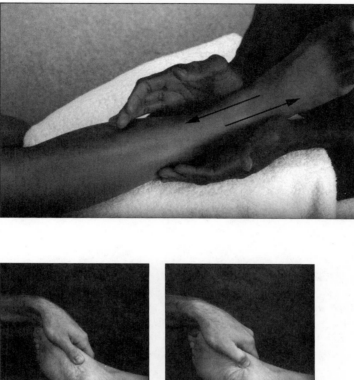

Figure 14-3:
This move is
called
"cradling,"
and it feels
most
delicious.

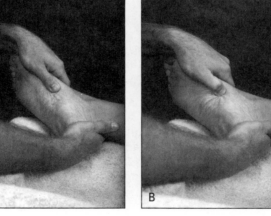

Figure 14-4:
Start with
your thumb
in the posi-
tion on the
left (a); then
inch your
thumb for-
ward while
bending it
to wind up
in the posi-
tion on the
right (b).

A   B

Index finger technique

Sometimes (for example, when you're working on the sides and tops of your
partner's feet), using your thumbs is just plain awkward. That's when you can
use the length of your index finger to slide next to the ankles and between the
long bones that run from the heels to the toes, for example, as shown in
Figure 14-5a.

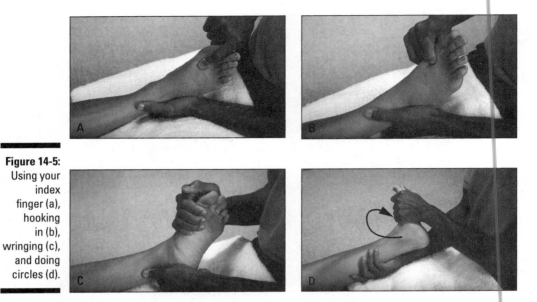

Figure 14-5:
Using your index finger (a), hooking in (b), wringing (c), and doing circles (d).

Hooking in

Using the tips of the thumbs or index fingers, bend slightly at the last knuckle and "hook in" at the point you're targeting (see Figure 14-5b). This technique allows for some pinpoint pressure on the bony, intricate surfaces of the foot.

Wringing the foot

Because the arch of the foot corresponds to the spine in reflexology, this technique is like giving a chiropractic adjustment to the foot. Grasping your partner's toes with one hand and her heel with the other, give a gentle twist in opposite directions as if wringing out the arch of the foot (as shown in Figure 14-5c).

Ankle circles

Holding your partner's ankle in one hand, circle her foot around in both directions (clockwise and counterclockwise) for several seconds, stretching the muscles and tendons in the area, and warming up the ligaments (see Figure 14-5d).

Step-by-step

Begin by getting into the most comfortable position, as mentioned earlier, and then do this warm-up:

- Cradle the ball of the foot.
- Cradle the ankle.
- Do ankle circles.
- Stretch the toes back and forth.
- Squeeze the foot.

Now you're ready to move into the 15-step foot massage routine that follows, which is based on the work of Claire Marie Miller in North Carolina.

TIP

Remember to start on the left foot, complete the entire routine, and then repeat the process on the right foot. Refer to Figure 14-1 if you need help.

1. **Head: Your head is filled with lots of important anatomical highlights, such as the brain. It's worth spending a few extra minutes here as you begin your reflexology routine.**

   To affect the reflexes of the head, do some small, focused, thumb walking in three lines down the big toe and three lines across the bottom of the big toe.

2. **Neck: The neck can be an area of nagging pain. Sometimes working the reflex areas for the neck can help bring relief.**

   Do thumb walking back and forth along the base of the big toe, right where it attaches to the foot. To specifically treat the region at the base of the back of your skull, "hook in" with your thumb on the lower, inside part of your big toe, between it and the second toe. This is often a key point for relieving headaches and neck tension.

3. **Face: Yes, even the face has a reflex on the foot, which is perhaps why it seems so easy to put your foot in your mouth.**

   Do thumb walking across the top of the big toe, then "hook in" right at the base of the toenail.

4. **Sinuses: The sinus cavities are hollow areas in your head, behind your face. Keeping them clear and healthy helps you breathe more easily.**

   The points for the sinuses can be found on the bottoms of all of the little toes. To stimulate them, do three lines of thumb walking down the bottom of each toe, and "hook in" right in the center of each toe for a couple seconds.

5. **Ears/eyes: The ears and eyes have reflexes by the base of the middle toes. Stimulating those reflexes may help you keep your senses of sight and hearing keen and alert.**

Using your knuckles or both thumbs, press in on the spots on the bottom of the foot between the second and third toes (for the eyes) and between the third and fourth toes (for the ear reflexes). You can press both areas at the same time. The spots are on the very edge of the bottom of the feet, almost on the webbing between the toes themselves.

6. **Lungs/chest: The area around the balls of your foot reflects your air passages, bronchial tubes, lungs, and chest muscles. If you stop breathing, you may run into some serious problems, and so you will benefit by paying attention to the healthy functioning of your lungs.**

   Use the index finger technique for this reflex, sliding the length of your finger between the long metatarsal bones on top of the foot and pressing in against them. You can also switch your hand around and slide your finger between the same bones from the bottom.

7. **Diaphragm: The diaphragm (discussed in more detail in Chapter 7) is the muscle at the bottom of your lungs that is responsible for keeping you breathing. So, if you like breathing, try to keep this muscle happy.**

   Pushing the toes up toward your partner's head with one hand, use the thumb of the other hand to walk back and forth along an imaginary line at the base of the ball of the foot, approximately two inches from the toes.

8. **Spine: Many people experience back pain, and many of those same people seem to have pain in the arches of their feet as well. A coincidence? Not when you know that the arches of the feet correspond in reflexology with the spine.**

   Do thumb walking up and down the reflex for the spine, which is basically the arch of the foot. You may want to switch thumbs when you're moving up the arch and back down, which will make this technique less awkward.

   Then "wring" the spine out by twisting the arch of the foot. Hold the heel with one hand and the toes with the other, while twisting gently in opposite directions.

9. **Inner organs: The center of the bottoms of the feet correspond to several of your internal organs, and this is the area where you can easily get confused. You may want to study the chart in Figure 14-1 quite closely as you go about stimulating the reflexes here. The internal organs are where you take the outside world in and transform it into your body. Important digestive and filtering processes take place here.**

   When you're working on the left foot, do thumb walking in the center below the lung and diaphragm reflexes, where you'll find the areas corresponding to the stomach, the pancreas, the spleen, and the heart. Then walk your thumb from left to right across the center of the foot and down the outside, which corresponds with the last half of the large intestine.

When working on the right foot, walk the thumb in the same area, but as you do, you'll be stimulating the liver and gallbladder instead. Then walk your thumb up the outside edge of the heel and across the center of the foot to stimulate the first half of the large intestine.

Understanding the large intestine reflex is easier if you consider both feet together. Picture the large intestine going up the right side of the abdomen, across the upper abdomen, and down the left side (because this is what it actually does). Now you can imagine how you're affecting this reflex by walking your thumb up the outside of the right foot, across the center of both feet, then down the outside of the left.

10. **Small intestine: "A man is only as happy as his digestive tract." This ancient saying, which I just made up this minute, highlights the importance of healthily functioning intestines.**

    Using your thumbs to walk helter-skelter in all directions, crisscross back and forth over the bottom of the heel, which corresponds to the lengthy loops of the small intestine.

11. **Hips/knees: Your hips and knees are your foundation, and stimulating these reflexes can help keep you in balance.**

    Walk your thumbs along the upper part of the foot toward the outer edge, midway between the toes and the heel, moving in all directions around the general area of the *cuboid bone*, which is the little protuberance that sticks out the farthest in the middle of your foot on the outside edge.

12. **Sciatic: The largest nerve in your body, the sciatic can be the unfortunate victim of a proportionally large amount of pain.**

    Using the thumb and index finger, pinch all along the back of the base of the heel, then up a couple inches along the Achilles tendon toward the calf. Repeat several times.

13. **Reproductive organs: Men and women, as you've undoubtedly noticed by now, have different reproductive organs. But, as it so happens, the associated reflexes are located on the same areas of the feet for both sexes.**

    Halfway down from the center of the ankle bones, toward the bottom of the heels, you'll find the reflexes for the reproductive organs. The inner ankle points correspond to the uterus or prostate, and the outer ankle points correspond to the ovaries or testicles. Use your thumb or the tip of your index finger to "hook in" for a few seconds on these points. You can also walk your thumb up over the top of the ankle from one point to another, which stimulates the fallopian tubes.

What to do if you find a problem

While you're exploring the various reflex areas on your partner's foot, you may come across a very specific spot that is significantly more tender than the rest. You'll be able to tell you've hit a tender area, because your partner will suddenly jerk her foot out of your hand and shout, "Whoa, what's *that* spot?" When this happens, consulting your reflexology chart, discovering the corresponding reflex, and immediately proclaiming the presence of a life-threatening disease in that area of the body is *not* a good idea. Feel free to tell your partner which part of the body the tender area represents, but that's all you should do. This is not a time to show off

your newfound knowledge of foot anatomy and proclaim yourself a medical expert.

Rather than diagnosing her "illness," tell her that if the pain persists in that spot, she should consider consulting with her physician and get a general checkup. You actually may have stumbled upon a viable health concern here. Then again, your partner may have stepped on a tack the day before, in which case, the tender spot you're hitting in the center of her left foot is simply a boo-boo, not the sign of a diseased spleen.

Stimulating the reproductive organ reflex points for pregnant women is said to help induce labor. Although I've never heard of a woman going into premature labor due to a massage to the foot, just to play it safe, stay away from this area completely if your partner may possibly be pregnant. Some people skip foot reflexology altogether on potentially pregnant people for this reason.

14. **Bladder and kidneys: Save these reflexes for the end of the routine, because they're organs of elimination, and stimulating them promotes a cleansing reaction.**

    Starting near the heel, use thumb walking up and back along the arch of the foot, almost up to the ball of the foot. This line is a little more onto the bottom of the foot than the spine reflex (explained in Step 8). Repeat twice.

15. **Overall squeeze of the foot: Never finish a foot without saying good-bye to it first. You may want to reapply some of the warm-up moves from the beginning as a cool-down here. Reflexology can be rather intense, and leaving your partner with some nice, pleasurable sensations at the end is a good idea.**

    Finish with an overall squeeze of the foot, very quickly touching all the areas you've worked on before, cradling a little bit, and generally being nice. Some people like to apply a soothing skin cream at this point. Cooling mint preparations feel especially good, and you can find plenty of mint cream options at popular bath stores.

Part V
Living the Good Life: Massage for Every Body

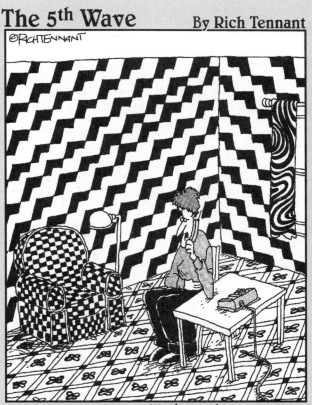

The 5th Wave   By Rich Tennant

"I've tried massage, meditation, and aromatherapy
but nothing seems to work. I'm still feeling dizzy
and disoriented all day."

In this part . . .

Alright, you can confess. You've finally gotten all the way to Part V, and still there's a nagging little voice in the back of your head saying something silly like, "Massage really isn't for me, at least not on a consistent basis. Sure, maybe as a novelty once or twice it's great, but how am I supposed to take advantage of it in real life? Isn't it just for the rich and famous, after all?"

No, no, no! Don't get so down on yourself like that. There are lots of ways that you can enjoy massage in many areas of your life, areas that perhaps you hadn't thought of before. That's what this section is all about.

You don't need to be rich and famous, for example, to take part in the luxury spa lifestyle you've seen on TV. Chapter 15 shows you how to simply and inexpensively recreate those experiences for yourself, your friends, and your family. Or say you're a weekend warrior looking for a way to stay limber and uninjured while pursuing your part-time passion for sports. Then the massage moves and stretches in Chapter 16 should be perfect for you.

And how about if you have a new baby? Or if you're pregnant? Or 96 years old? Chapter 18 provides easy-to-use tips and techniques made exactly for you. Of course, if you're "in the mood" and you're with that special someone, you can use massage as a sensual prelude to your encounters, as explained in Chapter 19.

Finally, if you find that people are calling all hours of the day and night asking for massage, telling you you're a "natural" and that you have "great hands," Chapter 20 offers some tips on going pro and creating a successful career for yourself based on helping others feel better.

Whether you're an athlete, an infant, a road warrior, a hedonist, a sexy octogenarian, or expecting triplets, you'll find something here that can improve many levels of enjoyment, pleasure, and health in your life. Massage truly is for every body.

Chapter 15

The Spa Lifestyle: Massage, Youth, and Beauty

*E*ver notice how some people seem like they were born with a silver-plated bottle of Evian water in their mouths? They're the ones out there living it up at expensive luxury spas, getting all the massages, right? Not!

Over the past decade, the household income of the average spa-goer has dropped from around $500,000/year down to about $50,000/year. That one "0" makes a lot of difference. Today, spas are for everybody. If you're not making $50,000/year, don't despair. With the advent of *day spas,* which I describe in this chapter, the experience of luxury is becoming even more accessible to people from all walks of life. And, if you're steadfastly opposed to spending money, this chapter also contains a few tips and techniques to turn your very own home into a luxury spa, almost for free.

Spas: More than Just a Pretty Jacuzzi

Spas are not, as commonly believed, just a kind of Jacuzzi. Although the word *spa* has become interchangeable with *hot tub,* a spa can also be a really cool place where all kinds of exciting things take place, like chardonnay grape massages for instance.

Back in the good old days of King Louis' court in France (it may have been Louis XV, or XIV, or perhaps VIP . . . I'm not sure), certain ladies-in-waiting found themselves waiting around so much that they began feeling jaded. "Another typical almond-oil massage from our love slave, Gregory?" said one lady to the next. "How boring."

So, they came up with a new idea. Their servants filled huge vats with smashed chardonnay grapes, and the ladies proceeded to jump in *au naturel* for a total-immersion aromatherapy experience. The sensation was so new, and the positive effects of the grapes on their skin so pronounced, that they decided to make it a tradition.

Thus was born an early version of a spa treatment that can still be experienced today. At the Meadowood Spa in Napa Valley, California, for example, they offer a treatment based on this theme (ladies-in-waiting not included). The distilled essence of chardonnay grapes is infused into the massage cream used by the massage therapists there.

Choosing a Spa

Today, whether you plan to immerse yourself in grapes, or to simply try to lose a few pounds and look your best, you can choose from a large array of spas to visit. They range from super-luxurious to down-home rustic. So how do you decide where to go?

Spas = H$_2$O

What is a spa anyway, and what does the word spa really mean? Originally, it was a Latin acronym from the words, Sanitas *Per Aqua,* meaning *health through water.* This was a phrase favored by the Romans, who took those three words with them everywhere they went, including a town in modern-day Belgium that had healing hot spring waters bubbling out of the ground. They called this town Spa, perhaps also in reference to the Latin words *'espa'* (meaning "fountain") and *'sparsa'* (from *spargere,* meaning, "to bubble up").

You can go to Spa, Belgium, and immerse yourself in the waters there. Visit 209.41.63.136/spa/spa.htm on the Web to find out more.

First, knowing what kinds of spas are out there helps. Spas fall into three basic categories:

- ✔ **Destination spas:** This is the King Louis kind of spa, the type of place you go when you want a super special experience. They're called *destination spas* because they are dedicated to the spa experience and nothing else. When people visit them, the spa is their final destination, and they usually stay for several days to a week.

- ✔ **Resort spas:** Becoming more and more popular, these spas are an important part of a larger resort. Guests may travel to the resort for other reasons, but many of them take advantage of the spa while they're there.

- ✔ **Day spas:** The fast food joints of the spa world. Day spas are places to go to receive spa treatments, massages, and more, and you don't have to travel far or stay overnight to do so.

Visiting the spa down the street

These days, you can probably find a day spa available right in your very own neighborhood. Several multimillion dollar day spas have opened recently, but the majority existed first as hair salons that expanded into spa services. Some good massage is going on at day spas, because many skilled massage therapists are finding work there.

Although the true origins of the term *day spa* are somewhat shrouded in mystery, the term is generally attributed to a business woman and spa owner from Connecticut named Noelle DeCaprio. She started her day spa in 1978 and is credited with being the first person to classify her establishment in this manner.

Want to give your Aunt Minnie in Cleveland a spa surprise for her birthday but you don't know how to set it up? Just call 1-888-SPA-WISH (888-772-9474) and order a gift certificate that's good for massages, facials, and other treats at nearly 800 day spas across the U.S. And check out the coupon at the back of this book to receive a discount!

Choosing a spa that's right for you

Spas range from rugged adventure outposts in the desert to the most puffy pampering palaces on the planet. You have almost unlimited choices when you're deciding where to go, which is great, but the number of choices may also make your decision kind of difficult.

Some spas, such as the Green Valley spa in St. George, Utah, offer rock climbing on the menu right alongside their massages. Some spas expect you to join in on every exhausting 6 a.m. mountain hike they offer. Others leave you alone to steep in herbal baths all day.

So, how do you choose?

First, decide what's important to you and what you want to accomplish on your spa trip. This can usually be broken down into a few basic categories: fitness, healing, spirituality, relaxation, or some combination of these.

Next, talk to someone who's been there before, or get the details from a reliable source. Here are three sources that may help you make the right match with a spa:

- Get in touch with Spa Finders travel agency and check out their magazine by calling 800-ALL-SPAS (800-255-7727) or visiting www.spafinders.com.

- Pick up the spa travel guide, *Fodor's Healthy Escapes* (Fodor's Travel Publications), by Bernard Burt, which lists great spas of all types in many parts of the world.

- The International SPA Association (ISPA) has a Web site, the Global Spa Guide, at www.globalspaguide.com, which may help you find the right place for your spa trip.

Spa Treatments

So what do people actually do at spas all day, other than get massages and douse themselves in crushed grapes? Believe it or not, they are also in pursuit of improved health. Yes, that's right. And the way they achieve it is to eat spa food, follow a spa exercise program, and receive what are known as *spa treatments,* all of which are good for you in one way or another. Spa treatments include:

- Scrubs
- Wraps
- Hydrotherapy
- Facials
- Mud, seaweed, and other messy things

If you don't want to travel to one of the three types of spas to receive these treatments, you can create them at home for yourself and your family. The advantages of this approach are obvious. First, if you're like most people, you live right in your own home, so you won't have to travel far to get there. Also, having your husband or wife or best friend wrap you in herb-infused sheets is a lot cheaper than paying a professional wrapper to do it.

If you're like most people, a 10-day spa vacation in Maui is a little out of reach, except perhaps as a once-in-a-lifetime dream vacation. But you can still take advantage of your local day spa a few times a year, and create some spa experiences for yourself at home, each and every week. Each type of spa treatment I list below includes a version you can try at home, and, as you can see, they're not that difficult.

For the following treatments, you need a very specialized piece of equipment. Don't worry — it's very inexpensive, and you can find it in the spa department of your local drug store. It looks amazingly like a simple 6-pack cooler, but I call it a *spa thermal unit*. Use it to store the hot moist towels that you need to wipe off spa goop from your partner's body.

Scrubs

During their stay at a spa, many people sign up for an exfoliation, which is a word that comes from that ancient spa language, Latin. It means "to strip away dead leaves." In other words, it's a fancy name for a body scrub.

Body scrubs are good for you because they slough away dead skin cells, allowing your skin to breathe again and preparing your pores to absorb all those enriching ingredients like massage oils from India and mango bath salts from The Body Shop.

If you don't have the time or patience to create the entire body scrub experience that follows, try using a pair of *scrub gloves*. You can find them in beauty supply stores, drug stores, and gift shops. These textured gloves do the exfoliation for you while you simply rub the skin. No water, soaps, or other ingredients are needed.

Body scrub ingredients

Body scrubs are very easy to do. You need just a few simple ingredients:

- Loofah sponge
- 4 cups of warm water in bowl
- 4 hot, moist, wrung-out hand towels in an ice chest

- Washcloth
- 2 bath towels
- Body bath
- Exfoliant (1/2 cup sea salt with approximately 3 tablespoons of water and 3 drops of essential oil added)

The exfoliant itself is quite simple. Mix the sea salt with water a little at a time until you have a batter-like consistency, and then add a few drops of your favorite essential oil. Any of the many over-the-counter skin scrubbing products you can buy at the beauty store or department store will work quite nicely, too.

You may not want to do this treatment on your new $800 silk carpet from Turkey, because drips and drops of salt and other ingredients do tend to find their way onto whatever surface you're using.

Step-by-step body scrub

The following steps show you how to create a body scrub that's as nice as one you experience at a spa. Just make sure to keep your partner warm because wet bodies cool down fast. You can cover the areas you're not working on with a towel.

1. **With your partner face down on a bath towel, moisten her back and the back of her legs with a washcloth.**

2. **Place a dab of exfoliant in one palm and use circular movements to scrub your partner's skin.**

3. **Use a hot, moist towel from the cooler to wipe off the exfoliant.**

4. **Dip the loofah sponge in the bowl of water, squeeze a dab of body bath onto it, and then go back over your partner's skin again with circular movements.**

5. **Use your second hand towel to wipe the skin.**

6. **Have your partner turn over and repeat Steps 1–5 on the front of the legs, torso, and arms.**

   Never use sea salt or body exfoliants on the face. You can purchase exfoliants made specifically for the face in the cosmetics departments of most major department stores.

7. **When you've finished exfoliating the front of the body, apply some massage lotion to the skin.**

   You can either do this application of lotion quickly, or you can linger and perform an entire massage, depending upon your mood and your partner's mood.

8. Have your partner turn over once more, replacing the damp bath towel beneath her with a dry one, and apply skin lotion to her back and the backs of her legs.

9. Touch your partner's skin (or have somebody else touch it) gingerly, exclaiming, "Ooh, aah, you feel *so* smooth!"

Facials

As you may know, the cosmetics industry is big business, with lots of expensive products out there for you to buy, but all you need in order to give yourself or a partner a very nice facial treatment is a little bit of aloe and a ripe papaya. You never knew it could be so easy, did you?

Facial ingredients

You have to have just a few things ready in order to perform a fun and effective facial:

- ✔ 3 hot moist hand towels in your cooler
- ✔ Cotton pads
- ✔ Facial toner
- ✔ 1/2 ripe papaya (no seeds or skin) blended with 1 teaspoon aloe vera gel
- ✔ Skin cream

Step-by-step facial

Follow the steps in this section to create a relaxing, rejuvenating facial.

1. **Cleanse the face with skin toner and remove any makeup.**

2. **Place a hot, moist towel on the face and hold it in place for 2 minutes, allowing the pores to open.**

    Remember to leave an opening for the mouth and nose if you want your partner to be able to breathe through this procedure.

3. **Remove the towel and apply the papaya/aloe blend in a thin smooth layer over the face, using your fingers.**

4. **Place another hot towel over the face to keep the mixture moist.**

5. **Massage your partner's hands while the face is covered.**

6. **Exchange the towel for a warm one after a few minutes and continue massaging the hands.**

7. **Remove the towel, wiping off whatever's left of the papaya/aloe mixture with it.**

8. **Using a face cream, do the face massage routine in Chapter 11.**

Remember to always stroke upwards when you're giving a facial, like professional estheticians do, so you won't pull down on the delicate collagen fibers which give your skin its tone.

Wraps

Some people think that body wraps are only good for losing inches. And certain wraps *can* help you slip into that red dress that's been hanging for years in the closet. But, as you've probably been told (by everyone except the manufacturers of the wraps), what you're really losing is water weight, which will, unfortunately, come back.

Serious health spas use wraps that detoxify the body, usually known as *herbal wraps.* And they work by tricking your body into thinking it has a fever, causing it to purge itself of internal toxins. While working as a wrapper at big spas, I used to routinely unwrap people and find the sheets permeated with the smell of nicotine and other products that the client's body was purging.

Other types of wraps, like aromatherapy ones, for example, are available, but my favorite is the herbal wrap, because it is the most deeply detoxifying, so that's the one I describe for you here.

This treatment is a bit more involved than the others, so only attempt it if you're in a truly experimental mode and want to learn by trial and error.

Herbal wrap ingredients

Get ready for a fun production in your kitchen as you prepare the herbal wrap, and don't be discouraged if the wrap is not as warm as you'd like the first time you try. This treatment takes a little practice to do well.

- ✔ 3 ounces of herbs — the fresher the better (Try a combination of chamomile, rosemary, lemongrass, and eucalyptus.)

- ✔ A little bag or piece of cheese cloth in which to tie up the herbs for soaking (Even a clean sock will do in a pinch.)

- ✔ A sheet for soaking and wrapping

- ✔ A big pot to heat water in and make the herbal solution

- ✔ A pair of rubber gloves handy so you don't scald your fingers

✔ A rubberized sheet, or space blanket, or piece of plastic (like a drop cloth)

✔ A wool blanket

Herbal wrap step-by-step

Follow these steps to create a do-it-yourself herbal wrap similar to the type given at great luxury spas.

1. **Place the herbs in the cloth, basically creating a big tea bag, and drop it in a big pot of hot (not boiling) water.**

   Maximum temperature should only be around 165 degrees Fahrenheit. Soak the herbs 20 minutes. Then add the sheet to the pot of hot tea and let it soak for a few minutes.

2. **While the sheet is soaking in the herbal tea, lay the wool blanket down, then place the plastic or rubberized sheet on top of it.**

3. **Wring the sheet out *very well,* remembering to wear your rubber gloves.**

   Lay the sheet down on top of the plastic and have your partner lie down on it. In order to make the herbal wrap work best, have your partner sit in a hot bath, Jacuzzi, or sauna before getting wrapped.

4. **Wrap around your partner the hot sheet, then the plastic wrap, and then the wool blanket.**

5. **Make sure your partner is comfortable.**

   You can put something beneath his knees and head for support, if desired, and give him a sip of cool water through a straw. Leave him wrapped for about 20 minutes, keeping an eye on him. And, if he asks, scratch his nose for him (wrapped people often complain of itchy noses).

6. **When you unwrap him, give him some more water and help him sit in a comfortable chair where he can relax for another 20 minutes, letting the herbs dry naturally on his skin.**

Hydrotherapy

Hydrotherapy is a word that means, obviously, therapy with fire hydrants. Just kidding . . . but that description is actually quite close to the truth. Would you believe, for example, that people pay good money in spas to stand naked against a tile wall while a hydrotherapy expert sprays a blast of cold water at them from a pressure hose? It's true (this is called a *Scotch Hose treatment*).

Hydrotherapy treatments in luxury spas can also involve the use of super-expensive *hydrotherapy tubs,* which look like a cross between a bathtub and a Jacuzzi. You don't need to be in one of these tubs to experience hydrotherapy. In fact, your own bathtub or shower at home will do just fine.

Here are a few ideas for taking advantage of your own water source to do a little hydrotherapy at home:

✔ **Bathe someone.** For most of us, the last time we were bathed was in early childhood by our mothers, and we've forgotten how soothing it is. Using a pitcher, pour warm water over your partner's head, shoulders, and back in the bath. Then wash her slowly and luxuriously.

✔ **Take a cold plunge.** Many spas have what's known as a cold plunge, which is a pool kept at a shockingly low temperature. Patrons jump in after being heated up in saunas and whirlpools. You can simulate the extremely invigorating effects of this activity by drawing a cold bath and immersing yourself for 30 seconds (or as long as you can stand it).

✔ **Share a bath with a friend.** First, make sure the friend wants to share the bath with you. After you determine that, slip into a tub of warm water with 10 drops of aromatherapy oil added, and see what happens next. It may not be entirely therapeutic, but it certainly will be fun.

Exercise . . . a day of pleasure

The spa lifestyle is for everyone — unless you're the type who disdains pleasure and health, like the flagellant monks of the Middle Ages, for example, who used to wander around the streets beating themselves with sticks. If that's your idea of fun, definitely stay away from anything to do with spas.

If, on the other hand, you have what it takes to treat yourself to some healthy enjoyment in life, why not plan an entire day of spa pleasures? The sultans used to do it, and so did Cleopatra with rose petals a foot thick on the floor of her love chamber. But how about you?

You can recreate a day of luxury just like the ones people experience at spas. Trade each treatment with a lucky partner and spend the day together. Then go out and celebrate your indulgence with a healthy meal at a restaurant.

The whole exchange (not including dinner) takes about 5 hours. Just follow these simple steps:

1. **First, start with a body scrub to cleanse the skin and prepare you to absorb the healthy effects of the oils and other ingredients to follow.**

2. **Take turns soaking in a bath (or soak together if you're so inclined), with a dozen drops of your favorite aromatherapy oil or a few ounces of healing herbs added.**

3. **Exchange long luxurious massages, following along with the step-by-step instructions in Chapter 11.**

4. **Give each other a spa facial to prepare yourselves for reentry into the world.**

Mud, seaweed, and other messy things

Other kinds of spa treatments work, too, but I don't go into them here, because if you tried them at home you may mess up your furniture or carpet. These treatments involve the use of such products as mud, seaweed, and clay — and they can be really messy! If you do experiment with these products (many of which are available at cosmetics counters and in beauty supply stores), try to confine your activities to the bathroom, where you're less likely to stain things.

Massage-O-Matic Specialty Stores

When you're searching for items to create your own spa or massage environment at home, try checking out a new type of outlet known as the *massage specialty store*. Until recently, this type of store didn't even exist, but now they're popping up in many locations. If you ever find yourself near one of them, you really should pay a visit, because they're quite cool. And don't be intimidated by the New Age feel at some of these places. Everyone is allowed inside, not just crystal-toting members of the massage avant-garde.

Three basic types of massage-oriented storefronts exist:

- Manufacturers' outlets
- Ergonomic specialists
- Massage-o-matics

Manufacturers' outlets

Some of the companies that manufacture equipment such as tables and chairs for massage pros have also begun experimenting with selling their wares directly to the public. These companies are still concentrated in that global hotbed of massage innovation, California, although they exist elsewhere as well. Their number will grow quickly as these items become more popular, and in the meantime you can find some quality massage products in a number of other stores, too, such as the Sharper Image. (See the "Massage Gizmos" section in Chapter 10, which explains the use of many massage devices.)

Check these massage stores out, if you have the opportunity:

✔ **The Massage Company:**

- 1714 Lombard Street, San Francisco, CA 94105 (telephone: 415-346-7828)
- 1533 Shattuck Ave, Suite A, Berkley, CA 94709 (telephone: 510-704-2970)

✔ **Bodywork Emporium:**

Call 800-TABLE-4-U (800-822-5348 or 310-394-4475 extension 14) for a free, 48-page catalogue

✔ **Massage Central:**

12235 Santa Monica Boulevard, Los Angeles, CA 90025 (telephone: 310-826-2209)

✔ **New Life Massage Equipment:**

2853 Hedberg Drive, Minnetonka, MN 55305 (telephone: 800-852-3082 or 612-546-4100)

✔ **Best of Nature:**

176 Broadway, Long Branch, NJ 07740 (telephone: 800-228-6457, or 732-728-0004)

You can find a lot of massage equipment on the Web as well. Go to www.mtswarehouse.com, for example, to find good prices on professional massage tables, and www.massagematters.com for a few, select, high-quality massage items.

Ergonomic specialists

Some stores are not primarily massage outlets, but they do offer massage items and other tools that make our working and living environments more ergonomically correct. *Ergonomics* is a fancy term for the science concerned with designing and arranging things (like pieces of furniture) so that people interact with them most efficiently and safely.

One store in particular, Relax the Back, has created the mother lode of ergonomically designed furniture to help you prevent injuries and keep you healthy. It also sells several massage items that you can choose from. The philosophy of Relax the Back is that an ounce of prevention is worth a pound of cure. Call 800-290-2225 to find a store near you, or look them up at www.relaxtheback.com on the Web.

Massage-o-matics

Believe it or not, places exist where you can just pop in off the street and get your back rubbed for ten minutes. This kiosk take on the massage phenomenon is ideal for people traveling through airports or rushing through big cities. Here are a couple of examples:

- ✔ **The Great American Back Rub (800-BACK-RUB or 800-222-5782):** This company has stores in New York City; Kennedy Airport (New York, New York); Dallas, Texas; Toronto, Canada; and Los Angeles, California — and it's always looking to expand.

- ✔ **The Stress Station:** This company has two locations in the Phoenix, Arizona, area, one in Scottsdale (480-990-1701), and one in Paradise Valley (602-692-9004), with plans to expand. It also provides outcall massage to your location.

In some areas, you may find independent massage practitioners who've set up shop on their own or in small groups in public places such as Central Park in New York City, The Champs-Elysées in Paris, or the beach in Bali or Southern Thailand. Approaching these people for a massage-o-matic experience is perfectly safe. Just follow the same words of advice found in Chapter 7 that you'd heed when receiving any kind of massage, especially the one that tells you to remember that "You're the boss." Declaring what kind of massage you want to receive from these public practitioners is perfectly acceptable, even if the massage only lasts five minutes. Don't let an overly enthusiastic street masseur pound your back until it's black and blue.

Chapter 16

Higher, Faster, Stronger: Sports Massage

*H*ey . . . you there . . . do I see you getting ready to put this book down and rush out to the local schoolyard for an impromptu ballgame? Yes, you. Are you planning on stretching much before you jump into that game? If you're like most part-time athletes, you're probably not guilty of over-stretching. Am I right? It's just such a hassle. Well, this is another arena where massage can come in handy. What could be better than having some-one stretch your muscles for you? That, and much more, is precisely what you can do with sports massage. And you get the lowdown on it in this chapter.

When the Going Gets Tough, the Tough Get a Massage

If you're a serious athlete, chances are pretty good you probably understand the benefits of massage already. Most competing athletes think massage is valuable to athletic performance. Just look at top Olympic competitors, many of whom have used massage for years to gain an extra edge. In fact, beginning in 1996, massage became an official part of the services offered to all athletes in the Olympic Village itself.

Athletes utilize massage in a number of ways:

✔ To rehabilitate after getting injured in their sport

✔ To recover from intense workouts and competition

✔ To maintain optimal muscle tone and flexibility on an ongoing basis

✔ To appear relaxed and cool getting their massages in front of the competition at big events

Good times to use sports massage

You can use sports massage any time you want, even right before church on Sunday morning, or at midnight after drinking margaritas all evening at the annual company Fourth of July party. But using sports massage right around the time you're going to be engaging in the sport just plain makes more sense, don't you think? And that basically boils down to three different occasions:

✔ **Pre-event massage:** As the name would imply, this type of sports massage is used by athletes directly before the event. And, contrary to popular belief, a massage at this time will not zone the athlete out to a state of zombiehood, but rather invigorate her further in preparation for competition.

✔ **Post-event massage:** Directly after an event (like just past the finish line at the Boston Marathon), is a place and time that athletes almost universally appreciate a good massage. Massage helps the muscles, not to mention the psyche, recover more quickly.

✔ **Ongoing training massage:** Getting massaged throughout the training cycle is more and more popular with many athletes. Some even receive massage every day.

Where to find sports massage

If you live in a large metropolitan area, chances are good that you have a sports massage clinic somewhere close by. If you live in a small town, try inquiring at your local osteopath or chiropractor's office. They may know someone who offers sports massage.

Massage pros go through a special advanced training in order to become certified sports massage therapists. You won't offend anyone by asking about their certification and where they got it. So if you're really looking for a qualified person, check out their qualifications. Makes sense, doesn't it?

Athletic trainers are quite often sports massage therapists also, or they can at least recommend one. Beware, though, of the trainer who thinks he's doing sports massage just because he knows how to give a few karate chops to your back. He may be doing you a disservice, and he probably doesn't understand that true professional sports massage is becoming a highly evolved discipline. The days of Rocky Balboa's coach giving him a shoulder rub along with a motivational speech before the big fight are over. "And if he gets up, hit him again!"

Call the American Massage Therapy Association (AMTA) at 847-864-0123, and they will provide you with the name of someone on their National Sports Massage Team (NSMT).

The Techniques

Sports massage, when applied by skilled practitioners, is an advanced form of massage therapy, with many involved maneuvers. The instructions here are not meant to make you an expert. They simply suggest a couple of moves that can help ease the strains of the weekend warriors in your life, including you. In other words, after reading this chapter, don't go out and announce yourself as a special trainer for Olympic marathon runners. That should be left to the pros.

Sporty moves

This section provides you with some basic sports massage moves. Notice how they're similar to regular massage moves? It's just that they're bigger and often deeper, and certain moves are used much more frequently during sports massage then, say, during a relaxation massage.

Compression

Often in sports, overworked and overtired muscles have to be pressed into submission. With this move, shown in Figure 16-1a, you can apply enough direct pressure to help relieve muscle spasms and provide a calming effect to the area.

Cross-fiber friction

You may remember the term cross-fiber from Chapter 10. Then again, you may not. And you may be thinking to yourself, what the heck is cross-fiber friction anyway? Don't fret: Cross-fiber friction is simply the use of some relatively intense rubbing across the opposite direction that the muscle fibers run in any particular area, as you can see in Figure 16-1b. This technique is especially good for muscle fibers that are put under strain during sports.

Deep pressure

People who work out a lot often end up creating some really sore spots along with the improved tone in their bodies. Pinpointing these sore spots can be tricky, but after you do, treat them to some direct deep pressure, as shown in Figure 16-1c, to help release knotted, cramped, and contracted muscle tissues.

Kneading

When you're kneading an athlete, you want to make sure your motions are big and strong, and that your hands grasp as much muscle tissue as possible. See Figure 16-1d, and refer to Chapter 10 for the three steps of kneading, which are squeezing, rolling, and pushing.

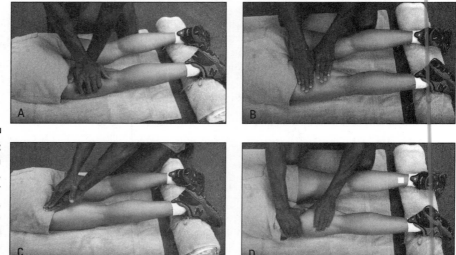

Figure 16-1: Compression (a), cross-fiber friction(b), deep pressure(c), and kneading(d).

Stretches

Stretches feel really good to people who've been using their muscles a lot in sporting activities, but be careful not to over-stretch people and possibly injure them. Always ask for feedback from your partner while you're performing the stretch, and always err on the side of not-enough stretch rather than forcing it toward too-much.

Hamstring stretch

With your partner lying on her back, lift one leg up, supporting it firmly at the ankle and on the hamstrings themselves, as you push the leg slowly and steadily back toward the head. Don't lock the knee during this maneuver. Hold the stretch for 5 to 10 seconds, and then release (see Figure 16-2a). You can add more impact by having your partner push back against your hands during the stretch, then release while you stretch the leg a little farther.

Quad stretch

The quadriceps muscles in the front of the thigh get especially tight on runners and other athletes. A good way to stretch them is to have your partner lie face down, raise her leg up to 90 degrees, then lift her foot straight up while also lifting beneath her knee with your other hand, as shown in Figure 16-2b. Only lift until you feel the natural resistance of her muscles. For an extra stretch on limber partners, bring the foot closer to the buttocks at the same time.

Calf stretch

When you stretch the calf, you stretch the Achilles tendon, too, which is extremely strong. So don't be afraid to give a deep stretch here by cupping the heel and pressing your forearm firmly against the bottom of the foot, moving the toes toward the head, as shown in Figure 16-2c.

Arm stretch

Lift the hand up over the head, pulling up slightly on the elbow, as shown in Figure 16-2d. This stretch is easier to do on a massage table, but if you don't have access to a table, just try bending your partner's elbow out to the side a little first until you get her arm into the correct position.

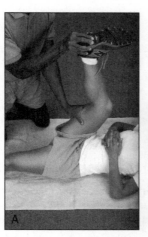
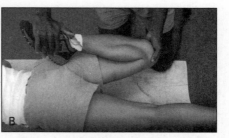
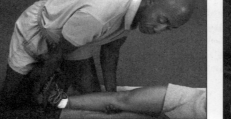
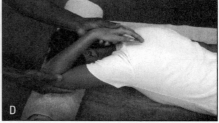

Figure 16-2: Stretches for the hamstring(a), quad(b), calf(c), and arm(d).

Routines

You can perform an entire sports massage routine, which is going to look similar to the regular routine you discover in Chapter 11, except that your partner will be wearing an athletic outfit instead of a towel! But that's not the only difference. You'll also be using a lot more cross-fiber friction, compression, and deep kneading, focusing on the muscles that have done the exertion. And some extra stretching aids in recovery, too. Other than that, though, don't be too surprised if sports massage looks amazingly similar to non-sports massage.

A Pain in the Elbow, a Pain in the Butt

Athletes run into all kinds of problems because they push their muscles to the limits, and certain sports are famous for causing certain pains. You've probably heard of tennis elbow, for example, and runner's cramps, both of which are problems that can be helped with sports massage.

Tennis elbow

Tennis elbow is a slow, creeping, debilitating condition that can really make you unhappy over a long period of time. This condition is a swelling of the tendons in the forearm near the elbow and an irritation of the muscles there caused by repetitive use. Of course, the best thing to do when you start noticing this type of pain is to stop doing what's causing it (namely, playing tennis). Some people don't want to stop playing tennis, though. In that case, try taking a break just for a few days, using ice to reduce soreness in the area. Also, a physician may be able to help by prescribing anti-inflammatory drugs, so check with your doctor.

A little sports massage can help tennis elbow, too. Remember to do some gradual warm-up massage moves first before digging straight in with these two rather intense maneuvers. Also, apply ice for 5 to 10 minutes beforehand to reduce inflammation. Then follow these steps:

1. **Supporting the arm at the wrist, with the elbow resting on the floor or massage table, grasp your partner's forearm and slide your hand down *slowly* from her wrist toward the elbow, as shown in Figure 16-3a. Repeat this move several times with your hand in different positions so your thumb presses against the entire forearm.**

2. **Using the tips of your fingers or thumbs, apply cross-fiber friction to the muscles on top of the forearm near the elbow, as shown in Figure 16-3b.**

   This is the area most directly affected in tennis elbow, so take it easy on your partner, using more ice if necessary to lessen discomfort. Apply more squeezing, gliding, and a little kneading afterwards to help smooth things out.

Figure 16-3:
Squeeze the forearm muscles and push slowly down toward the elbow(a); then apply deep friction to the fore-arm muscles near the elbow(b).

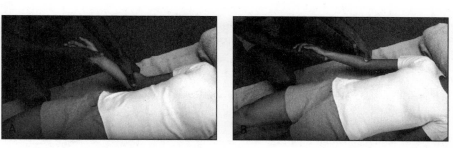

Runner's cramps

Runners often get muscle cramps in their calves, hamstrings, quads, or buttocks after pushing themselves to the limit. If you've ever been the victim of runner's cramps, you know that they are not fun at all. These cramps take over your leg like an invading alien from the latest episode of *Star Trek,* and they show no mercy. If you're standing at the time the cramp starts, you begin limping around and screaming like a maniac. And if you're lying down, the cramp is even worse. The following techniques may help the next time someone you know falls victim to a charley horse.

For over a century now, runner's cramps have also been known by the term *charley horse,* which originally came from the world of baseball. No one knows for sure who Charley was, or why he had a lame horse, though some people say he was a groundskeeper at a Sioux City ballpark.

Make sure the athlete drinks plenty of fluids to counter the cramping effects of dehydration. And after the massage, try placing some ice on the area for a few minutes to further reduce soreness.

When a cramp strikes, follow these steps to help ease the athlete's pain:

1. **Get the person to lie down comfortably and apply direct compression to the area, as shown in Figure 16-4a.**

2. **After a few seconds, release the pressure and apply a stretch to the muscle that is cramping, as shown in Figure 16-4b.**

3. **Grasping at the far end of the muscle on either side of the spasm itself, push the muscle fibers in toward the middle, as shown in Figure 16-4c.**

   Hold for several seconds.

4. **Have your partner contract the opposing muscles, which in Figure 16-4d are the muscles in front of the lower leg, near the shin.**

   This technique will have the effect of further loosening the cramping muscle.

5. **Stretch gently one more time.**

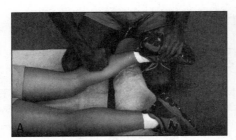
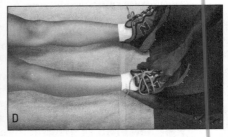
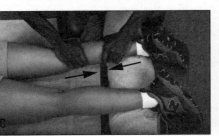

Figure 16-4:
Relief for a
cramping
muscle.

Chapter 17

Taking It With You: Massage On the Go

- -

In This Chapter

▶ Receiving massage around the world

▶ Getting massaged while on the road

▶ Using massage to relax while flying

- -

*W*herever your hands can go, massage can go, too. And there's no limit to the strange and wonderful environments you can find yourself in when seeking out professional massage or exchanging one with a traveling partner.

The only problem is, you have to get to your destination in order to enjoy the massage offered there, and the getting-there part often causes quite a bit of tension. That's why I share a coach-class massage with you at the end of this chapter, to help make getting there a little less of a pain.

One World, Many Massages

If you travel around much and receive massages in different parts of the world, one thing you'll notice pretty quickly is that each culture has its own distinct attitudes about massage and its own unique ideas about what a massage should be. In Turkey, for example, the massage you receive in a traditional *hamam,* or bathhouse, may include a tremendously vigorous rubdown in a big steamy chamber by a silent giant who is apparently indifferent to your discomfort, or your bliss, for that matter. On the other extreme, a massage on a cruise ship sailing the warm waters of the Caribbean may be an airy-light, soothing experience given to you by a sensitive and delicate English woman.

Just say the word

Wherever you are in the world, people often appreciate it if you attempt a few words of their language. And what better opportunity to practice your language skills than when seeking a massage in Madagascar, a backrub in Bangalore, or some reflexology in Rotterdam? With that in mind, I include a list of phrases in several different languages in the following table, all of which will get you the same result no matter where you are in the world — a massage!

Language	Phrase
German	Ich möchte eine Massage.
Spanish	Me gustaria un masaje.
French	Je voudrais un massage.
Portuguese	Gostaria de uma massagem.
Chinese	Woa Yao ANN MOU.
Japanese	Messeji wo uketoritai.
Italian	Gradirei un massaggio.
Thai	Chan yahk die maw newad pan bow lan.
Greek	Thelo ena massage.
Hindi	Mujhe massage chahiye.

In Thailand, you can enter one of the public pavilions at a sacred temple to receive your massage on a low, wide bed, while dressed in loose-fitting pajamas.

The Japanese take their bathing and their massages seriously, and they've developed a very elaborate system of hot spring resorts called *onsen*. If you visit one, you'll get to immerse yourself in a series of ever-hotter baths and receive a massage directly afterward.

And, in Mexico, you may find yourself in an adobe enclosure up in the mountains where white-robed massage therapists try to attune you to the inner rhythms of the surrounding environment.

You get the idea — massage can be found almost anywhere you go these days, even in the places you least expect it. I have a client who was on a trip through the Yucatan, visiting ancient Mayan ruins, when she received a message about massage from a very unexpected source.

She had heard of a spiritual healer who lived in a remote Mayan village, and she wanted to meet this woman. After traveling for hours on a dirt road, she was escorted into the healer's hut. This ancient woman, way out in the jungle, took a close look at her and said (through a translator), "You need to get a massage. And not just any massage. Special massage! Many many special massages." Sure enough, my client has been on a quest to receive as many massages as possible ever since, and the massages have helped her recover from a number of injuries.

Massage on the Road

You don't have to travel by Jeep to a remote Mayan village to have someone tell *you* to get lots of massages, right? No, you've probably already figured that one out for yourself. And when you travel, chances are you're much more likely to receive your massage-on-the-road in a hotel room rather than in the Yucatan outback.

Hotel rooms, even though they're often expensive and advertised as luxurious getaways, offer their own distinctive brand of discomfort. They are, after all, not home. Massage is the perfect antidote for hotel discomfort. Chapter 8 shows you what to do to get a professional massage while staying in a hotel and how to deal with the hotel concierge. In this section, I offer a few words of advice for exchanging massages with each other in hotel rooms.

The most important thing about on-the-road massage is to bring along your own traveling *inner chamber* like the one described in Chapter 9. That way you can transform almost any blah hotel space into your own personal massage sanctuary. Then simply follow the instructions from Chapter 11 as you trade massages with each other.

To create your traveling inner chamber, remember to pack:

- ✔ Massage oil
- ✔ A little massage gizmo (see Chapter 10)
- ✔ A portable CD player with mini-speakers
- ✔ Candles and matches
- ✔ A familiar photograph
- ✔ Incense
- ✔ A bathrobe

In a pinch, you can always try *magic fingers,* if it's available in your room. Magic fingers is a rather hokey-looking device installed in the beds at many hotels and motels. When fed with coins, it vibrates the entire bed, and can be actually quite pleasurable. As singer/songwriter Jimmy Buffet says, "Put in a quarter, turn out the lights, magic fingers makes ya feel all right."

18-wheeler massage

All around the world, the people who probably put in the most hours traveling are truckers. Day after day, for thousands of miles, with their butts glued into high-bucket seats, they roll across the countryside, their necks, shoulders, and backs getting more and more tense as they go.

You can't get much tougher than truckers. They're not the type to complain, but recently even they, too, have seen the light about massage. The Triple T Truck Stop in Arizona now offers therapeutic massage to the guys and gals hauling goods in their big rigs across the U.S.

If you've ever had any thoughts along the lines of, "I'm too tough for massage. That's for wusses who can't stand pain," just consider the example of the truckers.

If they see the value of massage therapy, it's good enough for me — and for you!

Massage in Coach Class

The toughest thing about travel is that it involves an awful lot of moving around, often in air-tight steel tubes hurtling through the upper atmosphere. Air travel is one sure way to get stressed out. Whoever uttered that famous phrase, "Life is a journey, not a destination," probably wasn't sitting in coach class on a transoceanic flight at the time.

Although there's just no way to get what you need the most on flights (namely, a hot shower and lots of fresh oxygen), you can still offer yourself or your traveling companions a little relief with a coach-class massage. By the way, this technique works equally well in first or business class, although it may not be quite as necessary.

The coach-class self-massage

Imagine yourself sitting in your coach-class seat like a good little passenger, all packed in like fruitcake in a tin, when suddenly the thought strikes you that you are, indeed, exceedingly uncomfortable, and you need to do something about it. You've already stood up twice to stretch, climbing all over other passengers to do so. Nothing seems to help.

The time to try massage has arrived. The five-step routine shown here is especially good for relieving tension in your sinus area, which can become sore due to cabin air pressure changes and dehydration. Just follow these steps and take a look at Figure 17-1:

1. **Lean forward slightly (not too far, or else you'll bang your head into the tray table of the seat in front of you), and hook your thumbs into the tender neck muscles just below the bony ridge at the base of your skull. Press in here, making little circles with your thumbs as you apply firm pressure, as shown in Figure 17-1a.**

2. **Use your thumbs to press in to the upper inner corner of your eyes, right next to the nose, as shown in Figure 17-1b.**

   Pressure against the nose bones can help relieve sinus soreness. If you're wearing glasses, take them off first. And if you're wearing contacts, don't press directly against them through your closed eyelids.

   This move can be done very discreetly, but if you end up sitting next to someone who looks at you strangely, just smile, point at your own head, and say, "Sinus trouble. If I don't do this my eyes will fall out."

3. **With firm pressure, make fingertip circles on your temples, moving the skin and muscle over the bone below while keeping your fingers firmly anchored to one spot on the skin (see Figure 17-1c).**

4. **Press straight in on the temples and hold for 5 to 10 seconds (as shown in Figure 17-1d).**

   You may also try moving your jaw around a bit at the same time, which will allow you to press at slightly different depths into the muscles.

5. **Press the heels of your hands into both sides of your head, above the ears, compressing the junction between your *parietal bones* and your *temporal bones* (as shown in Figure 17-1e).**

   Hold this for up to 30 seconds. It often helps reduce headaches and take pressure off your poor skull in those pressurized airplane cabins.

Be careful not to wallop the passengers on either side of you with your elbows when performing this maneuver.

A couple extra tips

Try stretching your legs out a little and pushing several points along the outside of your thighs (being careful not to kick the person in the seat in front of you and cause a mid-air scene!). Then bend forward a bit and reach underneath your knees to massage the upper calves.

If you have stuffy sinuses, and nothing else has helped, try doing what the scuba divers do: Pinch your nose shut and blow gently into it (be careful not to blow too hard). This simple technique often equalizes pressure inside and outside your head.

Ah . . . relief.

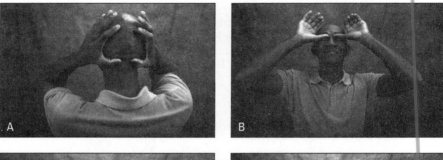

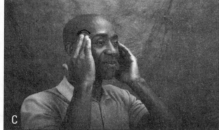

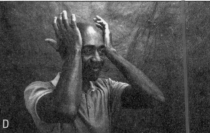

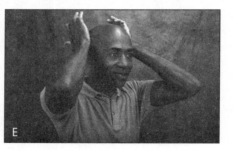

Figure 17-1:
Your coach-
class
massage.

Chapter 18

Massage for the Whole Family

• •

In This Chapter

▶ Sharing massage with your whole family

▶ Massaging your baby

▶ Enjoying massage during pregnancy

▶ Giving massage to seniors

• •

*W*elcome to the mom-and-pop chapter of this book, the one that gives you that warm and fuzzy feeling inside. Yes, you can include everybody in the family in your newfound passion for massage, from newborn babies right up through Grandma and Grandpa. All it takes is a little creativity on your part, and the willingness to share your newfound skills.

All in the Family

Elaine, a sales manager from Living Earth Crafts massage manufacturing company in California, put it best: "The family that massages together, stays together."

That makes sense. If you can't share massage with your family, who can you share it with, right? But just how exactly do you go about sharing it? Often, getting your family members to lie still for massage isn't that easy. And getting someone to *give* a massage is even harder. People all have their own agenda, their own time schedule, and their own feelings about physical contact. You are the person interested in massage, and you're the one who is reading this book. So, if you want to introduce massage into your family, you have to use certain stealthy techniques to get everybody thinking the same way you do.

Here are a few techniques you can use to get your family into massage, even if they don't seem interested at first:

▶ Give a foot massage to the couch potato while he's watching his favorite team in action.

- Use massage as a reward for children who complete their homework.

- Offer the family chef a massage in return for preparing a special meal.

- Make the idea of massage non-threatening by offering the simple, seated, back and neck massage (fully clothed) from Chapter 12.

- If someone says no to massage, respect that person's feelings, but offer a tidbit of information that may help, such as the location of the headache-reduction massage point in the webbing between the thumb and index finger (see Chapter 13).

- When a family member does agree to receive his or her first-ever massage, start out easy, with very light pressure, so you don't turn them off to the idea. Do some gentle warmups first, and then use more intense maneuvers after the person is used to your touch.

- Be willing to be the first one to offer massage and to continue offering it even if the favor is not reciprocated for a while.

Massaging my father

My father went to Emory University Hospital once for heart surgery, because his arteries were blocked. The entire family was scared.

My mom and sister and I accompanied him, and we watched as they wheeled him into the operating room, which was filled with high-tech, expensive equipment that we didn't understand. Hours later, he came out okay, but the nurses had to strap him to his hospital bed so he wouldn't accidentally roll over on the tubes and wires that sprouted from his body.

I stayed by his side all night, watching his pain and discomfort increase until he asked me to try to do something about it.

"Would you mind giving me a little massage, Son?" he asked.

I agreed, and then slid my hands along the hos-pital mattress under his back until I could curl my fingers up and work on his knotted muscles. The operating table had been as hard as a block of concrete, and being strapped in one position for hours turned out to be the most painful part of the operation.

"You know, Steve," he said, his face just inches from mine, "After what I've been through, it feels great just to be alive. And what you're doing feels indescribable."

So, every hour or so during the night, I awoke from sleep in the chair beside him, stretched my fingers beneath his back again, and offered the best massage I could. We didn't speak many words, but the father-son communication between us had never been stronger. It's an experience that bonds us to this day.

Sometimes, other people just plain aren't into massage. Don't force your family members into it if they're not comfortable. More commonly, they'll be ready and willing to experiment with massage, but only on the receiving end, leaving you perpetually in the role of giver. If, no matter what tactics you use, you still end up being the only person in your family wild and crazy enough to give massages, I say go ahead and do it! You'll be creating a closeness that wouldn't be there otherwise, and your family will eventually express their gratitude in other ways.

Baby Massage

"Where touching begins, there love and humanity also begin — within the first minutes following birth." — Ashley Montagu

My wife and I were waiting in line at the grocery store one day with our four-month-old son sitting in his stroller. Suddenly, the woman behind us reached over and started massaging his toes. "Massage is very good for babies," she said, "especially here on the big toe. If he's depressed or angry, this will make him feel better." We were amazed, and it must have shown on our faces, because she looked up at us and smiled reassuringly. "Don't worry," she said, "It really works. I saw it on TV!"

Regardless of how you feel about strangers touching your child's feet in supermarkets, this story does point to the widespread acceptance of baby massage and child massage by people everywhere.

Cultures from around the world embrace the concept of baby massage:

- ✔ People from India have massaged their babies for centuries.
- ✔ Eskimos and native people from East Africa have long histories of using baby massage, too.
- ✔ In Bali, children are held in constant physical contact for the first six months of life, and only then are their feet first allowed to touch the ground.

Touch is part of the fabric of life, from the moment we first emerge from the womb into our parents' arms. Unfortunately, the more "civilized" and technologically advanced we become, the less time we seem to have to touch our babies, and that's why spending some quality time massaging babies is so important.

Why baby loves massage

If you spend a little time around babies, you may start to think to yourself, "Hey, babies are different than normal humans. They seem hyper-sensitive. Every little touch is magnified a hundred times. Is it just me, or do babies feel things differently than we do?"

Babies do indeed feel things more intensely than adults. This is caused by an abundance of special touch-sensing organs in the skin called *Meissner's corpuscles*, which are five times more prevalent in children three years old and younger than they are in adults. Babies have 80 Meissner's corpuscles per square millimeter of skin versus 20 per square millimeter for adults and 4 per millimeter for seniors.

Meissner's corpuscles are especially good at detecting light, fleeting movements across the skin, and so this type of movement is especially effective on babies.

Also, researchers at the Touch Research Institute (TRI) in Miami have found that massage can actually help premature infants grow faster and leave the hospital sooner. Touch is a lifesaver for infants, who crave it as deeply as they crave oxygen, or light. So, when you add to that the pleasure it provides, it's no wonder babies love massage.

Baby massage moves

One thing about babies: They're really, really small. You can tell how small they are when you try to massage them and one of your hands covers their entire back. Besides, most of the time they're either squirming around like tadpoles or lying fast asleep. So, what techniques are you supposed to use on such tiny, wriggling creatures?

Here are a few pointers to get you started:

- Choose a time when the baby is tranquil to give the massage, perhaps after a bath, shortly after waking up, or right before bedtime.
- Use light touch to stimulate the Meissner's corpuscles in your baby's skin, providing extra pleasure that makes him want to stay in one place longer.
- The massage may only last one or two minutes before the baby squirms away, but that's okay. Just give as much as you can.
- Don't be afraid to make firm (but not hard) contact. Babies are more resilient than they look and like a nice, solid, reassuring touch. If you use only very light, tickling touch, the baby misses some of the benefits of massage.

Baby massage routine

The following moves are easy to do, as you can see from Figure 18-1. The hardest part will probably be getting your baby to sit still for them.

1. **With the baby lying face up, run your fingertips lightly up over his abdomen, chest, and face, and then bring them back down again, as shown in Figure 18-1a.**

   Remember: This move is just to stimulate the Meissner's corpuscles, so it doesn't need to be firm at all. You can add some extra effectiveness to this move by saying "Whoooosh!" as you bring your fingers up over the baby's body. After a little practice, your baby begins to anticipate this deliciously pleasurable move and smile when you approach him with outstretched fingers.

2. **With your hands on the baby's sides, sweep your thumbs up over his abdomen, moving them outwards. Then lightly brush the thumbs back over the skin and repeat four to five times.**

   This is a calming stroke that's good for the internal organs. *Note:* This move (shown in Figure 18-1b) requires relatively firm pressure, and you may need some oil or lotion, as well.

3. **Using your thumbs, make little circles with moderate pressure into the fleshy area of baby's little tush, as shown in Figure 18-1c.**

   He may try to squirm away from you while you're doing this move, but you may catch him smiling as he does so. This move feels great.

4. **Apply an itty-bitty version of kneading to the baby's chubby little thighs, as shown in Figure 18-1d.**

   Babies appreciate a little attention to these muscles, especially as they become more active and stand on their legs longer.

5. **Help your baby stretch his legs by grasping his lower leg, pushing his knee up toward his chest, and then gently stretching the leg out straight toward you (see Figure 18-1e).**

   Repeat this move three to four times. Support his opposite hip with your other hand to keep him steady while you do this move. Babies naturally love to stretch, just like dogs and cats, so this move feels especially good.

6. **If you can get him to sit still long enough, you can apply a light (and very quick) version of the reflexology moves from Chapter 14 to your baby's feet.**

   Babies are born with a complete set of reflexology points on their feet, and, in general, they love to have them stimulated, especially those little toes (see Figure 18-1f).

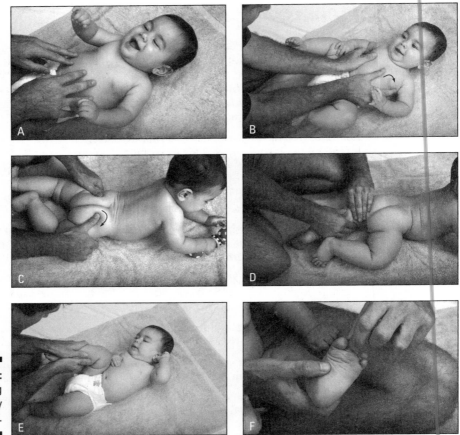

Figure 18-1:
Massaging
Baby
Capellini.

Baby massage training

Babies don't need any special training to begin enjoying massage, but mommies and daddies can certainly benefit by learning a few tips from baby massage experts. Some good videos are available on the subject, and classes are given in many areas for parents, foster parents, grandparents, and anyone else interested. The massage techniques taught are not just for newborns either. Toddlers enjoy massage, too.

If you really get into it, you can become a certified baby massage instructor yourself. Some good training programs in the U.S. are offered by a woman named Vimala Schneider McClure, who experienced baby massage firsthand in India and brought it back to the U.S. She founded the International Association of Infant Massage, which now has over 2,500 members, and she wrote *Infant Massage: A Handbook for Loving Parents,* (Bantam Doubleday Dell Publishing Company).

Contact one of the following numbers or visit the following Web site if you're interested in baby massage:

- ✔ International Association of Infant Massage (IAIM); contact person: Vimala Schneider McClure; telephone: 800-248-5432

- ✔ Cinnabar School, P.O. Box 34326, Westbrook, Calgary, AB, Canada T3C 3W0; telephone: 403-246-6720; www.babymassage.com

- ✔ Tender Loving Touch; contact people: Elain Weisberg and Rita Day; Louisville, KY, telephone: 502-458-7007

Not for Women Only

Massage can be enjoyed equally by men and women, of course, but there are certain circumstances in which women definitely receive a little something extra from the experience. I'm talking about that trio of specifically female conditions:

- ✔ Pregnancy
- ✔ PMS
- ✔ Menopause

When a woman receives a massage during any of these times in her life, it not only benefits her, but all the people she lives with as well. Keeping females happy with massage is especially important for all males who live anywhere in their approximate vicinity.

And who are the women closest to you? Usually they're related to you in one way or another. Mothers come to mind right away, for example. Massage is one of the best things you can do for your mother, whether it comes directly from your hands or as a gift (check out the coupons from Spa Wish in the back of the book for an easy way to purchase massage gifts for your mom, regardless of what city she lives in). Wives and girlfriends deserve special massage attention, too, because they have the ability to instantaneously cut off a man's supply of something that he loves very much indeed — his happiness.

If a lot more women received a lot more massage, there would be a lot less strife in a lot of families. Think about it.

Massaging mommy-to-be

If you are living with a pregnant woman, you can't do too many things for her that would make her happier than a nice massage. In fact, she'll absolutely love you for even offering.

Labor day massage

I was once asked by a client to accompany her into the labor room and assist with some massage during delivery. This sounded like a good idea, so I read up on the subject and consulted with several experienced colleagues. When the big day came, however, things didn't turn out exactly the way we all expected.

A few minutes after arrival in the hospital birthing suite, I reached down to massage my client's feet between her rather powerful contractions.

"Don't you touch me!" screamed my normally demure client in a voice that reminded me of Linda Blair in *The Exorcist.*

Perhaps I was the wrong gender. For centuries, women have stuck together at the crucial time of labor, offering each other the support and understanding that only *they* know how to give. A man, even with the best of intentions, often just can't seem to get the touch right at moments like that.

About half an hour later, standing a respectful few feet away, I watched with amazement as my client's daughter made her appearance in the world. The massage could wait for another day.

Doulas

Some women blend the lines between working as a massage therapist and a childbirth assistant. In many countries, women calling themselves *doulas* go through the process of labor with a woman, offering encouragement, support, and often touch.

If you'd like more information or are interested in becoming a doula or childbirth assistant yourself, contact the Association of Labor Assistants and Childbirth Educators, P.O. Box 382724, Cambridge, MA 02238; telephone: 617-441-2500; e-mail: alacehq@aol.com; Web: www.alace.org.

Pregnancy massage pointers

Giving massage to a pregnant woman is perfectly safe, and there are even special massage tables with big holes in the center (so the woman can lie down on her stomach) made especially for that purpose, but there are a few points you should keep in mind for safety's sake:

- A pregnant woman should not lie facedown on her abdomen but rather faceup or on her side (unless a special table like the one described in this section is used).

- In the later stages of pregnancy, she should not lie facedown or *faceup*, but only on her side, because the extra weight of the fetus can put pressure on her aorta and cut off circulation when she's on her back.

✔ Make sure that she's comfortably supported at all times, using pillows and other cushions beneath her legs and head.

✔ Use only very light and soothing touch directly on the abdominal area.

✔ Stay away from the points near the heel that correspond to the reproductive organs in reflexology, because they're supposed to help induce labor. Refer to Figure 14-3 for the location of these points.

For more information on this topic, see the sidebar in Chapter 10, "Pregnancy: A contraindication?"

With these guidelines in mind, you can confidently offer massage to your favorite pregnant person. A high percentage of pregnant women report back pain, sciatic pain, leg cramps, swelling of the ankles, and other problems that massage can help ease. So, she will definitely appreciate your efforts.

To find out more, a good book on the subject is *Mother Massage: A Handbook for Relieving the Discomforts of Pregnancy,* by Elaine Stillerman (Delta Books).

PMS (Please Massage Soon)

Few people realize that the real words behind the acronym PMS are "please massage soon." The phrase was coined back in the 1970s when some men started noticing that their wives or girlfriends periodically seemed to need an especially large share of love and attention. Massage was the perfect answer, and so many a man offered his sweetie some tender touch at those times when she seemed to need it the most.

If your honey comes to you looking stressed-out or on the verge or tears for no apparent reason and asks you for a massage, do not ask any stupid questions. Just start massaging. Immediately.

Meno-possiblities

All kinds of crazy things start happening with a woman's hormones about the time she's going through menopause. Many of these things have an effect on the way she looks and the way she feels.

Massage can help create continued possibilities for health, good looks, and pleasure as a woman enters this stage of life. Massage is extremely beneficial at this time, because the increased circulation and the actions of the oils and creams used are good for the delicate collagen and elastin fibers that are beginning to break down, causing wrinkles. You're not going to rub away the wrinkles, but you can definitely add a healthy glow to gracefully maturing skin. The emotional reassurance and comfort given through caring touch do a lot to renew a woman's balance, too.

The facial and the full day of spa pleasures I outline in Chapter 15 are sure to be appreciated by menopausal women, as well as a massage.

Senior Massage

As Art Linkletter once said, "Old age is not for sissies." All sorts of things start to happen to a body after it's been around for a while. In addition to the expected stiff joints and achy muscles, many seniors feel a deeper pain as well, the pain of loneliness.

Massage can help with the stiffness. It can help with the aches. And sometimes it can even help with the loneliness. Massage treats the little things that eventually become the big things. A little stiffness, for example, could lead to the awkwardness and lack of coordination that eventually ends up causing a fall. When seniors feel more relaxed and coordinated after a massage, they are less likely to fall.

Little daily doses of touch can make the difference between a lonely life and a more fulfilled one. We are each born yearning for touch as babies, and, as we age, the need for contact is still there, though we often suppress it.

A new movement is afoot for seniors these days. As the population in industrialized countries gets progressively older, people are not taking to the idea of retirement like they used to. A few years ago, the word *retirement* used to mean "ready to die." Now it means, "twenty more years of activities and then maybe slowing down a little." Massage can play a big part in keeping seniors vital and healthy during those years.

In Chapter 5, I mention one of the world's favorite seniors, and a great fan of massage, Bob Hope. He's had a massage almost every day of his life for over 50 years, and he says it's been an important part of what's kept him going. As of this writing, he's nearing the 100-year mark. Maybe we could all learn a few things about aging from him.

Reach out and touch someone older

You can easily extend massage to seniors. Most are extremely grateful for the contact. All you really need is a tiny bit of courage to take that first step. Go ahead . . . reach out and touch someone older. Try these suggestions to get started:

- ✔ Visit a senior citizen neighbor and spend a little time with her. Offer to give her a light shoulder and neck rub.

- ✔ Visit a retirement home and volunteer to make the rounds and talk to the residents. When you do, hold each one by the hand, making simple contact.

- ✔ Self-massage is great for seniors, too. If the opportunity is there, go ahead and teach the self-massage moves in Chapter 13 to a special senior. This is also a great way to share your enthusiasm for massage with your own parents or grandparents.

You should follow a few guidelines when massaging seniors:

- ✔ Seniors are generally more frail than younger folks, so use gentler movements when giving them a massage.

- ✔ They're not made of porcelain, however, and you don't need to treat them like they're going to break at any second. Start off softly, and progressively increase the vigor of your massage until you reach a comfortable level.

- ✔ Make extra sure to ask for lots of feedback so you know what you're doing is okay.

A chance to give back

In studies conducted at the Touch Research Institute, it was found that seniors received almost as much benefit from giving massage as they did from receiving. Teaching seniors how to massage their grandchildren, for example, is a wonderful way to help them feel involved and in touch with the younger generations.

You may be surprised how good the simple act of giving a massage can make someone feel. The contact is what counts. If you think Granny's a loner who enjoys being off in a corner, give her another chance and have her help you massage the baby. You may be surprised.

Professional senior massage

If you're headed in the direction of becoming a massage pro yourself, and you think you may want to specialize in offering your services to seniors, special organizations and trainings are available just for you. Contact the Day-Break Geriatric Massage Project in California (call 707-829-2798 or visit them on the Web at www.daybreak-massage.com). They have books, videos, trainings, and a symposium for massage therapists who specialize in senior massage.

Final contact

A friend called once and asked me to come over to give a massage to his father, who had recently suffered a stroke. It took both of us several minutes working together to get his father up on the massage table, because he was weak and partially paralyzed. The stroke had also taken away his ability to speak.

For almost an hour, I did the best I could to help relieve some of the stress and fear that this man was going through. His muscles quivered. His eyes looked directly into mine. Near the end of the massage he reached his hand out and held onto my arm, and I felt a powerful silent communication pass between us through the touch. For 10 seconds, 30 seconds, a minute, he just held me.

The next day I was scheduled to come massage him again, but that morning I received a call. He was gone. Now, several years later, I can still feel the strength of his grip on my arm.

Massage can offer some serious help for older people suffering from Parkinson's Disease, stroke, poor blood circulation, and other conditions. In some cases, patients have avoided amputations and terminal disability through the massage they've received. Many seniors, such as widowed people for example, are seldom touched, yet they're the people who need it the most. Massage can help.

Touch at the end of life

Massage can offer much needed reassurance for those people near the end of their lives. Some massage pros have specialized in this type of work, giving massage in hospitals and hospices. A sizable number of clergy, members of the National Association of Bodyworkers in Religious Service (NABRS), are also involved.

You can learn more about offering this type of massage in the book *Compassionate Touch: Hands-On Caregiving for the Elderly, the Ill and the Dying*, by Dawn Nelson (Talman Company).

Chapter 19

The Lover's Touch: Massage and Intimacy

*L*et's face it: Sometimes, massage can just plain be sexy. Regardless of how therapeutic it is. Regardless of the fact that it was recommended centuries ago by ancient respectable guys like Hippocrates. Regardless of how favorably many physicians think of it today. Regardless of the way it's used by superstar athletes in smelly locker rooms. And regardless of the hundreds of thousands of professional practitioners out there who help heal millions of people through their non-sexual touch.

As a practitioner of therapeutic, non-sexual massage myself, I am amongst those who would like to convince you that there's a *big* difference between sensual touch and therapeutic massage. But that doesn't mean sensual touch can't be therapeutic. In fact, the famous musician Marvin Gaye sang a song on that very topic. You guessed it — "Sexual Healing."

 This chapter offers a few basic ideas to get you started with some sensually oriented massage. You can take many of the suggestions from the rest of this book, too, and add a little spice to them. Be careful who you use your sensual healing techniques on, though, because they can be quite powerful.

Sensual Touch

You need a few important ingredients in order to create a great sensual massage. These include the following:

- A naked supermodel
- A gallon and a half of musk-scented massage oil from ancient Persia
- Any CD by Barry White

Just kidding! Actually, having any of those ingredients on hand may indeed improve your chances of experiencing the ultimate sensual massage, but they're certainly not necessary. The following are the three things that you definitely need for a good sensual massage:

- The right intention
- Spontaneity
- Sensitivity

The right intention

So how do you go about being sensual with your chosen partner after you've decided you'd like to share a sexy massage together? The trick is to change your *intention*. You can tell the difference instantaneously when someone has a sensual intent with their massage moves. You may be surprised how the very same moves performed on the very same part of the body can have incredibly different effects, depending upon who's giving the massage, and what his or her intention is. You can feel it in the touch.

A fine line lies between sensual and sexual massage, and believe it or not, sometimes sensual is better. Sensual massage is more relaxed. It doesn't expect anything. Sex is something that gets done, while sensuality just *is*.

Once in a while, simply enjoy the touch without thinking about where it may lead. Relax there in the arms of sensuality for a time, taking some pressure off of you and your partner. You may like what you find.

Spontaneity

Perhaps the most important rule for sensual massage is, "Go with the flow." If you feel like the most appropriate place for the massage is out on the beach at midnight, then take your bottle of oil and head outside. Then again, the kitchen floor can become an exotically sensual environment when you lie down on it with your partner. Wherever you are, look around for items that can enhance your experience. You're bound to be able to use something that you have on hand — a texture, a sound, or a taste — like a big, juicy, ripe strawberry, for example.

Sensitivity

With sensual massage, you have to be especially sensitive to your partner's emotions during the session. Envelope him or her in a sense of warmth, caring, and safety. You don't have to beat your partner's tension into submission or accomplish anything at all really. Just *be there* with him or her.

Soft hands

In sensual massage, the idea is not so much to soothe your partner's sore muscles, but to enchant him. So, you don't need to use as much pressure or strength as you do in a regular massage. Practice using *soft hands*, letting your fingertips and palms drift over the surface of the skin without trying to achieve any therapeutic purposes. This technique changes the massage mood, making it more sensual.

A massage called Tantra

You may want to know about a special, sensual, energy-raising technique called *Tantra*. This technique combines meditation and lots of interesting activities you can use to change sexual energy into sensual/spiritual energy. You and your partner can engage in sensual massage, for example, to heighten your experience of togetherness, instead of rushing straight into the whole sex thing and then rolling over and falling asleep afterward.

If you're into enhancing your sensual life, you can choose among many workshops, videos, and books. Pick up one of the books by Mantak Chia, for example, which you can find on the Web at www.tantra.com. And while you're there, you can have fun discovering other aspects of Tantra, such as art and instructions from the *Kama Sutra,* an ancient text on sensuality. Plenty of couples workshops on the subject are available, too.

Have fun!

Setting the Sensual Mood

Sensuality is all about creating a sensual mood, right? So, it follows that your inner chamber, as I describe in Chapter 9, is especially important during a sensual massage. But just how exactly are you supposed to make it sensual? You can use candles and incense, but how about something a little more daring?

You may want to check out a few of the items listed below to help you and your partner get into the appropriate sensual mood. After all, you don't have all day to lie around waiting for the proper mood to strike. You're a busy person, and you have lots of other things on your mind. If you're feeling adventurous, try the following suggestions, and see what happens.

Flavored massage oils

Okay, I admit it . . . flavored massage oils are a little on the hokey side. But you can't knock it till you try it, right? These days, there are flavors for every taste. You can even find, believe it or not, a cappuccino-flavored massage oil, which must be for those times you need a quick pick-me-up and don't want to suffer the extreme embarrassment of falling asleep with your tongue in your partner's navel.

Of course, the idea here is to enjoy the flavor of the oil while you're licking it off, but be careful not to get addicted to this pastime. Don't swallow whole pints of the stuff, because it could jeopardize your health. Like all oils, edible ones have a lot of cholesterol and fat, too. And nothing would be worse than gaining weight by licking your mate, which can lead to the worst of all excuses for not giving your honey a sensual massage: "I'm on a diet."

If edible oils interest you, check out the Wild Syde on the Web at wildsyde.com or call 800-433-6459 or 732-714-0306.

Little devices

Little devices that buzz and vibrate can be quite a pleasurable addition to a sensual massage experience. You can purchase such devices guilt-free at trendy shops in cities around the world these days, or you can order them through the mail.

Videos

All kinds of sensual massage videos are out there for you to use to help get you in the mood, but they share one big problem: The models are too good looking. For most people, watching one of those videos without feeling a little inadequate is difficult. If you do watch them, just keep reminding yourself that those people spend ten hours a day exercising, seven days a week. When they're not exercising, they're at the tanning salon, or the local health food restaurant having a bowl of lettuce for lunch, dressing on the side.

Sensual Moves

Here are a few moves that you can use when you're creating your sensual massage together. You may notice that some of these moves are not really moves at all, but attitudes. In a sensual massage you take more liberties with your partner. You drape yourselves over each other more, coming closer and dissolving the giver/receiver barrier.

Creating fuller contact

In therapeutic massage, you usually bring just your hands and arms into contact with your partner, for the most part. In sensual massage, on the other hand, it doesn't matter how much of your body comes into contact with your partner. In fact, the more contact the better, as shown in Figure 19-1. For massage maneuvers applied to the back, the neck, and the head, sit right down on your partner's tush. Just make sure not to rest all your weight on him, though, because you may cut off the circulation.

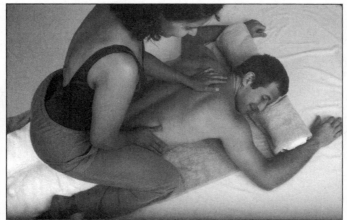

Figure 19-1:
Sitting on top of your partner is great in sensual massage.

Limb draping

When you're massaging your partner's limbs, let the entire leg or arm rest across your body. This creates a sensation of support and intimacy, especially when you combine it with light, lacy moves with your fingertips on the inner thigh area, as shown in Figure 19-2. Ooh la la!

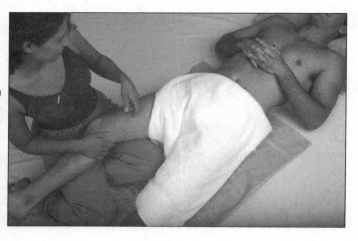

Figure 19-2: Sensually draping your partner's limbs over your body adds to the experience.

Hair gliding

The fine ends of your soft, silky hair can be instruments of exquisite pleasure. Simply let your hair hang down and brush lightly across your partner's skin anywhere on his body while you're giving the massage, as shown in Figure 19-3.

Do not attempt this move if you have a buzz cut or a spiky Mohawk hairstyle, because you could inflict serious damage.

Belly touching

Ever notice how you instinctively cringe and protect your chest and abdomen when danger is present? You do this because the front of the human body is incredibly vulnerable and sensitive. This vulnerability is bad for self-defense from attacking wolverines, but it's great for sensual massage. Simply use a series of light, gliding strokes all up across the abdomen and chest, as shown in Figure 19-4. These moves are not meant to affect the muscles, as the chest massage moves in Chapter 11 are, but rather just to stimulate the skin (and the mind) of your partner.

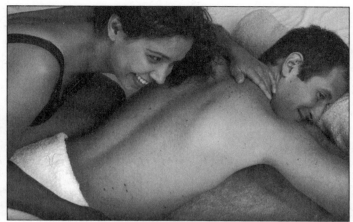

Figure 19-3: In sensual massage, using your hair is part of the fun.

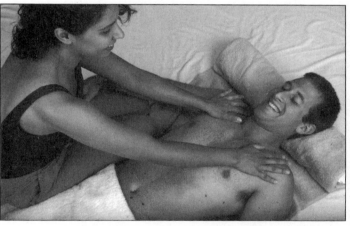

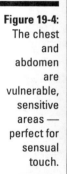

Figure 19-4: The chest and abdomen are vulnerable, sensitive areas — perfect for sensual touch.

The most sensual organ of them all

Simply rubbing your hands and fingers over a person's erogenous zones can be, well, erotic, but it's not the only game in town. If you've been with your partner for a long time, you may want to explore some newer, less obvious zones.

One particular organ is too often neglected, and it can be the most sensual one of all. On all humans, it's found in the same area. Everybody responds to stimulation there in a different way, though, making seduction and sensuality an endless surprise.

Of course, I'm talking about the brain. If you can get inside your partner's imagination, you can lead him on an infinite number of new erotic experiences without ever leaving the safety of your house. Try it the next time you're sharing a sensual massage together.

Fantasizing is okay

If you find yourself repeatedly imagining that you're receiving your massage from a naked movie star on a beach in Tahiti, don't worry. That's normal. In fact, you may even use the fantasy to make the sensual massage more sensual.

Encourage your partner to share a few juicy morsels from her fantasy life while you're applying these sensual moves. You may be surprised how the combination of your familiar touch and the fantasy of an exotic, unfamiliar situation adds to your experience.

The ultimate aphrodisiac

I once had the pleasure of massaging Dr. Ruth Westheimer, and I'll never forget what she said to me at the end of the massage. Still lying on the table, she glanced up at me with her trade-marked mischievous grin, and said, "Don't you want to ask me a question?"

"A question?"

"Yes, you know, about love, or sex?" Her eyes twinkled.

I couldn't pass up the opportunity for some free expert advice, and so I asked Dr. Ruth what the most powerful aphrodisiac in the world was. Oysters? Ginseng? Bark from the yohimbe tree in Africa?

"Whatever works for you, works!" said Dr. Ruth, and the phrase has rung true all the years since she spoke it. You and your partner can create the ultimate, personalized sensual massage experience that's right for you. Just remember Dr. Ruth cheering you on from the sidelines, which should put a smile on your face, and then go for it!

Chapter 20

Have Hands, Will Travel: Doing Massage for a Living

*S*o, now, after practicing your new techniques and discovering the incredible benefits of massage, you may be thinking to yourself, "Hey, all this massage stuff is just *too much fun*. I'd like to find out how I can spend a large percentage of my own time making others feel better like all those fantastic professional massage therapists I've been reading about. And besides, it may help to pay the rent."

May I then shamelessly take this opportunity to suggest to you a fantastic book on exactly this subject, a book that was, coincidentally, written by me? The book is *Massage Therapy Career Guide for Hands-On Success*. It is packed with over 300 pages of essential information for the person who is seriously considering a walk down the massage career path, and for the person who has already begun that journey.

Right here in this chapter, you're going to get enough information to make a sound decision on whether massage therapy may be the right career choice for you. You also find several tips and connections to get you going in the right direction.

Is This the Career for You?

The first thing you should do when considering a career in massage is ask yourself a series of tough questions to determine your true motivations and chances for success. Answering the following questions, excerpted from *Massage Therapy Career Guide*, may give you a good preliminary idea about how well suited you are to this profession.

The ten traits of a born massage therapist

1. Do people swoon and tell you that you have "great hands" when you simply place them upon their neck and shoulders and squeeze a little? Yes/No

2. Do you feel sympathetic pain someplace in your own body when someone else tells you about their own pain? Yes/No

3. Do you feel very comfortable with your own and others' bodies? Are you free from excess inhibition and body image hang-ups? Yes/No

4. Do you have the ability and desire to work several hours a day at a very physical endeavor requiring significant stamina? Yes/No

5. Is it easy for you to remain in silence for an entire hour (or several hours in a row), without indulging in conversation if a client doesn't wish it? Yes/No

6. Have people ever told you that your presence makes them feel peaceful or calm? Yes/No

7. Do you take your own health seriously by exercising, watching what you eat, and using moderation? Yes/No

8. Does the idea of changing your lifestyle and livelihood seem exciting rather than horrible? Yes/No

9. Is the human body a source of wonder and intrigue for you, making you want to learn more about how it works through intensive study? Yes/No

10. Are you willing to invest a significant amount of time and money for schooling, supplies, association memberships, and equipment? Yes/No

Count up the number of "Yes" responses and compare your total with the following:

- 9–10 Head to the nearest massage school to enroll.

- 6–8 Begin serious investigation about the possibilities; send away for more information from massage schools.

- 3–5 Seek the advice and inspiration of established massage therapists in your area who may be able to give you some insight about what daily life in the massage field is really like.

- 0–2 Consider more deeply what your needs and motivations are for looking into massage as a career.

An honest look at yourself

Before you take the plunge, you really need to stop and ask yourself: Am I really into touching all those strangers all day long for the rest of my life?

This is not a career for everybody. It takes a certain kind of person to be a massage therapist. And if you are that kind of person, what you may discover, after a short while, is that those "strangers" you may be touching are not really strangers after all, but fellow human beings whom you can relate to on a meaningful level through your newfound skills.

Massage gives us an acceptable avenue for empathy. Practicing professionals can touch others in a caring, compassionate way, helping them with their problems, easing their stress, and letting them know they're not alone. Massage therapists are paid to *be there* for people.

That's no small thing.

So take an honest look at yourself. Does that deep desire to help and empathize with others outweigh whatever reservations you may have regarding the nitty-gritty reality of dealing with the not-always-wonderful public? If so, maybe you have quite an adventure ahead — a massage adventure.

The Massage Adventure

After you make this fundamental choice and decide to pursue your career in massage, then you have to prepare yourself for your new role in society. Yes, people may look at you with different eyes when they see you carrying around one of those big massage tables that look like padded suitcases. How will they react? What will the neighbors say?

It's strange to think of yourself as this new person, isn't it? It's almost like becoming a police officer or ship captain or any other profession that involves the wearing of a uniform. You're on display as what you are, and it may be uncomfortable at first.

These sensations gradually fade away, though, as you begin to associate more and more with other people who make a similar career decision. The first place you begin to meet your fellow travelers is usually in massage school.

Getting trained

Chances are that you already know somebody who knows somebody who has taken up massage as a career. It's ever more popular, with people from many different backgrounds.

There are over 800 massage schools in the U.S., where training usually lasts about 6 months. In some areas, though, you can get certified in as little as a hundred hours, and in others you need more than 1,000 hours, which can take up to a full year. Other countries can require significantly more training, such as Canada for example, with schools that have 2,000- or even 3,000-hour programs, lasting up to three years. Most schools offer part-time classroom hours for those students who work another job, and some even have Saturday classes once a week for extended periods.

Here are some of the things you explore in massage school:

- ✔ Anatomy
- ✔ Physiology
- ✔ Massage (duh!)
- ✔ Applicable ethics, history, law, and so on.
- ✔ Hygiene
- ✔ Allied therapies, such as hydrotherapy
- ✔ Professional conduct and ethics
- ✔ And much more

Sounds like an actual academic program, doesn't it? That's because it is. Massage school is not just rubbing and relaxing all day, but that doesn't mean it isn't fun. Most graduates have very fond memories of their massage school days. And, just like in other schools, you establish new friendships, possibly spark romance, and change life paths.

Choosing a school

All massage schools are not created equal. And the one you choose may play an extremely important role in your overall experience of massage. Some schools have a very grass-roots feeling, and attending them makes you feel like a part of the massage revolution as it unfolds across the globe, touching people's spirits, as well as their bodies, in many important ways. Other schools are more interested in providing their students with a no-nonsense, technically oriented approach to massage based more strictly on a medical model.

All schools let you attend an open house or a class to see whether the school's "personality" is the right match for you. Take advantage of this opportunity, and make sure to ask plenty of questions when you meet past and present students.

Another way you can check the standards of a school is to see whether it is accredited by an official organization. In the U.S., for example, schools accredited by the Commission on Massage Training Accreditation/Approval (COMTAA) or the Integrative Massage and Somatic Therapies Accreditation Council (IMSTAC) had to meet some very strict guidelines. You can be rest assured of the quality. Information about these accrediting organizations is available from the American Massage Therapy Association and Associated Bodywork and Massage Professionals.

The prospect of attending a massage school may excite you, but you have no idea how truly valuable the experience is until you go through it yourself. Some of the high points include:

- ✔ Camaraderie
- ✔ Increased knowledge and self-confidence
- ✔ Exposure to new techniques and systems
- ✔ A return to the stimulating, youthful lifestyle of the student
- ✔ Credentials you can travel with
- ✔ Self-transformation (See the sidebar later in this chapter.)

Chapter 21 lists ten of the best places to study massage.

An information-packed book about massage schools is available from Associated Bodywork and Massage Professionals (ABMP). It's called the Touch Training Directory, and you can order it by calling 800-458-2267 or 303-674-8478 or by visiting www.abmp.com.

Determining cost

Massage school may cost anywhere from several hundred dollars a semester at a vocational technical school up to around $15,000 at some of the top schools, with the average seeming to hover in the $5,000 to $6,000 range. Schools in countries outside the U.S., based more on a medical education framework, can cost quite a bit more.

As you can see, massage school usually entails a substantial investment. And that doesn't include the equipment and supplies you need to get started after you finish school. You need things like a massage table, business cards, and so on. So you need to think long and hard before plunking down that much dough for an education in touch therapy. This thought process is good. Think

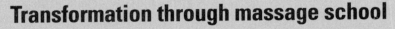

Transformation through massage school

It's a rare person who can go through massage school and not be transformed on some fundamental level. What makes this so, you ask? Several things:

✔ Everybody there is making a change of some sort in their lives, which makes for a lot of very open people, ready to share themselves with you, and ready to have fun!

✔ People enrolled in massage school are there to take charge of their own lives in an entrepreneurial sense and a health sense, too, so you're likely to do some important networking with kindred spirits. Many business relationships have been forged in the classroom.

✔ Many students are often scared out of their wits that they won't be able to support themselves after they graduate; this makes them feel vulnerable, and vulnerability is a

very endearing quality in most people. It lets you all communicate on an honest level.

✔ School offers you a time-out from the race you've been running in your life up to now. It gives you time to take stock of what's most important, of where you've been and where you truly want to go.

✔ When you begin literally touching people on a daily basis, as you will in school, you quickly get back in touch with what's real, and what matters. Life matters. Health matters. People matter. What you're doing is important, and as you realize this more and more each day, your life may transform.

Attending massage school is no guarantee for a changed life, but it's a pretty good bet that you may come away with some insights and direction that you never even considered before you began. Just stay open.

of it as a filtering system that keeps the less-than-serious from getting into the profession. Even with the costs, many tens of thousands of new massage therapists enter the worldwide market every year.

Obtaining licensing and certification

After you graduate from school, you receive a certificate stating that you passed the course. Then, in many areas, you have to take that certificate and apply to take yet another exam to get your license. The license legally allows you to practice massage in your area. You never thought it would be so complex, did you?

The laws regarding licensing can indeed be confusing, and they're different everywhere you go, so the best advice I can give you is to do some thorough research into the regulations in your own area. Just a little accidental slip-up could turn you into an outlaw massage rogue, which would not be good for your professional reputation.

Discovering your new lifestyle

Freedom at last! After you make it through schooling, certification, and licensure, you're out there in the real world massaging real people — for real money. This new lifestyle you create for yourself is nothing like the boring 9 to 5 routine at your old job. But with your old job, you knew when you were working and you knew when you were off. Now, it seems like you're always either coming back from giving a massage, just about to give a massage, or thinking of ways you can get more people to sign up for massages.

Ah, there's the real rub; there's never an end to the massage work that needs to be done.

When you work for yourself doing massage, you have to create some new rules and boundaries, like any self-employed person, so that your work life doesn't swallow you whole. Whether you work in a spa, a clinic, a doctor's office, or in your client's homes, you're going to need new boundary rules (see the sidebar about boundary rules in this chapter).

So how much will you make? (the real story)

Many would-be massage therapists add up the numbers. "Let's see, 50 dollars per massage, doing just 5 massages a day, 5 days a week, makes $1,250 per week, times 50 weeks . . . oh my god! I'm going to be rich. Rich, I tell you!"

As a result of such calculations, many unsuspecting people have found themselves several months later sitting in a classroom studying the function of the gluteus maximus muscle. They bide their time, going through the motions, just waiting for their chance to graduate and become massage millionaires.

Well, it doesn't always work out exactly that way. In fact, it seldom ever does. The average annual salary of a massage therapist in the U.S. is under $20,000 per year, according to one association's statistics, and the number of massage school graduates who end up not working in the field at all is surprisingly large as well.

The truth is that, like any business, the massage business is a hard business. It may be a little more "romantic" than some other fields, but the day-to-day reality of it includes an awful lot of good old-fashioned hard work, combined with many things you may not have thought you would need, like marketing savvy, business plans, self-promotion, and managerial skills.

You can, indeed, make a very good living doing massage, and that may continue to be the case as more and more people worldwide realize the benefits that massage offers. But don't do it just for the money. You need to have another, deeper, reason, too, or you may end up like certain old rock-and-roll stars and massage therapists, eventually burning out.

Boundary rules

The rules you come up with for yourself as a massage therapist are completely personal. No two massage therapists need follow the exact same guidelines. The important thing to remember is to stick by whatever rules you set. This increases your self-esteem, makes life a lot easier for you, and lets your clients know that you're serious about your business.

The following are just a few suggestions of potential boundary rules. Yours may be much different. Practice saying your new rules out loud in front of the mirror a few times to yourself, as if you were talking to a client. Eventually, they seem natural.

- I don't work on weekends.
- I don't work after 8 p.m.
- I only take new clients by referral.
- I don't accept tips/I do accept tips.
- I have a 24-hour cancellation policy or the massage must be paid for in full.

The tip of the iceberg

You may have heard stories about massage therapists who get incredible tips from wealthy clients, and you may have wished that you, too, could receive such large gratuities. This is very natural. Yet, some people say that if you receive tips for massage, you do a disservice to the industry. They say tipping turns massage into a service (like a waiter serving food to your table) rather than a treatment (like a doctor helping you find relief from a particular problem). You wouldn't consider tipping your doctor, would you?

The problem here is just the tip of the iceberg, so to speak, of a larger underlying issue about how we want others to perceive massage. In the end, it's up to you whether to receive tips or not. It's hard to turn down that cash staring you in the face as someone hands it to you. Believe me, I've accepted a few whopper tips myself over the years. There's really nothing wrong with it, in the right circumstance, but it's also good to be aware of the larger issue. (See Chapter 8 for more information.)

Becoming a real pro

After you're out there and actually making a living giving massage, you may soon find that there's more to the job than just the hours spent working hands-on. In order to become a real pro, you need to network your way into the industry and become a part of it, just like you would become a part of the telephone industry, say, or the music industry. And that means . . . going to parties!

That's right. You have to go to some organized massage parties, also known as conventions, that are held every year in various locations. Speaking of associations, it's a great idea for you to join one of them, at least for a year on a trial basis, to see how the contacts, information, and sense of community can help you get going with your new career.

Make sure to subscribe to an industry magazine or two, and read each issue from cover to cover. This may help you feel like an insider as you become familiar with all the people, places, and history that make massage what it is today.

Where the Profession Is Headed

In a nutshell, up. Yes, up is the direction the profession of massage therapy is heading. And I'm talking on a worldwide scale here. If you're looking to get in on a growth industry, you really couldn't pick a better one than this, because the number of human bodies out there available to be massaged is growing at a tremendous rate. Sometime around the publication of this book, for instance, world population is going to surpass the 6 billion mark. So there's no shortage of clients. And there's more wealth now than there ever has been before, so many people can afford to pay for massage. An even bigger trend, though, and one that has already started, is that insurance companies may pay for massage because it's a cost-effective, health-care alternative.

That's right — in the future, as a massage therapist, others may respect you as a part of the evolving medical field, and your services may be paid for through insurance billing. This is already happening, but it may soon become more common.

And in addition to the respect and success that you can claim, there's a "certain something" that makes massage special, too. It's in the simple human act of touching — of contact. That's our true specialty, and let's hope it never changes, no matter how successful we become.

Where you can go as a massage therapist

If you spend the time to gain some expertise in massage, people may eventually be seeking you out for your services, rather than the other way around. Believe me, this feels very good. It is the exact opposite of sitting in your underwear on Saturday morning searching through the want ads hoping there's someone out there who can appreciate your abilities.

After you work to establish yourself as a massage therapist, you may be at an entirely different place than you have ever experienced up to now. A good place. It's a place that often leads to other places, as those who gain success turn around and teach their skills to others in a variety of ways.

Many massage therapists compound their success by turning to teaching at massage schools, at weekend workshops, and in books and videos that they create for other massage therapists. Some massage therapists even go on to become consultants, speakers, and sought-after health experts.

And just think, it all starts when you make that simple, profound decision, to reach out and touch other people. Through massage you can do that.

The gift beyond price

If you decide to pursue massage, you may discover some things about life and about yourself that you never would have guessed otherwise. You will literally "get in touch" with your own existence in a new way. You change. You grow. This is the most valuable gift you receive, and it comes to you when you start to dedicate yourself to giving to others. What a concept.

Go ahead! Give it a shot! It is truly a path worth pursuing.

Best of luck to you.

Part VI
The Part of Tens

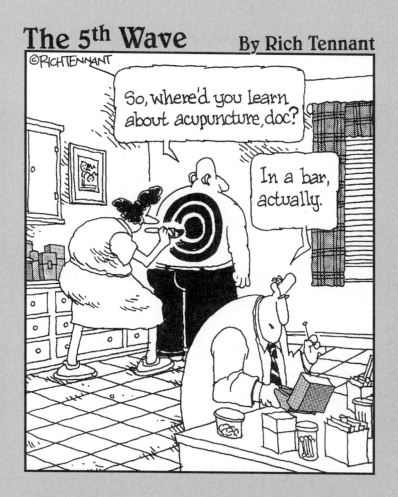

In this part . . .

Even with all the nifty photos and detailed instructions in this book, there still might be times when you'd rather just have somebody else make the massage decisions for you. Instead of figuring out all the moves for yourself, for example, wouldn't it be nice to slip away to one of the most fantastic spots on the planet and have a professional give you a massage? You'd probably like me to suggest the top ten places to do just that, wouldn't you?

And, in the same vein, wouldn't it be convenient if I were to cut to the chase and say to you, "Okay, here are the ten simplest massage moves you can perform on anyone (including yourself), anywhere, anytime, to relieve stress"? That would take a lot of the work out of learning massage. I bet you'd like that, wouldn't you?

Ah ha! I thought so, but you're not lazy. It just means that you've been reading for a long time now, and you're a little tired. You'd like some understanding here, a little compassion.

So that's what this last section is all about. Here in The Part of Tens, I relieve you of your burden of figuring things out and just go ahead and list things for you. In the process, you'll discover the answers to such burning questions as "What's the best place to get a massage in Morocco?" and "How can I massage my cat's ears?"

In addition, you are made privy to a short list of top places to study massage professionally so that you can go out and wow the world with your newfound healing gifts. I even help take the pressure off you on birthdays, Mother's day, anniversaries, and other special occasions by listing ten ways to give massage as a gift.

Who's your buddy?

Chapter 21

Ten Top Places to Study Massage

*I*f you decide that, after reading this book, there is absolutely no way that you can go on with your life without rushing out to become a professional massage therapist, I would just like to say . . . congratulations! You have made a very wise and dynamic career decision. One of the very first places this decision may take you is a massage school of some kind or another. Massage schools each have their own personality, history, reputation, strong points, weak points, and so on. Choosing the right school to spend some important, life-transforming time in over a period of several months or a year is not a decision you should enter into lightly.

In the same way that you end up making friends with the people you are physically close to (in school, at work, as part of white house internship programs, and so on), you usually end up choosing a massage school that is somewhere in the vicinity of your house or apartment. However, if you have the luxury of mobility and can consider schools in a variety of locations, I have compiled a list here that may help. Keep in mind that these schools are some of my personal favorites as well as those recommended by colleagues. There are many other fine schools around. In the U.S. alone, approximately 800 massage schools dot the landscape, and that number just keeps growing.

If you'd like to see a much more extensive list of schools, I suggest the *Touch Training Directory,* published by Associated Bodywork and Massage Professionals. It costs about $15, and you can get it by calling 800-458-2267 or 303-674-8478 or visiting www.abmp.com.

Massage Schools in the U.S.

And now, if you'd like to consider some really dreamy places to attend massage school in the U.S., check out the following suggestions.

Keep in mind that you can go experience a weekend workshop or a week-long intensive class before deciding to commit to a full course of study at many of these listed schools. This is a highly recommended way to get to know your prospective fellow students, faculty, and the facility itself. Call each school to receive a catalogue of workshops.

Atlanta School of Massage, 2300 Peachford Road, Suite 3200, Atlanta, GA 30338; 770-454-7167; www.atlantaschoolofmassage.com.

Like many massage schools, the Atlanta School of Massage started out as a small dream in the minds of people who really liked doing massage themselves. Then it grew. And grew and grew. Now it has a management board of its own, and a large, full-time staff. In addition to traditional training programs in Swedish massage, sports massage, and so on, ASM developed one of the first extensive spa therapy training programs offered at any massage school. Students can receive certification for specialties in spa services (see Chapter 15 for more info on spa treatments).

California Healing Arts College, 12217 Santa Monica Blvd., Suite 206, Santa Monica, CA 90025; 310-826-7622; www.chacmassage.com.

This school, run by a very together woman by the name of Lucinda, has a great referral system and graduate internship program. Students here get one of the best opportunities anywhere to transition themselves into the actual workplace, which is often a shock after spending several months in the rarefied and idealistic air of the massage school environment. The school takes advantage of its urban location in L.A. to get students ready for the real world.

Down East School of Massage, P.O. Box 24, Waldoboro, ME 04572-0024; 207-832-5531; www.midcoast.com/~dsm.

Imagine a private reserve in the woods of Maine, complete with a pond and one dirt road called Moose Meadow Lane. Then add a modern, three-story school building, a devoted, caring owner, and a topnotch, fully accredited massage training program. You then have the ingredients for an intense yet tranquil massage learning experience in one of the most beautiful settings anywhere.

Educating Hands, 120 SW 8th Street, Miami, FL 33130; 305-285-6991; www.educatinghands.com.

This is another school I'm rather biased about, right here in my own hometown. Educating Hands has been around for many years, and owner Iris Burman has dedicated herself to graduating students who use their hands to express their hearts. It's a fun, yet comprehensive, fully accredited program, and the beach is only ten minutes away.

Esalen Institute, Highway 1, Big Sur, CA 93920; 408-667-3000; www.esalen.org.

As touted in Chapter 2, Esalen can be considered a kind of epicenter for massage consciousness in the U.S. Situated on the dramatic northern California coastline, it acts as a magnet for some of the best teachers in the world. Instructors have developed their own particular massage style there (not surprisingly called Esalen Massage), which you can learn while in residence. Not a bad way to spend your school days.

Heartwood Institute, 220 Harmony Lane, Garberville, CA 95542; 707-923-5000; www.heartwoodinstitute.com.

"A school that is more accurately lived than simply attended" is the way this campus set on 240 acres of rolling mountains, meadows, and forests is described. Located way, way, way up in northern California, this is the place to go if you want to experience the "whole enchilada" during your massage training experience. There's organic food, fresh air, stunning views, and a comprehensive holistic philosophy that permeates your time there, making it one of the most unforgettable episodes in your life.

Kripalu Center for Yoga & Health, P.O. Box 793, Lenox, MA 01240; 413-448-3400; www.kripalu.org.

Set on a hill overlooking a lake in the Berkshire Mountains of western Massachusetts, Kripalu has had a long, illustrious history of training massage practitioners, especially those interested in the "spiritual" side of massage. Instructors at this residential facility practice a lot of yoga and meditation, making them the perfect peaceful practitioners to teach stressed-out folks from the big city. You may want to test the waters at this somewhat eclectic place before you commit, though, especially if chanting in Sanskrit at 6 a.m. is not your cup of tea.

Scherer Institute of Natural Healing, 935 Alto Street, Santa Fe, NM 87501; 505-982-8398; www.schererinstitute.com.

If you're going to go to massage school someplace, why not gorgeous New Mexico, where you can hike, ski, soak in hot pools in the desert, and eat some of the best Mexican food anywhere? The Scherer Institute has had nothing but rave reviews from the press and from friends who've gone there. Now with a second facility in Taos, they offer a holistic experience that is unsurpassed.

Suncoast School of Massage, 4910 Cypress Street, Tampa, FL 33607-3802; 813-287-1099.

All right, I admit it, Suncoast is my alma mater, and the owners, Dan and Telka Ulrich, are long-time friends. I may indeed be somewhat biased about this school, but that doesn't mean you shouldn't consider going there, because it's excellent. The program has consistently turned out highly skilled and competent massage therapists, some of whom even go on to write books about massage.

Swedish Institute, 226 W. 26th Street, New York, NY 10001; 212-924-5900.

Okay, so spending months out in the splendid beauties of nature at some massage school in the mountains eating nothing but organic fruit is not your idea of a good time. Perhaps you would prefer the fast pace and abundant nightlife of a major metropolitan area instead. What metropolitan area is more major than New York City? In fact, one of the oldest massage schools in the country is located right in the heart of New York City. This doesn't mean you can spend all your time pursuing that acting career or goofing off, though. The program is quite comprehensive and takes 1,224 hours to complete.

International Schools

Therapeutic massage is growing in popularity outside the U.S. — perhaps even faster than it is inside — as many people around the world come to see the value of "alternative" therapies. The following are some neat schools in several countries.

Australian School, 104C Warrigal Rd, Burwood VIC 3125, Queensland Australia; tel. 03 9830 0555.

Many massage schools in Australia receive extra assistance from the government so people can afford to get a massage education there. The Australian School of Therapeutic Massage offers a good basic course and is recommended by an Australian massage association.

Clare Maxwell Hudson's Massage, 87 Dartmouth Road, London, England NW2 4ER, UK; tel. 00 44 181 450-6494.

Clare Maxwell Hudson has written a number of popular books on massage, and she has a well-known school in London as well. The school started out with basic courses in 1984 and has since evolved into a full-fledged training institute. Much of the class work can be completed part-time, on weekends, to allow for the schedules of busy professionals. Owner Hudson believes one of the most valuable parts of her training is the work placement in hospitals that students are offered each semester. This is a good place to get hands-on guidance from an internationally recognized expert.

Federation of Masseurs, 24 rue des Petits Hotels, 75010, Paris, France; tel. 01 44 83 46 00.

The Federation of Masseurs Kinesitherapeutes is not actually a school. It's an organization that can lead you in the right direction when you're seeking massage training in France. Things are different in France for massage therapists because their training is a part of the medical system, and graduates, known as *kines* (key-nays), are highly respected professionals within the medical community. If you're planning on studying at one of the schools in France, you need a keen desire to work in medical settings, and, of course, it helps if you know how to speak French.

Federazione dei Massofisioterapisti (F.N.C.M.), Massofisioterapisti Via Aosta 16, Trento, 38100 Rome, Italy; tel. 03 94 61 915 499; www.geocities.com/CapeCanaveral/Lab/2521.

This is another network of people teaching and developing massage techniques. Working with the ministry of health to uphold professional standards, the FNCM also lists classes in many different massage modalities given throughout Italy.

Institute of Thai Massage, 17/7 Morakot Road, Hah Yaek Santitham, Chiang Mai, Thailand; tel. 66-53-218632; www.infothai.com/itm.

If you're like most people, the first time you receive a Thai-style massage, you immediately want more, and you may even feel the desire to share the great pleasures and health benefits of this ancient art, called Nuad Bo-Rarn in Thailand, with others. Maybe that's why so many people make the pilgrimage to Chiang Mai to study with Master Chongkol Setthakorn, head teacher at the Old Medicine Hospital there since 1985. Five levels of courses are available, each lasts five days for a total of 180 hours.

Karlsbad Spa Training, Czechoslovakia, contact Dr. Jonathan Paul DeVierville, The Alamo Plaza Spa, 204 Alamo Plaza, San Antonio, TX 78205; U.S. tel. 210-223-5772; www.karlsbadspa.cjb.net.

Dr. Jonathan Paul DeVierville, Ph.D. is a veritable fountain of information about water. In fact, he knows so much about water and hydrotherapy that he has decided to dedicate his life to sharing the healing message of spas. Each year in May he takes a small group of lucky students to Czechoslovakia with him to study the traditional forms of hydrotherapy and other healing methods used in the spas there.

Northern Institute of Massage, 100 Waterloo Road, Blackpool, England FY4 1AW; tel. 44 1253 403548.

This school has been around since 1924, and they have graduated over 35,000 students (many of whom are still alive). The students spread out across the English-speaking world to ply their hands-on trade. In the past ten years, the school has seen an upsurge in activity as more and more people in the U.K. become interested in alternative therapies. The school has even opened branch offices in other countries — two in Ireland, and one in the Caribbean. Call if you're interested in schooling, or even if you're a visitor just traveling through — workshops are open to everybody.

South Australia Health Education Center, 38 Currie Street, Adelaide, Australia SA, 5000; tel. 08 8410 1975; www.massage.net.au.

If you'd like a massage school experience down on the south coast of Australia, and you want to study with people serious about their massage (the principal and several instructors were invited to the Commonwealth Games to offer sports massage to the athletes), this is the school for you.

Sutherland-Chan, 330 Dupont Street, Suite 400, Toronto, Canada; tel. 416-924-1107; www.sutherland-chan.com.

If you'd like a multi-cultural, multi-ethnic, cosmopolitan experience while studying massage, in a peaceful, laid-back Canadian city, Toronto may be the place for you, and the Sutherland-Chan School & Teaching Clinic may be the perfect school. It's located right in the middle of downtown Toronto, which features excellent housing and actual humans walking around at night. Sutherland-Chan has been around since 1978. The program is a hefty 2,200 hours, and fully 70 percent of the students already have a college degree when they arrive. What really sets the school apart is its intense clinical outreach program. In order to graduate, every student performs supervised clinical work in area hospitals.

West Coast College of Massage Therapy, 555 West Hastings Street, Vancouver, Canada V6B 4N4; 888-449-2242; www.collegeofmassage.com.

You have to get ready for some serious schooling if you study massage in Canada, which requires between 2,000 and 3,000 hours of training, depending on which province you live in. The direction and emphasis of training at the West Coast College is based on the medical model approach to healthcare, according to Ron Garvock, dean of massage therapy at this school in Vancouver. This three-year program costs $25,000 Canadian dollars, which perhaps makes it the highest standard in massage education in North America. They also have campuses in the Toronto area and are expanding into Victoria and Niagara as well.

Chapter 22

Ten Outstanding Places to Receive a Topnotch Massage

In This Chapter

▶ U.S. massage spots

▶ International massage spots

You're going to get double your money's worth out of this chapter because it actually includes not ten, but twenty, spectacular places to receive a massage, ten in the U.S. and ten in other countries. How can we afford to do this, you ask? Well, we spare no expense when it comes to letting you know about potentially the most spectacular massage experience of your life.

Let's face it, just about anywhere you are when you're receiving a massage is an outstanding place. Close your eyes and off you go to paradise. But trust me on this, your experience may be enhanced if you manage to make your way to one of the many truly incredible environments that are waiting for you out there. Any one of the following locales may set your imagination soaring and stimulate your sense of the beautiful in life. You may also find it quite an adventure getting to some of these exotic spots, so buckle up and get ready for some of the most pleasurable explorations of your life.

U.S. Massage Spots

Here are some great places to go in the U.S. when you're seeking your next fabulous massage experience.

Enchantment, 525 Boynton Canyon Road, Sedona, AZ 86336; 800-826-4180; www.arizonaguide.com/enchantment.

This is one place I'm almost reluctant to name because it's such a special secret hideaway, but because you were kind enough and smart enough to buy this book I suppose you deserve to find out about it. First, go to Sedona, a small town two hours north of Phoenix, Arizona. Then follow Boynton Canyon Road a few miles out of town where you enter a spectacular valley sacred to the Native Americans who once lived in cliff dwellings there. The massage you receive in the spa is more than a massage. Be prepared for an exchange of energy between you, the massage therapist, and the powerful vibrations of the canyon itself. It's filled with something mystical.

Esalen Institute, Highway 1, Big Sur, CA 93920; 408-667-3000; www.esalen.org.

This is the only spot to make it onto both the ten top schools list and the ten top massage spots lists. This place deserves it. Some people say that the consciousness of the entire planet has been shifted in a positive direction by people who receive massages on Esalen's deck overlooking the Pacific. Here, a bunch of talented, sensitive people practice a form of massage that is meant to fine-tune your body and your awareness to an entirely new level. And you experience the whole thing while listening to the majestic fury of the Pacific Ocean pounding the rocks hundreds of feet below. I think you should go there and check it out.

Green Valley Spa, 1871 West Canyon View Drive, St. George, UT 84770; 800-237-1068; www.ishopper.com/greenvalley.

Just a two-hour drive from gaudy Vegas, Green Valley is a true oasis in the Utah desert — a magical place. To receive your massage, you enter a womb-like inner chamber where it's hard to tell whether you're inside or outside. All the ingredients used on your skin are plucked by hand from the surrounding hills, and every detail of the environment is chosen to create a special experience, down to the color of the fruit in the water you drink. I personally cannot say enough good things about this place.

Harbin Hot Springs, P.O. Box 782, Middletown, CA 95461; 707-987-2477; www.harbin.org.

Well, this spot is not for everyone. There are, after all, dozens of naked hippies walking around, seemingly oblivious to the fact that there are lots of other people in close proximity who are not naked hippies. Harbin can indeed feel like a throwback to the sixties or seventies, but the sublime waters gushing from the underground spring are more than enough to make up for the funky surroundings. Take turns dipping your body (naked or not, no one will judge you) into the hot spring and then the cold stream for some intense stimulation before heading into the massage center for your hour-and -a-half appointment with bliss.

Kohala Spa, 425 Waikoloa Beach Drive, Kona, HI 96738; 808-886-1234; www.kohalaspa.com.

Ever wanted to receive a therapeutic massage from a native Hawaiian healer in preparation for a swim with the dolphins in a natural lagoon pool immediately outside the massage room door? Me too. Well, the Koala spa is where you can do just that, and you can also enjoy the amenities at one of Earth's finer resorts. This could be one of the greatest things you may ever experience, in the realm of massage or any other realm.

Little Palm Island, 28500 Overseas Highway, Little Torch Key, FL 33042; 800-343-8567; www.littlepalmisland.com.

If you're in the Florida Keys and you're searching for a secluded resort on its own private island where you can receive a massage in a mangrove tree house, then Little Palm Island is probably the place for you. This is Gilligan's Island gone upscale, with about two dozen thatched-roof bungalows, a pool, a bar, water sports, and an incredible gourmet restaurant. What else do you need?

Nemacolin Woodlands Resort & Spa, 1001 LaFayette Drive, Farmington, PA; 15437; 800-422-2736; www.nemacolin.com.

Tucked away between silos and cow pastures in the Laurel Highlands out near West Virginia, you will find a surprisingly beautiful place called Nemacolin Woodlands Spa that would be considered a jewel in even the most exclusive areas. The newly renovated spa was designed by the well-known artist Clodagh, who has created more of a spiritual experience than a building. Within its walls, you'll discover an opportunity to commune with the harmonious elements that have been brought together — water and wood, stone and light, sophistication and earthiness. After you're thoroughly relaxed in these surroundings, request to receive your massage from a massage therapist who's been on staff for a few years, long enough to have been trained by one of the country's premier massage instructors, Bob King. Nemacolin flew Mr. King in for a special private training, which is indicative of the way they do just about everything — first class.

The Peaks, P.O. Box 2702, Telluride, CO 81435; 800-789-2220; www.thepeaksresort.com.

Swoosh down the slopes in this incredible alpine valley, straight into the embrace of a topnotch luxury spa where a squadron of massage pros wait to take care of you. Telluride's a lovely place in the summer, too. The only downside to receiving a massage here is that you may be lying down for an hour with your eyes closed instead of out exploring the spectacular countryside

Spa of the Rockies, 1 Crystal Park Road, Manitou Springs, CO 80809; 719-685-1198.

This is a little-bitty place, but it has a big heart, and it's really cool. You can find it up a side street in the old mining town of Manitou Springs, near Colorado Springs and spectacular Garden of the Gods Park. Try to visit in the winter so you can soak outside beneath the chilly night sky in a big hot tub;

then come inside to the sauna where your massage therapist joins you, beats you with wet oak branches, and covers you with organic honey before leading you to the massage room. Now I call that service!

Ten Thousand Waves, 3451 Hyde Park Road, Santa Fe, NM 87501; 505-992-5000; www.primenet.com/spareporter/waves.htm.

Besides offering a long list of very talented massage therapists on staff, Ten Thousand Waves gives you that all-too-rare opportunity, a chance to wear a kimono in public! Yes, they hand you a kimono when you check in at the desk. Next, you're off to the lockers, then out to a clothing-optional hot tub environment that is surrounded by breathtaking mountain scenery. After saunas and soaking, your massage therapist takes you to a light-filled chamber for some high-quality bodywork. As an added bonus, you can head into Santa Fe afterwards for some of the best green chili on the planet.

International Massage Spots

It's true, the world is big, and there are thousands of tremendous massage experiences waiting out there for you, but the following list at least offers a few good places to get started.

Amandari, Kedewatan, Ubud, Bali, Indonesia; tel. 011 62 361 975333; www.amanresorts.com/dari_m.html.

So, say you're bored. And you have an extra $25,000 or so burning a hole in your pocket. Why not come to Bali and live for several weeks at the incredible Amandari Resort? Locals believe the area to be a spiritual place, with nearby paths meandering through the jungle valley down to a sacred pool. While you're there, you can partake in the spiritual atmosphere yourself during a one-hour Amandari massage. During this sublime procedure, you will recline beneath a thatched-hut structure out by the tranquil lotus pool while being anointed with indigenous Indonesian oils by a highly skilled native practitioner. It doesn't get much better than this anywhere on Earth

Camp Eden, Currumbin Creek Road, Currumbin Valley, Queensland, Australia, 4223; Tel. 61 (7) 5533 0333 or (800) 074 157; www.campeden.com.au.

If you don't mind getting a leech stuck on your big toe, as I did when running the fitness course through the rainforests of lush Camp Eden, then you may surely enjoy a visit to this remote-yet-close health retreat. Camp Eden is near Surfer's Paradise along the east coast of Australia, where the weather is lovely, the people magnificent, and the massage therapists' fingers as strong as those of a man wrapping his hand around a can of Foster's lager after a long day herding sheep in the outback.

Casa del Sol, Av. Gral. Diego Diaz Gonzalez #31, Col. Parres, 62550 Cuernavaca, Mexico; tel. 52 (73) 21-0999, toll-free 01-800-999-9100; www.misiondelsol.com.mx.

Ethereal beings clad in white escort you through a complex of buildings con-structed of the most natural materials available: clay, wood and stone. You are ushered into inner chambers for your massage, which is more than a mas-sage, because at the same time you are surrounded by the philosophy of Mision del Sol, which attempts to bring your internal environment into total harmony with an ecologically balanced external environment. The end result, hope the resort's owners, is to increase human consciousness to a universal level. At the very least, you get a killer massage.

Charlie's Spa at San Souci, Box 103, Ocho Rios, Jamaica; 800-203-7456.

This is the place to go if you're the type who would like to receive a massage in a picturesque little gazebo out at the end of a walkway surrounded on all sides by the aquamarine waters of the Caribbean. All the while, you hear faint strains of reggae music wash up from the distant beach bar, and a giant sea turtle named Charlie floats effortlessly by in a nearby fresh water grotto. If you're the type who would like this experience, definitely call this spa.

Javana Spa, Plaza Bisnis Kemang, Building 2, Kemang, Jakarta, 121730, Indonesia; tel. 011 62 21 719-8327; www.javanaspa.com.

Up in the cool hills outside of hectic Jakarta, you find a tranquil, spectacular place — Javana Spa. The altitude (1,200 meters) makes for fresh air and a feeling of escape from the humid tropical world of mere mortals below. Hike through forests to hidden waterfalls, then head back to the spa for your mas-sage that includes natural oils and ingredients found right on this Pacific island. If you're feeling brave, ask for their traditional Indonesian massage, an intense experience that is "not for the faint of heart" as one resort official put it. Also, make sure to book your appointment in one of the rooms facing out toward the rainforest. The lush sights and sounds of tropical wildlife provide an exotic backdrop for your experience.

La Mamounia, Avenue Bab Jdid, Marrakech, Morocco; (212-4) 44-89-81, fax (212-4) 44-46-60; www.mamounia.com.

This resort, often described as the best hotel in Northern Africa, was the haunt of Winston Churchill, and it was one of the few places where he felt serene and removed enough from world affairs to practice his favorite pas-time, watercolor painting. To receive your massage, you enter the *hamam*, or Turkish bath. There an entire ceremony takes place in a beautiful white mar-bled, Moorish-tiled steam room that is perfumed with natural, delicately boiled herbs. You're scrubbed with a natural paste, then bathed and toweled before the massage, which is also done in the steam room. The whole process takes about two hours, and afterwards you may feel like a character out of a romantic international novel.

Les Thermes Marins, 2 Ave de Monte Carlo, BP 215, Monte Carlo, France; 98004; tel. 377-92-16-40-40.

If you're feeling kind of ritzy, put your Ray Bans on, hop in your yacht, and head to Monte Carlo for Les Thermes Marins, a spa with a sea view. And it's not only a view you get, but sea therapy as well. After a soak in a natural sea-water bath, request an hour-long massage before heading out to the casinos for the evening. This retreat has been called "the most luxurious thalas-sotherapy center, or seawater spa, in the world," but the price for a full day including four treatments won't drain your bank account.

Spa Deus, Via Le Piane 35-53042, Chianciano (SI) Italy; 39-(0) 578-63232, www.spadeus.it.

If you come under the spell of the Tuscan sun and can't wait to start your Italian getaway, but don't know where to begin and would like to get a massage while you're thinking about it anyway, definitely book an appointment at Spa Deus. They offer a good blend of European and American philosophies, and if you ever tire of the fine massages and healthy lifestyle choices there, you can head out in your rented Fiat for a little tour of the magnificent countryside.

Spiritual Massage, Angela Moraes, Rio de Janeiro, Brazil; tel. 5521 274-5195; e-mail: solgavea@mandic.com.br.

If you happen to be in Rio de Janeiro and you want a spiritual experience, call Angela Moraes, who offers something called Massagem Espiritual, which is Portuguese for spiritual massage. You may not know this, but Brazilians are famous for their spiritual inclinations, as well as their more, um, worldly inclinations. Just being in Rio is a kind of spiritual experience in itself. Call Angela to make it extra special. She has a healing center in a gorgeous area near mountains, beaches, and forests, but still right in the city.

Wat Po Temple, Bangkok, Thailand

If you're in Bangkok, just ask anybody where Wat Po is, and they may be able to tell you. It's kind of hard to miss sprawling temples with massive golden Buddhas, right? The massage you receive there has a reputation of being "intense," but in a good way, of course. And it won't be in a darkened private room with flute music playing, like you may expect, but in an open public pavilion with several beds all together, and you wear loose-fitting clothing. And be warned, the massage is so wonderful, and the price so affordable, you may end up here for hours!

Chapter 23

Ten Inventive Ways to Give Massage as a Gift

In This Chapter

▶ Creating great massage gifts

*I*f you really want to get on somebody's good side, here's a little secret: Give them a massage gift. You don't necessarily have to give the massage yourself (in some cases this could even be inappropriate), but you do have to put forth the effort to create the massage gift, arrange for it, pay for it, and so on. You may be surprised at how incredibly warm a reception your gift receives. Massage, ultimately, is always a gift for the person who's receiving it. Even if you're paying for it yourself, there's something very special about the physical act of receiving the massage. It's natural to respond as though it were a gift. The giver works so hard, on such an intimate level, that you can't help but feel connected to him, and grateful. Try some of the suggestions that follow to accentuate this quality of the massage you offer to others.

Spa gift certificates

Purchase a gift certificate that's good at over 700 great day spas in the U.S. and give it to a deserving individual. To order your certificate, call 888-SPA-WISH, and make sure to check out the coupon in the back of this book, because it gets you a discount! Way cool.

The massage birthday gift

For that special someone's birthday, your anniversary, or any other special occasion, hire a professional massage therapist to come over as a surprise gift. This could lead to some major gratitude immediately following the massage, so make sure you have a bottle of champagne chilled just in case.

The spa date

With so many spas around these days, it's possible for many people to get away to one for a night or two. Arrange in advance for a "spa date" on which both of you get multiple massages by a pro. Pack a good book, a bathing suit, and you're all set.

The royal treatment at home

Drop the kids at grandma's house and head home to cook your partner's favorite meal, arrange flowers, light candles, and warm the aromatherapy oil. Then put the skills you attain from this book to good use by giving a great massage. This is good for major brownie points in your favor.

B&B and massage

Take a trip to a quaint and charming little bed & breakfast and trade massages with your partner in this new, romantic environment.

Leave a little rub behind

When you're a houseguest, leave behind a massage gift certificate from a local massage therapist to show how much you appreciate your host's hospitality.

Massage for charity

Buy a gift certificate from a local massage therapist and offer it as a door prize for your church or community club auction.

Wedding day rub

Buy a massage for (or better yet, give a massage to!) a friend who is getting married. I received a massage on my own wedding day and have given massages to friends on theirs. You can always manage to make that extra hour appear on the big day, no matter how hectic things seem to get, and it really helps to calm the nervous bride or groom.

The massage economy pack

Negotiate with a local massage therapist to purchase a whole series of massages at a discount, and then share them with your partner, family, friends, business associates, and anyone else you can think of.

You're the gift

After you read this book, offer free massages to all of your friends and each person in your family. Do this even if you think you're not "good enough" at giving massage yet. If you give from your heart, people may respond accordingly. It's the gift that counts, not the wrapping.

Chapter 24

Ten Massage Techniques That Your Dog or Cat Will Love

In This Chapter

▶ Pleasing your pet with massage

You don't have to be a highly trained expert in several esoteric massage techniques in order to make your dog Sparky roll over in ecstasy when you rub his belly. However, maybe there are a few tricks here you haven't experimented with before. Your pet is sure to be overjoyed that you've read this book (and this chapter in particular) and are now ready to spend quality time trying out some new maneuvers. In fact, Sparky may have been the one who slipped that bookmark onto this page when you weren't looking.

Animals can teach us humans a thing or two about massage. Just watch a cat, for instance, over a period of five minutes (when it's not asleep), and you'll see what I mean. They are "in the moment" all the time, responding to their inner "call of the wild" to do whatever comes naturally. You can follow their lead with these massage moves. Yes, that's right, go ahead and get crazy with your techniques, letting your instincts take over as you bond and communicate with that special creature in your life. I limit the discussion to cats and dogs here because those are the most popular pets, but there's no reason you can't try these moves out on hamsters, gerbils, or Vietnamese pigs as well.

Paw pressure

Some people reserve their paw petting just for the furry tops of the paws, which is a big mistake. If you slide your fingers into the webbing of the paw pads underneath, you reach some areas that are hard to get to otherwise. Ever see your pets vigorously nibbling away at their own feet? This is the area they're trying to get, and if you help them out, they'll appreciate it.

Outer ears

Too many pet owners content themselves with a cursory scratch of the ears, when what your pet really wants is an all-out assault on the base of the back of the ear where it connects to the head. This seems to be an area that can never get enough intense rubbing. Use the tips of your index and middle fingers, really digging into the cartilage there that makes up the ear.

Inner ears

Inside the ear is a gold mine of prospective massage points, and it would be silly of you to stay away just because the inside of the ear is pink and potentially "yucky." Go ahead, promise yourself you'll wash your hands immediately afterwards, and then rub away on the little ridges and rolls within the cavern of the ear, exploring for new areas of pet pleasure.

Belly rub

The ever-popular belly rub is quite simple for most of us to perform. Just start rubbing, and your pooch keels over, kicking his paws up in the air in animal surrender. Experiment until you find the exact spot that causes the most frenetic paw movements. This is "ground zero" in belly-rub territory.

Watch out if you use belly rubbing on a cat because it will quite likely try to grasp your arm with its front paws and start clawing you with the back paws. This is the natural feline "disemboweling" reaction, meant to eviscerate any unlucky little rodents it catches out in the yard.

"Knee" kneading

Did you know that what we usually think of as the "knees" on our pets are actually the wrists? It's true, and it's also true that this is a little-known area of intense pet-massage satisfaction. Just try massaging your own wrists for a few seconds. Feels good, right? Animals love it, too. Use your fingertips to rub little circles in all directions around the joint, down onto the paw a little bit, and back up onto the leg slightly, too. Pinch in between the bones and tendons, and do a few joint movements while you're at it.

Chin wedgies

Just at the tip of the jutting underside of your dog or cat's chin you'll find the spot where the two sides of the jaw come together. The little triangle of soft tissue that you'll find there is a site of supreme sensitivity. Use your pinkie finger if necessary to reach into this area and rub back and forth with firm pressure. If you do the maneuver correctly, your pet becomes your slave and may do anything you ask it to, as long as you continue to provide such pleasure.

Tall tails

Right on top of the base of the tail, where it connects to the back, is a magical spot. Grind into it with enough finger pressure, and your pet's tail will begin to rise (cats) or wag (dogs). A "tall tale" is a sure sign that they like this very much.

Underarms

We tend to not pay that much attention to human armpits, often skipping them altogether during full-body massages. This is understandable, because some armpits are not places most of us would want to go, but it's also sad for our pets, whose armpits are licked clean on a daily, if not hourly, basis. You can give a good massage into this area by using all four fingers held flat. Slip them between the leg and the body and rub your fingertips into the many tendons, muscles, and ligaments you find attached there.

Nose nudgies

Press straight down onto the front of the nose with firm pressure and rub up and down just slightly, avoiding the nostrils. Try pushing until your pet pushes back and you begin to get into a little dance with each other, leading your pet around by the nose, which is kind of cute. At least it's cute for about 30 seconds or so.

Doggy and kitty chiropractic

Starting at the tail, use your fingertips to massage each vertebrae, working your way up the spine one bone at a time. Try mini-kneading maneuvers and some circular rubbing, making sure to get between the bones, too, into those little notches.

Chapter 25

Ten Quick and Easy Massage Techniques for Easing Stress

In This Chapter

▶ Achieving quick stress relief with massage

There are certain circumstances that are not completely conducive to giving or receiving hour-long full body massages complete with music, candles, and scented oils. Like when you're in a crowded elevator, for example, or if you're sitting at a departure gate at JFK airport. In places like those, it's important to remember not to take all your clothes off and start rubbing (either yourself or another person) because that may give massage a strange reputation.

Luckily for you, there are some quick little massage moves you can use every day in public places to help relieve stress. And none of them require you to embarrass yourself.

Easing Your Own Stress

The following are five quick and easy ways to ease your own stress with massage.

Eye hooks

This move feels better than it sounds. Hook your thumbs up into the inner upper corners of your eye sockets, pressing in against the nose bone and up against the ridge of the brow. Hold for 5 to 10 seconds. This is great for headaches and sinus congestion (see Chapter 17 for a photo).

Headache point

Known to shiatsu practitioners as Large Intestine 4, or LI4, this point is noted for helping to relieve headaches. It's located in the webbing of your hand between the thumb and index finger. The problem is that most people don't press exactly the right spot when they try to stimulate this point on themselves.

The spot is not directly in the center of the meaty part of the webbing, but rather in against the bone of the hand. To press here effectively, grasp the webbing between thumb and index finger with your opposite hand, squeeze it, and then move your thumb in against the side of the hand. See Chapter 11 for a look at this move.

Jaw circles

We all carry whole bunches of tension in our jaw muscles (yes, even you). One good way to alleviate this is to use your fingertips and make tiny little circles right into the center of your jaw muscles. Open and close your mouth slowly at the same time to increase the effect.

You may also want to try gently pulling your chin down until your mouth begins to open, relaxing the jaw muscles. You may be surprised at how tightly you hold your mouth closed, perhaps out of a fear of looking like a dufus. Go ahead, you're all alone; let your mouth hang open for a minute. It'll feel great.

Ear reflexology

According to the zone theory, each point on the bottom of your foot reflects areas in other parts of your body, as you find out in Chapter 14. Did you know that your ears also reflect every other part of the body? Yes, it's true. The Chinese even have an extensive system of treating many disorders with pressure on the ears.

You can give your whole body a boost by simply rubbing your ears with a vigorous little kneading movement between your thumb and first two fingers. Start at the lobe below and walk you fingers up around the outside to the top of the ear, giving little tugs outward as you go. Even if it does nothing for the rest of your body, it makes your ears feel great.

Foot drainage

Most everyone agrees that a foot massage feels great, but what if you're all alone and you only have a few minutes? Well, then try this one move to affect the bladder and adrenal reflex points on the bottom of the feet. It's a good way to stimulate detoxification and elimination while providing some stress relief at the same time.

With one foot up on the opposite knee, press in with your thumb, sliding it back and forth along the arch between the heel and midway up the foot. Check Figure 14-1 to see where this reflex is.

Easing a Partner's Stress

Following are five ways you can help others relieve their stress.

The vice grip

Tightly grasp the top of your partner's right shoulder (the area between the shoulder and neck, consisting mostly of the trapezius muscle) with both of your hands and have her turn her head very slowly to the left. Then have her hold the position at the extreme end of the turn for 10 seconds before slowly turning back. You can switch shoulders if you'd like or repeat on this side if only one shoulder is tight. This is an excellent way to help reduce major stress in the neck and shoulders.

Head squeeze

Although it may look like you're trying to squeeze your partner's head like a gigantic melon, you're actually doing him a big favor with this move, especially if he has a headache. With your elbows well out to the sides, press in with the heels of your hands, using very firm pressure against the sides of your partner's head, just above and in front of the ears. Hold for 10 to 15 seconds, asking your partner how the pressure feels. Discontinue if he experiences any discomfort. This is especially effective on tension headaches and has even been known to help with hangovers.

Hooking the skull

Standing behind your partner, place your thumbs at the base of his skull, on the muscles at the top of his neck. Then use a cat-pawing motion to dig your thumbs further into the muscles there, as if you were trying to hook your thumbs up under his skull. This will really loosen up the entire neck.

Make sure not to press directly into the spine with this move, as it may be uncomfortable. Stay about an inch to either side.

Scalp circles

Place your fingertips firmly against your partner's scalp and make little circles while pressing down. Make sure your fingers don't slip across atop the hair but remain firmly pressed against the scalp as you move the skin and thin muscles below. Then, after a few seconds, lift your fingers and repeat the circles on another spot on the scalp.

Wing lift

Have your partner bring one hand around to her lower back, which will lift her shoulder blade up a little. Then use your fingertips to hook into the muscles beneath the shoulder blade and pull steadily upward with light pressure on the blade itself, which will stretch the entire upper back and also have a loosening effect on the arm. Repeat on the other side.

Appendix

Massage Resources

• •

Massage, like any new field you're just getting into, can be a little confusing at first. There are so many resources you could use, so many directions you could search in. This appendix lists just a few of the many tools that could help you, but you'll find more than enough here to keep you busy for a long time.

Massage Books

There are lots of informative books on massage specialties. So, if you really feel the need to own another book besides this one, don't worry, you won't hurt my feelings. In fact, here are some suggestions:

Capellini, Steve, *The Royal Treatment: How You Can Take Home the Pleasures of the Great Luxury Spas*. New York, New York, Dell, 1997.

Claire, Thomas, *Bodywork: What Type of Massage to Get — and How To Make the Most of It*, William Morrow, New York, 1995.

Ford, Clyde, *Compassionate Touch*. NY: Simon and Schuster, 1993.

Knaster, Mirka, *Discovering the Body's Wisdom*, Bantam, New York, 1996.

Krieger, Dolores, *Accepting Your Power to Heal: The Personal Practice of Therapeutic Touch*, Santa Fe, Bear & Co., 1993.

Miller, Erica, *Day Spa Operations*. Albany, Milady, 1995.

Montagu, Ashley, *Touching: The Human Significance of the Skin*, Harper & Row, New York, 1971.

Nelson, Dawn, *Compassionate Touch: Hands-On Caregiving for the Elderly, the Ill and the Dying*, New York, Talman Company, 1993.

Pierpont, Margaret, *The Spa Life at Home*, Longstreet Press, Atlanta, 1997.

Thomas, Zach, *Healing Touch: The Church's Forgotten Language*. Louisville, KY, Westminster/John Knox Press, 1994.

Massage Magazines

In the U.S., there are three main magazines read by massage therapists. All of them include tons of information to help you get "plugged into" the massage world.

Massage Magazine: 1315 West Mallon, Dept. 50, Spokane, WA 99201-2038, 800-533-4263, ext. 50.

Massage Therapy Journal: 820 Davis Street, Suite 100, Evanston, IL 60201-4444, 847-864-0123.

Massage & Bodywork Quarterly: 28677 Buffalo Park Road, Evergreen, CO 80439-7347, 303-674-8478.

Massage on the Web

Given the velocity of change on the Internet, I can't absolutely guarantee that all of the following links will be completely current. However, you can rest assured that they will provide you with mega-amounts of information, more than you could possibly digest in one lifetime. So log on, start surfing, and prepare to launch into the World Wide Web of massage.

General sites

www.dharmanet.org/TBI/webring.html: This massage "Web ring" is a good place to start because it links together many sites all focused on massage therapy, and you can travel from place to place, always remaining within the ring. *Note:* especially helpful if you have a Web site on the subject of massage that you want to promote.

www.qwl.com/mtwc/guide/techniques.html: This site is known as "Massage Therapy Web Central," and you'll be able to find tons of links here for massage.

www.carpaltunnelmassage.com: Check here for insight into massage moves that can help with repetitive stress pain in the wrist.

www.babymassage.com: This is a site with a video available for instruction in (surprise!) baby massage.

www.childbirth.org: Here you'll find everything you could possibly want to learn about childbirth, including baby massage and massage for pregnant people.

www.daybreak-massage.com: This is thee site for people interested in offering massage to seniors (also called geriatric massage). They offer training and certification.

www.innerpeacemusic.com: This is thee site for Stephen Halpern, a musician who has devoted his career to providing healing through sound. Many massage pros choose his music to accompany their massage.

www.hometown.aol.com/ESMSatHome/schools.html: Check here for links to many horse massage schools.

www.NCBTMB.com: The site for National Certification Board for Therapeutic Massage & Bodywork (NCBTMB). This organization offers certification for massage pros in every state of the U.S..

Massage therapist locator sites

massagetherapynetwork.com: This site links therapists with customers and vice versa.

www.althealthsearch.com: This is a good place to find a practitioner in your area. It covers a lot of territory with over 180,000 listings.

www.massagenetwork.com: Look here for tons of info from around the world, locating therapists, etc.

www.massageresource.com: Travel to this Web site first if you're seeking therapists, schools, info, etc.

www.massagetherapyhomepage.com/directory.html: This page will help you find a school or therapist anywhere in the world.

Massage products

www.pressurepositive.com: This site has several massage products for sale, such as the "Backknobber" and others.

www.bodybalancing.com: This is the home site for the Body Balancer tool.

www.mtswarehouse.com: Here's a site for discounted massage tables of many makes and models.

www.monmouth.com/~bestofnature: This company bills themselves as a "massage supply superstore." The site definitely has a large number of products.

www.relaxtheback.com: These are the ergonomic experts with a large chain of retail stores featuring back-friendly furniture, tools, and some massage items.

www.wildsyde.com/kamamain.htm: This page on the Wild Syde Web site lists a sizable selection of edible massage oils, including the infamous "cappuccino" flavor.

www.massagetools.com: This is the Web site for the manufacturer of the Thumper vibrating massage device.

www.massagematters.com: A massage entrepreneur in the Atlanta area offers this special site featuring just a few well-chosen, high quality massage items.

Healing retreat and spa resources

www.spas.about.com: This may be the most comprehensive source of information about spas on the Web. Your experience here will be lead by a spa guide, Julie Register, who has spent many hours researching and cataloguing information as well as forging useful connections with many professionals in the spa industry.

http://209.41.63.136/spa/spa.htm: Check here for travel and related information about the original town of Spa in Belgium.

www.spawish.com: This is the 1-800-FLOWERS of the spa world. Get in touch with Spa Wish to order a gift certificate good at hundreds of day spas across the U.S.. Also, check out the coupon in the back of this book.

www.spadiscoveries.com: This is the International Spa of the Month Club Web site. This outfit will send you new spa products from top resorts every month.

www.spamagazine.com: This is the Web site for *Spa* magazine.

www.spafinders.com: This is the place to go when you're searching for spa vacations.

Equipment and Supplies

The following is a list of companies that make equipment for use by massage pros or the public, as well as some retail outlets where you can go to purchase massage items.

Living Earth Crafts: 600 East Todd Road, Santa Rosa, CA 95407, 800-358-8292, www.livingearthcrafts.com

Living Earth Crafts offers portable, stationary, and spa tables, plus oils, books, T shirts, videos, massage tools, and more.

Golden Ratio Woodworks: 2896 Hwy. 89 South, Emigrant, Montana 59027, 800-345-1129 or 406-333-4578, www.goldenratio.com

Golden Ratio offers a full line of tables, chairs, and allied products. They also made the extremely cool *Massage For Dummies* massage chair featured in some of the photos in this book!

The Body Balancer: Body Balancing Ltd., P.O. Box 51977, Palo Alto, CA 94303, 800-437-7004

This is where you can order the Body Balancer, featured in Chapter 10.

Natura Essentials: 2845 Harriet Ave South, Minneapolis 55408, 888-606-0055, www.naturaessentials.com

This company features an incredible collection of some of the finest aromatherapy products you can find anywhere, including candles, essential oils, diffusers, and more.

Trigger Point Co.: P.O. Box 391171, Anza, CA 92539, 800-763-2430.

This company manufactures the popular Thera Cane self-massage tool.

Educating Hands Bookstore: 120 SW 8th Street, Miami, FL 33130 305-285-0651 or 800-999-6991, www.educatinghands.com

This store-in-a-school near downtown Miami offers a great selection of books, videos, tables, chairs, massage muscle-builders, and accessories.

Downeast School of Massage Bookstore: 99 Moose Meadow Lane, Waldoboro, ME 04572, 207-832-553, www.midcoast.com/~dsm

This stores offers lots of books, study aids, charts, videos, models, music, lotions, oils, and accessories including the Thermophore moist heat pack.

Best of Nature: 176 Broadway, Long Branch, NJ 07740, 800-228-6457 or 732-728-0004, www.bestofnature.com

Billing themselves as "the largest massage supply superstore," Best of Nature offers tables, chairs, sheets, oils, accessories, creams, and more.

Inner Peace Linens: P.O. Box 940, Walpole, NH 03608-0940, 800-949 7650, www.innerpeace.com

What's the use of lying on an expensive padded massage table if it's covered with a cheap sheet? Contact Inner Peace for 100-percent cotton flannel massage table linens.

Massage Oils and Creams

Take it from me: if you're going to apply long firm massage strokes to the hairy leg of an Italian man, you'd better use some kind of lubricant, or you're going to have one angry Italian on your hands. You can find massage oils and creams at many health food stores and specialty shops, but in this section I've listed a few top-of-the-line products that the pros use.

Biotone: 4757 Old Cliffs Rd., San Diego, CA 92120, 800-445-6457 or 619-582-0027, www.biotone.com

This is a popular massage cream and oil manufacturer.

Heritage Products: Box 444, Virginia Beach, VA 23458, 800-TO-CAYCE, www.caycecures.com

Heritage produces the Edgar Cayce Aura Glow oil, the formula for which was inspired by the renowned healer.

Pure Pro Massage Oils: 955 Massachusetts Avenue, Suite 232, Cambridge, MA 02139, 781-933-8638, 877-373-5298, www.relaxu.com

These nice folks will send you a free catalogue if you ask for one nicely.

Tara Spa Therapy: P.O. Box 222639, Carmel, CA 93922, 800-552-0779 or 831-648-1932

Tara Spa Therapy carries Bindi Body Oil (my favorite). They also have a line of ayurvedic products, and much more.

Catalogues

These catalogues specialize in all kinds of products that are good for you and your body. Some also offer unique items like meditation pillows, prayer bells and such.

Harmony: 800-869-3446

This catalogue offers "products in harmony with the earth," and all the models look clean cut and happy.

Basic Massage Lines: 1207 W. Kingshighway, Paragould, AR 72450, 800-643-4751, www.bmlmassage.com

Like the name says, this company carries basic massage lines for pros and amateurs alike, offering one-stop shopping.

Inner Balance: 800-482-3608

This catalogue offers "natural solutions for health," and it has a number of massage related items.

Best of Nature: 176 Broadway, Long Branch, NJ 07740, 800-228-6457 or 732-728-0004, www.bestofnature.com

This is a no-frills massage, spa, aromatherapy, and body care product catalogue, mostly for the pros.

Self-Care: 2000 Powell Street, Suite 1350, Emeryville, CA 94608-1858, 800-345-3371, www.selfcare.com

Called "America's foremost specialty catalog of products for healthy living," this company carries large selection of health and wellness related products.

Explorations: 800-720-2114

A little bit on the "mystical" side, this catalogue offers great stuff for energy awakening, spirituality, relaxation, etc.

Organizations and Associations

Check out the organizations and associations listed here if you would like some information or you just want to chat with someone who knows what they're talking about.

American Massage Therapy Association (AMTA): 820 Davis Street, Suite 100, Evanston, IL 60201-4444, 847-864-0123, www.amtamassage.org

American Oriental Bodywork Therapy Association (AOBA): Laurel Oak Corporate Center, Ste 408, 1010 Haddonfield-Berlin Rd., Voorhees, NJ 08043, 609-782-1616, www.healthy.net/aobta

Associated Bodywork & Massage Professionals (ABMP): 28677 Buffalo Park Road, Evergreen, CO 80439-7347, 800-458-2267 or 303-674-8478, www.abmp.com

International Massage Association (IMA): 3000 Connecticut Ave. NW, #308, Washington, DC 20008, 202-387-6555, internationalmassage.com

International Institute of Reflexology: 5650 First Avenue North, Saint Petersburg, FL 33733-2642, 727-343-4811, www.reflexology-usa.net

International Spa Association (ISPA): International Spa & Fitness Association (ISPA), 546 East Main Street, Lexington, KY, 40508, 888-651-4772, 606-226-4326, www.globalspaguide.com

International Sports Massage Federation: P.O. Box 25983, Santa Ana, CA 92799-9610, 949-642-0735

National Certification Board for Therapeutic Massage & Bodywork: 8201 Greensboro Drive, Suite 300, McLean, VA 22102-3810, 703-610-9015, www.NCBTMB.com

National Association of Bodywork in Religious Services (NABRS): 337 Tranquil Avenue, Charlotte, NC 28209

Touch Research Institute: Department of Pediatrics, University of Miami School of Medicine, P.O. Box 016820 (Dept. - 820), 1601 NW 12th Avenue, Miami, FL 33101, 305-243-6781, www.miami.edu/touch-research

Get in touch with these organizations if you're searching for information, schools, and therapists in the U.K., France, Italy, and Australia.

Australia: Massage Australia, P.O. Box 38, Wentworth Falls NSW 2782 Australia, tel. 02 4757 3050 or 61 2 4757 3050, www.massageaus.com.au

The U.K.: The Institute for Complementary Medicine, P.O. Box 194, London SE16 1QZ, tel. 00 44 171 237-5165

Italy: Federazione Nazionale dei Collegi dei Massofisioterapisti (F.N.C.M.), Via Aosta 16, Trento, 38100 Rome, Italy, tel. 03 94 61 915 499 www.geocities.com/CapeCanaveral/Lab/2521

France: French Federation of Masseurs Kinesitherapeutes (FFMKR), 24 rue des Petits Hotels, 75010, Paris, France, tel. 01 44 83 46 00

Massage Specialties and Trainings

There are so many massage specialties and trainings out there that an entire book could be written just trying to explain all the different kinds. And in fact several books on that very topic have been written. This appendix is not here to confuse you about the subject, but rather to help if you're seriously interested in massage and bodywork as either a practitioner or a recipient and you'd like to start looking into some of the specialties that are available.

With each listing, you'll find contact numbers for trainings offered. These are by no means the only trainings available, but they represent some of the best. Also, if you're looking for a practitioner in a particular specialty, many of the training centers have lists of qualified people.

Note that some of the Web sites listed are not directly affiliated with the training centers but contain much relevant information.

Ayurveda

Many practitioners in the West are now offering massage and other treatments based upon this 5,000 year old system of natural healing from India.

Ayurvedic Institute: 11311 Menaul NE, Suite A, Albuquerque, NM 87112, 505)291-9698, www.ayurveda.com

Baby Massage

You don't have to be a massage pro in order to massage your own baby. Different types of classes are offered for therapists and novices.

Association of Labor Assistants & Childbirth Educators: P.O. Box 382724, Cambridge, MA 02238, 888-222-5223 or (617)441-2500, www.alace.org

Cinnabar School: P.O. Box 34326, Westbrook, Calgary, AB, Canada T3C 3W0, 403-246-6720, www.babymassage.com

Kate Jordan Seminars: 8950 Villa La Jolla Drive, Suite 2162, La Jolla, CA 92037, 760-436-0418, pregmassage@aol.com

Nurturing the Mother: 8703 Rollingwood Road, Chapel Hill, NC 27516, 919-929-4253

Chair massage

To learn how to give effective massage using the specially built massage chairs available today, contact these providers.

TouchPro Chair Massage Workshops: 800-999-5026

Seated Massage Experience: Touch 4 Productions, P.O. Box 260395, Tampa, FL 33685-0395, 800-868-2448 or 813-249-2911, www.seatedmassage.com

Connective tissue massage

These therapies usually "dig in deep" to re-pattern the way your body is held together by its basic glue, or connective tissues. They're great for changing poor postural habits, increasing energy, and improving physical function.

The Anatomy Trains by Tom Myers: 20 Roundabout Way, Scarboro, ME, 888-546-3747

The Rolf Institute of Structural Integration (Rolfing): P.O. Box 1868, Boulder, CO 80302, 800-530-8875 or 303-449-5903, www.rolf.org

Guild for Structural Integration (Rolfing): P.O. Box 1559, Boulder, CO 80306, 800-447-0150, www.rolfguild.org

Aston-Patterning: P.O. Box 3568, Incline Village, NV 89450, 702-831-8228, www.astonpatterning.com

Hellerwork: 406 Berry Street, Mt. Shasta, CA 96067, 800-392-3900, www.hellerwork.com

Energy work

Energy work is massage and bodywork that focuses on treating the invisible pathways of energy running in the human body. This energy has different names in different cultures. In Asia, it's known as *chi*, *ki* and other names. The following types of massage and bodywork deal primarily with this energy, affecting the entire body through that process.

Jin Shin Jyutsu: 8719 E. San Alberto, Scottsdale, AZ 85258, 602-998-9331, www.JinShinJyutsu.com

American Polarity Therapy Association: 2888 Bluff Street, #149, Boulder, CO 80301, 303-545-2080, www.PolarityTherapy.org

The Reiki Alliance: P.O. Box 41, Cataldo, ID 83810, 208-682-3535, www.reikicentrum.nl/reiki4all

Shiatsu: Ohashi Institute, 12 W. 27th Street, New York, NY 10001-6903, 800-810-4190, www.ohashi.com

Healing Tao: 1205 O'Neill Hwy, Dunmore, PA 18512, 717-348-4310, www.healing-tao.com

Therapeutic Touch: Nurse Healers & Professional Associates, 175 Fifth Ave, Suite 3399, New York, NY 10010, www.therapeutictouch.com

Freedom of movement massage

These techniques have been developed by people in the performing arts, sports, the medical professions, and other backgrounds. All of them open the body/mind to higher levels of freedom and expression, creating improved wellbeing at the same time.

The Alexander Technique: North America Society of Teachers of the Alexander Technique, P.O. Box 517, Urbana, IL 61801, 800-473-0620, www.alexandertechnique.com

Feldenkrais: The Feldenkrais Guild, P.O. Box 489, Albany, OR 97321-0143, 800-775-2118, www.Feldenkrais.com

Pilates: Physical Mind Institute, 1807 Second Street #28129, Santa Fe, NM 87505, 800-505-1990 or (505)988-1990, www.the-method.com

Pilates Institute: Sydney City Lvl 2, George Street, Sydney NSW Australia 2000, tel 02 9267 8223, www.pilates.net

Trager: The Trager Institute, 21 Locust, Mill Valley, CA 94941-2806, 415-388-2688, www.trager.com

Geriatric massage

If you would like to help senior citizens in a profoundly important and simple way, reaching out to them through massage is an excellent choice, and taking the training offered here is a good way to begin.

Daybreak Geriatric Massage Project: 216 Pleasant Hill Ave. N., Sebastopol, CA 95472, 707-829-2798, www.daybreak-massage.com

Horse massage

I know it may be hard for you to believe, but it's true: There are courses for people who want to learn how to massage horses, which is actually quite a big business these days.

Equissage: P.O. Box 447, Round Hill, VA 20142, 540-338-1917, www.equissage.com

Don Doran's Equine Sports Massage: 14735 SW 71 Avenue Road, Ocala, FL 34473-5102, 352-347-3747

Jack Meagher Institute of Sports Therapy: Equine Sports Massage, P.O. Box 1244, Concord, MA 01742, 413-772-1815

Mind/body/emotion massage

These methods work in a very profound way to help people uncover and deal with emotions and memories that might cause painful conditions.

The Rosen Method: The Rosen Method Center, 825 Bancroft Way, Berkley, CA 94710, 510-845-6606, www.mcn.org/b/rosen/default.html

Rosen Method Center Southwest: P.O. Box 344, Santa Fe, NM 87504, 505-982-7149, www.mcn.org/b/rosen/swrc.html

The Rubenfeld Synergy Center: 115 Waverly Place, New York, NY 10011, 212-254-5100, www.hometown.aol.com\rubenfeld\synergy\index.html

Pain relief massage

Although every style of massage can potentially help reduce pain, there are certain styles that specialize in pain reduction and reversal of trauma. The following a just a few of them.

The Bodywork Research Institute: 123 E. 8th Street, Suite 121, Frederick, MD 21701, 301-698-0932, trains people in massage techniques to relieve the painful symptoms of fibromyalgia.

Craniosacral Therapy: Upledger Institute, 11211 Prosperity Farms Road, Palm Beach Gardens, FL 33410-3487, 800-233-5880, www.upledger.com

Hoshino Therapy Clinic: Center for Biotherapeutics, 430 South Dixie Hwy, Miami, FL 33146, 305-666-2243

Neuromuscular Therapy Seminars: 1121 Prosperity Farms Road, #D-325, Palm Beach Gardens, FL 33410-3487, 800-311-9204 or 561-622-4334, www.iahe.com

Reflexology

International Institute of Reflexology: P.O. Box 12642, St. Petersburg, FL, 33733-2642, 727-343-4811, www.reflexology-usa.net

Spa therapy training

This category is for those people who would like to specialize in giving massage, hydrotherapy, and other treatments in the spa setting, as well as spa owners and managers.

The Bramham Institute & Spa: 1014 N. Olive Ave, West Palm Beach, FL 33401, 800-575-0518, www.spamastery.com

Thai massage

Many people make the pilgrimage to Thailand every year to learn the techniques of this traditional system, which includes a lot of stretching and moves similar to shiatsu.

Institute of Thai Massage: 17/7 Morakot Road, Hah Yaek Santitham, Chiang Mai 50300 Thailand, tel. (66-53) 218632, www.infothai.com/itm

Water massage

Some very interesting types of massage can be done in the water. The buoyancy helps to free people of chronic pain and ease certain fears.

Watsu: Massage School at Harbin Hot Springs P.O. Box 570, Middletown, CA 95461, 707-987-3801, www.waba.edu

Aquassage: 800-957-4808, www.massagetherapynetwork.com

A college degree in massage

If you want a college degree and a massage license, how about going to school where you can get both at the same time? At the New Center College, you'll earn an Associate of Occupational Studies (A.O.S.) degree with a major in Massage Therapy, the first of its kind in the United States.

The New Center College for Wholistic Health Education and Research: 6801 Jericho Tpk., Syosset, New York 11791-4413, 516-364-0808, ext.126, `www. newcenter.edu`

Index

• R •

rainforest, 24
ramus of the mandible, 52
range of motion, 133, 151
rashes, 131
rates. *See* cost
rectus abdominis, 56–57
rectus femoris, 54
referrals, seeking, 79–81
reflex arc, 35
reflexology
  baby massage and, 275
  basic description of, 229–240
  foot massage routine with, 232–240
  foot rollers and, 157
  quiz, 230–231
  training in, 337
reggae massage, 123
rehabilitative massage, 19–20
Reiki Alliance, 335
Relax the Back Corporation, 254
relaxation
  after a massage, 108
  giving up the responsibility for, 93
  increased, through massage, 13, 17–18
  massage techniques, 19, 70–71
  "staying loose" and, 92–93
Relaxation Response, The (Benson), 17
reproductive organs, 239. *See also*
    pregnancy
respiratory system. *See also* breathing;
    lungs
  basic description of, 62
  oils that are good for, 166
  skin and, 40, 43
retardation, 42
rhomboid, 57–58
ribcage, 188
ribs, 92, 188
robes, 105
rocking & rolling technique, 148–149
Rolf, Ida, 73
Rolfing, 73–74, 143, 334
rope analogy, 13–14

rose oil, 166. *See also* oils
rosemary oil, 166. *See also* oils
Rosen Method, 336
rubbing gloves, 159
rubbing technique, 145–146
Rubenfeld Synergy Center, 336
rules, for giving a massage, 166–167
runner's cramps, 263–264
Russell, Bertrand, 42
Rx (remedial) massage, 72–73

• S •

sacrum (tailbone), 172, 177
safety, feeling of, 97–98
Saint Francis, 120
Samurai warriors, 37
sandalwood oil, 166. *See also* oils
scalp, 180–182, 324
scents, 119–120. *See also* smell, sense of
Scherer Institute of Natural Healing, 305
schools, massage, 84, 303–306
  choosing, 294–295
  cost of, 295–296
sciatic nerve, 59, 177, 232, 239
scrubs, 246, 247–249
seaweed, 253
sebum, 42
secretion, 40, 42
self
  -confidence, 31
  sense of, 31, 70
Self-Care catalog, 331
self-massage
  basic description of, 213–228
  mini-routine, 214–222
  when traveling, 268–269
Sen, Wesley, 71, 170
sensitization exercises, 48–50
sensual pleasure, massage for, 22, 283–290
serotonin, 31
service bureaus, 83
sesame oil, 167. *See also* oils
setup, for massage, 162–163
sexual harassment, 69

FOR DUMMIES®

The easy way to get more done and have more fun

PERSONAL FINANCE

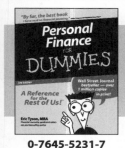
0-7645-5231-7

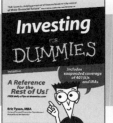
0-7645-2431-3

0-7645-5331-3

Also available:

Estate Planning For Dummies
(0-7645-5501-4)
401(k)s For Dummies
(0-7645-5468-9)
Frugal Living For Dummies
(0-7645-5403-4)
Microsoft Money "X" For
Dummies
(0-7645-1689-2)
Mutual Funds For Dummies
(0-7645-5329-1)

Personal Bankruptcy For
Dummies
(0-7645-5498-0)
Quicken "X" For Dummies
(0-7645-1666-3)
Stock Investing For Dummies
(0-7645-5411-5)
Taxes For Dummies 2003
(0-7645-5475-1)

BUSINESS & CAREERS

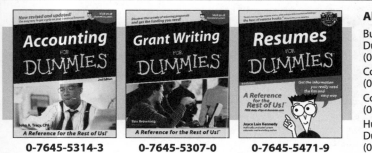
0-7645-5314-3   0-7645-5307-0   0-7645-5471-9

Also available:

Business Plans Kit For
Dummies
(0-7645-5365-8)
Consulting For Dummies
(0-7645-5034-9)
Cool Careers For Dummies
(0-7645-5345-3)
Human Resources Kit For
Dummies
(0-7645-5131-0)
Managing For Dummies
(1-5688-4858-7)

QuickBooks All-in-One Desk
Reference For Dummies
(0-7645-1963-8)
Selling For Dummies
(0-7645-5363-1)
Small Business Kit For
Dummies
(0-7645-5093-4)
Starting an eBay Business For
Dummies
(0-7645-1547-0)

HEALTH, SPORTS & FITNESS

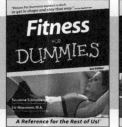
0-7645-5167-1

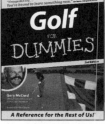
0-7645-5146-9

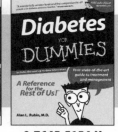
0-7645-5154-X

Also available:

Controlling Cholesterol For
Dummies
(0-7645-5440-9)
Dieting For Dummies
(0-7645-5126-4)
High Blood Pressure For
Dummies
(0-7645-5424-7)
Martial Arts For Dummies
(0-7645-5358-5)
Menopause For Dummies
(0-7645-5458-1)

Nutrition For Dummies
(0-7645-5180-9)
Power Yoga For Dummies
(0-7645-5342-9)
Thyroid For Dummies
(0-7645-5385-2)
Weight Training For Dummies
(0-7645-5168-X)
Yoga For Dummies
(0-7645-5117-5)

Available wherever books are sold.
Go to www.dummies.com or call 1-877-762-2974 to order direct.

FOR DUMMIES

A world of resources to help you grow

HOME, GARDEN & HOBBIES

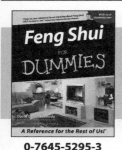

Feng Shui For Dummies
0-7645-5295-3

Gardening For Dummies
0-7645-5130-2

Guitar For Dummies
0-7645-5106-X

Also available:

Auto Repair For Dummies
(0-7645-5089-6)

Chess For Dummies
(0-7645-5003-9)

Home Maintenance For
Dummies
(0-7645-5215-5)

Organizing For Dummies
(0-7645-5300-3)

Piano For Dummies
(0-7645-5105-1)

Poker For Dummies
(0-7645-5232-5)

Quilting For Dummies
(0-7645-5118-3)

Rock Guitar For Dummies
(0-7645-5356-9)

Roses For Dummies
(0-7645-5202-3)

Sewing For Dummies
(0-7645-5137-X)

FOOD & WINE

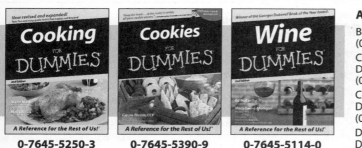

Cooking For Dummies
0-7645-5250-3

Cookies For Dummies
0-7645-5390-9

Wine For Dummies
0-7645-5114-0

Also available:

Bartending For Dummies
(0-7645-5051-9)

Chinese Cooking For
Dummies
(0-7645-5247-3)

Christmas Cooking For
Dummies
(0-7645-5407-7)

Diabetes Cookbook For
Dummies
(0-7645-5230-9)

Grilling For Dummies
(0-7645-5076-4)

Low-Fat Cooking For
Dummies
(0-7645-5035-7)

Slow Cookers For Dummies
(0-7645-5240-6)

TRAVEL

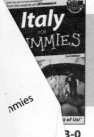

Italy For Dummies
3-0

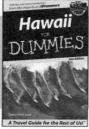

Hawaii For Dummies
0-7645-5438-7

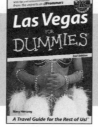

Las Vegas For Dummies
0-7645-5448-4

Also available:

America's National Parks For
Dummies
(0-7645-6204-5)

Caribbean For Dummies
(0-7645-5445-X)

Cruise Vacations For
Dummies 2003
(0-7645-5459-X)

Europe For Dummies
(0-7645-5456-5)

Ireland For Dummies
(0-7645-6199-5)

France For Dummies
(0-7645-6292-4)

London For Dummies
(0-7645-5416-6)

Mexico's Beach Resorts For
Dummies
(0-7645-6262-2)

Paris For Dummies
(0-7645-5494-8)

RV Vacations For Dummies
(0-7645-5443-3)

Walt Disney World & Orlando
For Dummies
(0-7645-5444-1)

e wherever books are sold. Go to www.dummies.com or call 1-877-762-2974 to order direct.

FOR DUMMIES®

Plain-English solutions for everyday challenges

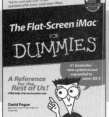

COMPUTER BASICS

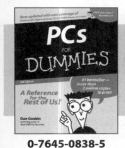

PCs FOR DUMMIES
0-7645-0838-5

The Flat-Screen iMac FOR DUMMIES
0-7645-1663-9

Windows XP ALL-IN-ONE DESK REFERENCE FOR DUMMIES
0-7645-1548-9

Also available:

PCs All-in-One Desk Reference For Dummies (0-7645-0791-5)

Pocket PC For Dummies (0-7645-1640-X)

Treo and Visor For Dummies (0-7645-1673-6)

Troubleshooting Your PC For Dummies (0-7645-1669-8)

Upgrading & Fixing PCs For Dummies (0-7645-1665-5)

Windows XP For Dummies (0-7645-0893-8)

Windows XP For Dummies Quick Reference (0-7645-0897-0)

BUSINESS SOFTWARE

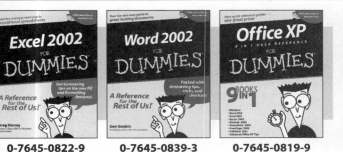

Excel 2002 FOR DUMMIES
0-7645-0822-9

Word 2002 FOR DUMMIES
0-7645-0839-3

Office XP 9 IN 1 DESK REFERENCE FOR DUMMIES
0-7645-0819-9

Also available:

Excel Data Analysis For Dummies (0-7645-1661-2)

Excel 2002 All-in-One Desk Reference For Dummies (0-7645-1794-5)

Excel 2002 For Dummies Quick Reference (0-7645-0829-6)

GoldMine "X" For Dummies (0-7645-0845-8)

Microsoft CRM For Dummies (0-7645-1698-1)

Microsoft Project 2002 For Dummies (0-7645-1628-0)

Office XP For Dummies (0-7645-0830-X)

Outlook 2002 For Dummies (0-7645-0828-8)

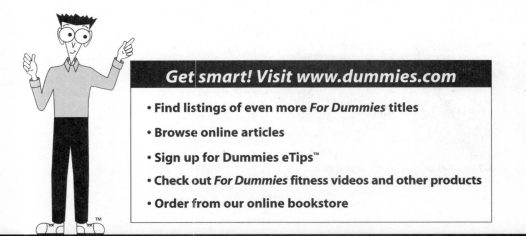

Get smart! Visit www.dummies.com

- **Find listings of even more *For Dummies* titles**
- **Browse online articles**
- **Sign up for Dummies eTips™**
- **Check out *For Dummies* fitness videos and other products**
- **Order from our online bookstore**

Available wherever books are sold. Go to www.dummies.com or call 1-877-762-2974 to order direct.

FOR DUMMIES®

Helping you expand your horizons and realize your potential

INTERNET

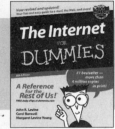

The Internet FOR DUMMIES

0-7645-0894-6

The Internet ALL-IN-ONE DESK REFERENCE FOR DUMMIES

0-7645-1659-0

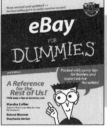

eBay FOR DUMMIES

0-7645-1642-6

Also available:

America Online 7.0 For Dummies
(0-7645-1624-8)

Genealogy Online For Dummies
(0-7645-0807-5)

The Internet All-in-One Desk Reference For Dummies
(0-7645-1659-0)

Internet Explorer 6 For Dummies
(0-7645-1344-3)

The Internet For Dummies Quick Reference
(0-7645-1645-0)

Internet Privacy For Dummies
(0-7645-0846-6)

Researching Online For Dummies
(0-7645-0546-7)

Starting an Online Business For Dummies
(0-7645-1655-8)

DIGITAL MEDIA

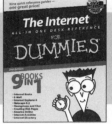

Digital Photography FOR DUMMIES

0-7645-1664-7

Photoshop Elements 2 FOR DUMMIES

0-7645-1675-2

Digital Video FOR DUMMIES

0-7645-0806-7

Also available:

CD and DVD Recording For Dummies
(0-7645-1627-2)

Digital Photography All-in-One Desk Reference For Dummies
(0-7645-1800-3)

Digital Photography For Dummies Quick Reference
(0-7645-0750-8)

Home Recording for Musicians For Dummies
(0-7645-1634-5)

MP3 For Dummies
(0-7645-0858-X)

Paint Shop Pro "X" For Dummies
(0-7645-2440-2)

Photo Retouching & Restoration For Dummies
(0-7645-1662-0)

Scanners For Dummies
(0-7645-0783-4)

GRAPHICS

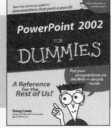

PowerPoint 2002 FOR DUMMIES

0-7645-0817-2

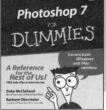

Photoshop 7 FOR DUMMIES

0-7645-1651-5

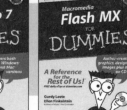

Macromedia Flash MX FOR DUMMIES

0-7645-0895-4

Also available:

Adobe Acrobat 5 PDF For Dummies
(0-7645-1652-3)

Fireworks 4 For Dummies
(0-7645-0804-0)

Illustrator 10 For Dummies
(0-7645-3636-2)

QuarkXPress 5 For Dummies
(0-7645-0643-9)

Visio 2000 For Dummies
(0-7645-0635-8)

Available wherever books are sold. Go to www.dummies.com or call 1-877-762-2974 to order direct.

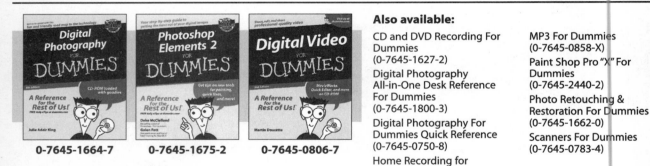